THE NHS AT
The State of UK Hea

Edited by
Mark Exworthy,
Russell Mannion
and Martin Powell

With a foreword by
Simon Stevens

P

First published in Great Britain in 2023 by

Policy Press, an imprint of
Bristol University Press
University of Bristol
1-9 Old Park Hill
Bristol
BS2 8BB
UK
t: +44 (0)117 374 6645
e: bup-info@bristol.ac.uk

Details of international sales and distribution partners are available at
policy.bristoluniversitypress.co.uk

© Bristol University Press 2023

British Library Cataloguing in Publication Data
A catalogue record for this book is available from the British Library

ISBN 978-1-4473-6859-5 hardcover
ISBN 978-1-4473-6860-1 paperback
ISBN 978-1-4473-6861-8 ePub
ISBN 978-1-4473-6862-5 ePdf

The right of Mark Exworthy, Russell Mannion and Martin Powell to be identified as editors of this
work has been asserted by them in accordance with the Copyright, Designs and Patents
Act 1988.

All rights reserved: no part of this publication may be reproduced, stored in a retrieval system, or
transmitted in any form or by any means, electronic, mechanical, photocopying, recording, or
otherwise without the prior permission of Bristol University Press.

Every reasonable effort has been made to obtain permission to reproduce copyrighted material. If,
however, anyone knows of an oversight, please contact the publisher.

The statements and opinions contained within this publication are solely those of the editors and
contributors and not of the University of Bristol or Bristol University Press. The University of
Bristol and Bristol University Press disclaim responsibility for any injury to persons
or property resulting from any material published in this publication.

Bristol University Press and Policy Press work to counter discrimination on
grounds of gender, race, disability, age and sexuality.

Cover design: Nicky Borowiec
Front cover image: ShutterStock/Ink Drop
Bristol University Press and Policy Press use environmentally responsible print partners.
Printed and bound in Great Britain by CPI Group (UK) Ltd, Croydon, CR0 4YY

FSC
www.fsc.org
MIX
Paper | Supporting
responsible forestry
FSC® C013604

Mark – to Sarah, Dominic and Finnian

Russell – to Judith, Lizzie and Catherine

Martin – to Annette

Contents

List of figures and tables

Figures

Tables

Notes on contributors

Pauline Allen, Professor of Health Services Organisation, London School of Hygiene and Tropical Medicine.

Anita Charlesworth, Director of Research, Health Foundation, London.

Kath Checkland, Clinical Professor of Health Policy and Primary Care, University of Manchester.

Amit Desai, Research Fellow, King's College London.

Mark Exworthy, Professor of Health Policy and Management, University of Birmingham.

Jon Glasby, Professor of Health and Social Care, University of Birmingham.

Ian Greener, Professor of Applied Social Sciences, University of Aberdeen.

Scott Greer, Professor of Health Management and Policy, University of Michigan, USA.

Jonathan Hammond, Senior Lecturer in Health Policy and Organisation, University of Manchester.

Ian Kirkpatrick, Professor of Public Management, University of York.

Mirza Lalani, Assistant Professor, London School of Hygiene and Tropical Medicine.

Russell Mannion, Professor of Health Systems, University of Birmingham.

Ross Millar, Reader in Health Organisation, University of Birmingham.

Catherine Needham, Professor of Public Policy and Public Management, University of Birmingham.

Martin Powell, Professor of Health and Social Policy, University of Birmingham.

Rod Sheaff, Professor of Health Services Research, University of Plymouth.

Nihar Shembavnekar, Economist, Health Foundation, London.

Sharon Spooner, Clinical Lecturer, University of Manchester.

George Stevenson, Economist, Health Foundation, London.

Ellen Stewart, Senior Lecturer & Chancellor's Fellow in Health Policy, University of Strathclyde.

John Stewart, Emeritus Professor of History of Healthcare, Glasgow Caledonian University.

Jennifer Voorhees, Clinical Lecturer, University of Manchester.

Justin Waring, Professor of Medical Sociology and Healthcare Organisation, University of Birmingham.

Giulia Zoccatelli, Research Fellow, King's College London.

Foreword

Simon Stevens
Lord Stevens of Birmingham, Kt, House of Lords
NHS Chief Executive, 2014-2021

It is relatively uncontroversial to argue that the past decade has been the NHS' toughest. Looking back, the NHS had emerged from the 2000s in comparatively good shape, having converted significant investment into radically shorter waits for routine care – at the time the public's biggest bugbear.

But by the early 2010s, the 'problem set' facing the NHS was rather different, and the policy mix of the prior decade was now misaligned with those challenges. The underlying epidemiological challenge was to improve outcomes for an ageing population with multiple long-term health problems. The resulting system challenge was in part to move closer towards what I labelled the 'triple integration' of physical and mental health, primary and specialist services, and health and social care. And the economic challenge was to try and do so at a time of deeply constrained revenue and capital funding. Because when the British economy sneezes, the NHS catches a cold, as Anita Charlesworth and colleagues show in Chapter 3 of this volume. The international comparisons are even starker. In the decade to 2019 it has been calculated that the UK spent on average £40 billion less each year than if we had matched average per-person health funding across the EU14. Indeed, the UK would have had to spend nearly a fifth more to match French per-person health spending, and nearly two-fifths more to match that of Germany (Health Foundation, 2022).

Yet despite these pressures, by the 70th anniversary of the NHS in 2018 there were some grounds for optimism. The NHS had just secured a more workable medium-term financial settlement, backed by broad consensus on its own long-term improvement plan. The government had agreed to replace the 2012 Health Act with a legal framework better aligned to population health and integrated care.

However, five years, three prime ministers and one pandemic later, the NHS turns 75 in a more uncertain position. So it is unsurprising that the debate on the NHS' future is again intensifying. Some argue that the chickens are coming home to roost from chronic political short termism that has repeatedly deferred long-term workforce decisions, underinvested in capital infrastructure and technology (even during a period of negative real borrowing costs), done little on prevention and stalled on social care reform.

But the public debate reaches wider than that, and is playing out across (at least) five frequently conflated, but conceptually distinct, questions.

First, how should care best be *organised and delivered*, including stimulating innovation and harnessing medical advances? Second, to what extent is pressure on the NHS a consequence of *wider public policy*, for example, on public health, social inequality and social care? Third, where there are access or quality problems, to what degree are they caused by an inadequate NHS funding *quantum*? Fourth, is UK healthcare in practice helped or hindered by relying on general taxation as its principal funding *mechanism*? Fifth, is UK economic *growth* helped or hindered by a tax-funded NHS?

As well as disagreeing on the answers to these individual questions, when evaluating the NHS' future prospects, commentators of different ideological hues also tend to disagree about their relative importance. Rudolf Klein and Ted Marmor have argued – in my view convincingly – that in predicting the outcome of contested health reforms it is ideas that matter, not just interests and institutions (Stevens, 2013). That is why this important new volume is such a timely and welcome intervention, bringing empirical and analytical rigour to this controversial terrain – on which the coming debate over the future of the NHS will likely be fought.

References

Health Foundation. (2022) 16 November https://www.health.org.uk/news-and-comment/news/uk-spent-around-a-fifth-less-than-european-neighbours-on-health-care-in-last-decade

Stevens, S. (2013) 'Contagious ideas: Marmor and Klein on transatlantic health policy and politics'. *Health Economics, Policy and Law*, 8, 407414. DOI:10.1017/ S1744133113000170

The NHS at 75: an unfolding story

Mark Exworthy, Russell Mannion and Martin Powell

Introduction

In its 75th year, despite the hallowed role that the NHS plays in the UK national psyche, the NHS found itself in a parlous position. Across a range of measures, the NHS was facing unprecedented pressures in 2023. First, public satisfaction with the NHS had fallen to its lowest recorded level – 29 per cent, falling 7 percentage points from 2021. Equally significant was the level of dissatisfaction with the NHS, at 51 per cent (Morris et al, 2023). Second, waiting lists were at an all-time high of 7.2 million (as of December 2022). Much of this can be explained by delayed care due to COVID-19 (a rise of 2 million since the start of the pandemic). This was despite the 'elective recovery plan' published in 2022 (NHS England, 2022). Third, there were 133,000 (full-time equivalent) vacancies in the NHS in September 2022, a vacancy rate of 9.7 per cent (Health Foundation, 2022). Vacancies in social care stood at 165,000, a vacancy rate of 10.7 per cent (King's Fund, 2023). Fourth, there was a wave of strikes among NHS staff. Members of the Royal College of Nursing went on strike for the first time in their history. They were joined by ambulance staff and junior doctors. NHS consultants had also voted for strike action. Fifth, while pay can explain some of the causes of these strikes, it is likely that high levels of stress and burnout were also significant factors. The 2022 NHS Staff Survey (published in March 2023) indicated that 45 per cent of staff were unwell due to work-related stress and 57 per cent had come to work despite feeling unwell. Overall, 34 per cent of staff felt burnout, with ambulance staff being especially prone (49 per cent) (Nuffield Trust, 2023).

The conditions prevailing in 2023 were the confluence of factors in the previous several years – financial austerity from 2010, the Brexit referendum vote in 2016 (and the consequent impact upon recruitment and retention of staff and pharmaceuticals) and COVID-19 pandemic (from March 2020). Arguably, the conditions were also the result of the NHS' politics, policies and organisational structure over the previous 75 years. So it is timely to reassess the contribution and state of the NHS in the past, in the present and in the future. It is, therefore, at a precarious time for the NHS that it reaches this important milestone anniversary with which this book is timed to coincide and commemorate.

We start this chapter by assessing the contribution of studies of previous anniversaries before outlining the analytical axes which will frame this book and examining the evaluative dimensions of the NHS as a health system.

The NHS through anniversaries

Previous NHS anniversaries have seen significant interest, and a wide range of books and articles were published to mark these events. For example, writing on the 60th anniversary of the NHS, Timmins (2008) noted that his brief history of the big anniversaries demonstrates 'plus ça change' – that many of the issues that the NHS is grappling with right now, and will continue to grapple with, always have been there. This book examines how these issues have evolved and transformed through the 75 years of the service. There have been many narrative or chronological histories of the NHS (see as follows). Chronological accounts come in many shapes and sizes. For example, Powell (1997, ch 4) covers the period 1948–1996 in some 25 pages. Probably the most readable account is that of Klein (2013) who covers the period over 60 years in 322 pages. The Official Historian of the NHS, Webster (1988, 1996) explores the period 1948–1957 in 460 pages and 1958–1979 in 971 pages respectively. Some accounts provide a periodisation, with the starting point of Bevan's NHS or the 1948 model or 1948 settlement (for example, Klein, 2013: c 146, 152). For example, Webster (1998) outlines three phases: creation and consolidation (1948–1964); planning and reorganisation (1964–1979); and continuous revolution (1979–). Powell (1997) examines the period largely in terms of decades. Klein (2013) suggests 'the politics of': creation, consolidation, technocratic change, disillusionment, value for money, the big bang, the Third Way, reinvention, transition and confrontation.

While this text cannot replicate the detail covered by some of these chronological accounts, it adds to them in three ways. First, many of the chronological histories do not cover the most recent period of the past decade or so. For example, Webster's (1988, 1996) 'Official History' ends in 1979, while his 'political history' (1998) ends with the NHS 50th anniversary of that year. Klein's (2013) narrative ends in about 2012, just before one of the biggest reforms in the history of the NHS. Second, it aims to provide an analytical approach that will set out broad themes of the book such as hierarchies, markets and networks; centralisation and decentralisation; public and private; and professional and managerial. Third, it aims to provide an evaluative approach which examines policy success in terms of temporal, intrinsic and extrinsic evaluation.

Analytical axes of health policy

We turn now to the four primary analytical axes which will be the lens through which we will examine the 75 years of the NHS. Each has its own theoretical and empirical context which we can only briefly summarise here. We will identify points where these axes intersect and examine the consequences that arise (Exworthy and Freeman, 2009).

Governing the NHS through hierarchies, markets and networks

The trilogy of hierarchies, markets and networks are different types of governance by which the NHS has been managed since 1948. Each type denotes a way in which the health system (including its constituent parts) is institutionally designed and governed. At any one time, these types will overlap in the NHS although different approaches have dominated at different times. It is, in effect, the 'operating system' for the NHS. Each type has its own coordinating mechanisms: 'If it is price competition that is the central coordinating mechanism of the market and administrative orders that of hierarchies, then it is trust and co-operation that centrally articulates networks' (Thompson et al, 1991: 15).

It has sometimes been argued that the British NHS has moved from a hierarchical and bureaucratic organisation to a market and then to a network, and then back towards a market (see for example, Exworthy et al, 1999). This is certainly a useful, if somewhat simplistic way to view the evolution of the NHS. This narrative claims that the NHS as hierarchy (which arguably ran from 1948 to 1979) regards the service as a form of top-down, relatively rigid command and control planning model, where decision-making was vested in elected officials at national level. Policies are transmitted from centre to periphery, with central parliamentary accountability summed up in Bevan's famous phrase: 'when a bedpan is dropped on a hospital floor its noise should resound in the Palace of Westminster'. The NHS as Market (1979–1997) asserts that the Conservative governments of 1979–1997 'marketized' the NHS, introducing the 'purchaser/provider split', the 'internal' or 'quasi' market, and contracted out ancillary services. The NHS as Network (from 1997 to the early 2000s) saw a brief period, where New Labour's 'Third Way' stresses collaboration and partnership (Goddard and Mannion, 1998). Labour rejected the old left and the new right in favour of a third way, where the 'new NHS' was not supposed to return to the old centralised command and control system of the 1970s, nor was it intended for there to be a continuation of the divisive internal market system of the 1990s. However, it has been claimed that Labour soon reintroduced marketisation in the shape of an enhanced Private Finance Initiative, greater choice for patients (including private hospitals) and Foundation Hospitals. This was also reflected in a shift towards more competitive cultures among NHS managers during the period 2000–2008 (Mannion et al, 2009).

The focus on the market was increased with the coalition government (2010–2015) and the Conservative government (2015–) with legislation such as the 2012 Health and Social Care Act (Exworthy et al, 2016). In many ways, market principles have continued to govern the NHS (such as through commissioning) in the past decade or so but, as the shortcomings of markets have become ever more apparent, there has also been greater emphasis on integration. Such integration is redolent of (professional/clinical, organisational and policy) networks, as in the case of Integrated Care Systems created in England in 2022.

However, these ideal types are too simplistic. They are not mutually exclusive and, as each does not exist independently of any other, it might be more appropriate to consider them as hybrid types. Exworthy et al (1999) argue that the three organisational forms have always co-existed. The early years of the NHS saw a weak centre with limited control over the periphery, where policy making was largely by exhortation, with ministers feeling that they lacked command and control (Haywood and Alaszewski, 1980; Klein, 2013). It could be argued that a more fully developed version of hierarchy only began to be established after the 1974 NHS reorganisation which introduced 'authority' into the NHS, as the existing 'Hospital Boards' and 'Management Committees' were replaced by 'Health Authorities'. Moreover, the period of so-called hierarchy co-existed with that of policy networks, and the NHS as collegiate system run by professional groups. This is consistent with Alford's (1975) structural interest theory, where professional monopolisers control the healthcare agenda despite the efforts of corporate rationalisers (for example, managers). Moreover, the NHS locally was largely dominated by medical networks.

The market narrative can also be contested. Despite the intentions of policy documents, competition on the ground was limited. This effect of marketisation was partial outside large urban areas as the geographical pattern of district general hospitals was designed to serve a catchment area. This meant that competition was possible only if patients were willing to travel rather than go to their local hospital. There is limited empirical evidence to suggest that patients were willing to translate their intention to travel into action (Exworthy and Peckham, 2006). Likewise, NHS commissioners and provider were not always willing to enact market principles in their entirety, seeking instead to work cooperatively. Such behaviour was also evident in Foundation Trusts whose senior staff generally did not exploit the autonomy of their organisational status, supposedly 'free' from hierarchy (Exworthy and Frosini, 2011).

Therefore, the market was never as 'red in tooth and claw' as favoured by its advocates or feared by its critics (Powell, 2003). One of the architects of the internal market, Alain Enthoven, considered that on a scale from 0 to 10, where 0 is a totally planned economy and 10 is the relatively free American economy, the internal market got somewhere between 2 and 3 for a year or so, and then fell back to more central control (in Powell, 2003).

It has also been claimed that hierarchy strengthened during the Conservative market period (up to 1997). The 'Working for Patients' document claimed that a clear and effective chain of command would be introduced for the first time (Secretary of State for Health, 1989: 13). Timmins (2017: 513) claims that the Conservatives introduced a 'line management that Stalin himself might have envied'. Jenkins (1996: 88) states that Bevan's bedpans were not just heard in the Palace of Westminster – 'they were picked up, emptied, cleaned, counted and given a numbered place on the Whitehall shelf'.

In their early years of government, New Labour advocated a third way of pluralism without competition, that retains the purchaser/provider split, but aimed to replace the market and competition with planning and cooperation. It reduced the number of purchasers and providers, moved to longer-term contracts and encouraged dialogue between purchasers and providers, who were no longer in a simple principal–agent relationship. In the words of Klein, Etzioni (famed for communitarianism) has replaced Enthoven (in Powell, 2003). However, after this brief period of rhetorical stress on partnership, Labour reintroduced choice and competition. It 'crossed the Rubicon' with a Concordat between the NHS and private medicine, leading to greater use of the private sector, and introduced 'Independent Sector Treatment Centres' (Gabbay et al, 2011). In other words, the internal market became an external market. It also embraced a different type of New Public Management (NPM) (for example, Ferlie et al, 2005) by increasing hierarchy through performance indicators and tight line management which reinforced central control.

With the Conservative/Liberal Democrat coalition government of 2010–2015, marketisation perhaps reached its high-water mark with the 2012 Health and Social Care Act. However, interpretation of subsequent events varies. On the one hand, some commentators point to more planning and even the end of the purchaser/provider split (for example, Timmins, 2017). On the other hand, other commentators argue that the recent Health and Care Bill 2022 will privatise the NHS (see Sutaria et al, 2017).

However, rather than periods based on sole archetypes, it is probably more accurate to point to a mix of forms, where later elements added to rather than replaced earlier landscapes, in the manner of geological sedimentation of rock formations (Jones, 2017). While the notion of sedimentation is helpful, the governance of the NHS has, for the 75 years, largely been shaped by the primacy or shadow of hierarchy (Durant and Warber, 2001; Heritier and Lehmkuhl, 2008), not least given the centrality of the NHS as a service funded largely by general taxation. Moreover, two of the elements require more detailed focus. We first examine the market in terms of the public and private or privatisation debates. Then we turn to explore hierarchy in terms of discussions about centralisation and decentralisation.

The public and private axis

Although the NHS is generally regarded as a 'state' system, it has never been a 'pure' version of this system. Powell and Miller (2013) claim that much of the academic literature on public versus private or privatisation makes empirical claims about privatiszation on the basis of absent or shaky definitions of the term, resulting in much of the debate on this issue largely being a 'nondebate', where opponents talk past rather than to each other. The term privatisation is multidimensional, and definitions and operationalisations of the term are often implicit, unclear and conflicting, resulting in conflicting accounts of the occurrence, chronology and degree of privatisation in the NHS, resulting in a Tower of Babel. They aimed to throw light on privatisation by applying the lens of the 'three-dimensional' approach (ownership, finance and regulation) of the mixed economy of welfare literature. This squares with the health systems typologies literature. In a review exploring the role of typologies as an analytical device in understanding both the theoretical and empirical manifestations of healthcare systems globally, Frisina Doetter et al (2021) point to three core dimensions – finance, provision and regulation.

In terms of finance, the NHS has always been largely funded by national taxation. However, there has been a gradual drift towards greater 'commodification' (Ungerson, 1997; Exworthy and Lafond, 2021). Some of the early battles about the NHS were concerned with imposing charges for prescriptions, dental and optical treatment, leading to the Cabinet resignation of the founder of the service, Aneurin Bevan. While charges (for example, for prescriptions) remain a relatively low proportion of NHS revenue, out-of-pocket expenditure by patients (that is, not through NHS funding or insurance funding) has increased in the past decade as restrictions of what services are covered by the NHS have increased. Such spending rose from 12.9 per cent of total health expenditure in 2010 to 17.1 per cent in 2019 (Anderson et al, 2022: 53).

Turning to provision, general practitioners (GPs), dentists and opticians are not salaried NHS employees, but 'independent contractors'. From this point of view, 'privatisation' (as follows) was built into the NHS at its inception. Moreover, the NHS has long made use of private and charitable facilities such as hospices and some mental health facilities. Finally, the degree of regulation has varied over time, but traditionally is one of the most important types of self-regulation by the professions through organisations such as the General Medical Council (GMC).

The 'public versus private' debate has been prominent for much of the period of the NHS. In the 1940s the British Medical Association (BMA) voted twice for its members not to serve in the new NHS, and Minister of Health Bevan was forced to give significant concessions on issues such as GPs being independent contractors, and allowing private practice outside the NHS and 'pay beds' within NHS hospitals. More recently in the era of marketisation after 1991 (see earlier), there has been a long debate about whether the NHS is being privatised. The three-dimensional account differentiates between provision/ownership and finance between state, market, voluntary and informal sectors. Greater privatisation results from an increase in any of the dimensions. The polar positions are represented by state funding and provision with high regulation to market funding and provision with low regulation. It is important to differentiate between different types of privatisation. For example, if we regard GPs as (private) independent contractors, then general practice has always been privatised (as opposed to the state nationalisation of the hospitals). Introducing the scope for charging by the 1950 Labour government represents an increase in private finance or commodification. The 'bottom-line' or minimalist definition implicitly adopted by most Conservative governments is that the NHS has not been privatised, as it remains (largely) free at the point of delivery. 'Privatise' seems to be an irregular verb in that recent Labour governments have stated that they have increased diversity in supply by using private organisations, but Labour oppositions have accused the Conservatives of 'privatising the NHS' for broadly similar activities (Powell and Miller, 2013).

While the wholesale transfer of the NHS into private ownership remains off the (political) agenda, there remains a policy rhetoric which emphasises corporatisation and commercialisation of NHS agencies (Veronesi et al, 2022). This has been accelerated during the past decade as a result of austerity (Exworthy and Lafond, 2021). Corporatisation refers to 'the transformation of governmental departments and units into semi-autonomous organisations, subject to private commercial law with independent revenues and managerial independence' (Hodgson et al, 2021) albeit with notional control by government.

The centralisation and decentralisation axis

By its very title, the *National* Health Service has national coverage and there is a degree of local administrative discretion and professional autonomy which creates variations between places. This might mean that services in one area are different in quantity and quality from another. Such a 'postcode lottery' somewhat undermines the notion of a standardised service but allows decision-makers to match local services to clinical need. Furthermore, the UK nations have each enjoyed a high degree of discretion which has, since political devolution in 1999, been widened further. Wales, for example, has no prescription charges unlike England.

While the public and private or privatisation debate is linked to the market, discussions about centralisation and decentralisation are linked to hierarchy. The NHS of 1948 was built on the tri-partite system. Hospitals were nationalised, and operated through appointed boards. Family practitioner services involving independent contractors were operated through appointed Executive Councils. However, until 1974, local authority services were the responsibility of elected local councils. This means that the NHS was composed of broadly nationalised/centralised and municipalised/decentralised services.

Although the NHS has often been seen as a 'command and control' model, the situation is more complex, with the circle of centre-periphery relations refusing to be squared (Klein, 2013: 35). For example, a 1950 report pointed bluntly to the 'fundamental incompatibility between central control and local autonomy' (in Klein, 2013: 35). It has been suggested that perhaps the 'hallmark of Ministry of Health policy-making in the 1950s: policy making through exhortation' (Klein, 2013: 37).

It has been argued that the early NHS was characterised by 'laissez faire', with little direct operational control over the implementation of most national policies. The 1960s saw increased central control as suggested by the 1962 Hospital Plan. While greater delegation was one of the professed objectives of the 1974 Re-organisation, one of its features was tight central control. Similarly, while the 1982 Re-organisation stressed decentralisation, it was followed soon afterwards by moves towards centralisation with a number of measures including central performance management, planning systems, 'circulars' and contracting out. Finally, although much of the rhetoric of the 1990 Act was decentralist, many of the implications were centralist.

In contrast to talking local but acting national, New Labour's 'Third Way' approach tended to stress both centralisation (national service; new central institutions and National Service Frameworks) and devolution (UK nations). Labour's second term showed a clear rhetorical trend to decentralisation and the 'new localism' (Greener et al, 2009).

In addition to differences between rhetoric and action, the definition and measurement of decentralisation is not fully clear (Peckham et al, 2005; Exworthy et al, 2010). The locus of decision-making may be decentralised, others are centralised and some may remain unchanged. This ambiguity and constant oscillation between the centre and the periphery/locality creates uncertainty in decision-making at different levels and so affects the decision space at each level (Klein, 2003; Anand et al, 2012).

Similar points can be made about the 'national-ness' of the NHS (Powell, 1998). While the characteristics of a national welfare state have rarely been discussed, it is possible to point to three main criteria that distinguish national from local services. First, in a national service there should be little autonomy and no democratic input at local levels. There should be a national chain of command: a transmission belt for implementing central policy. Second, there should be national as opposed to local funding, with the centre allocating money according to central criteria to secure horizontal equity in funding at the national level. Third, central control and funding should lead to provision which is equitable according to centrally determined standards in order to achieve in the words of Bevan, 'as nearly as possible a uniform standard of service for may be, with the same level of service' or to 'universalise the best' (in Powell, 1998). In short, the aim of a truly national service would be to make geography irrelevant.

A key manifestation of the centralisation/decentralisation axis was the introduction of Foundation Trusts (FTs) in England from 2004 onwards. With an emphasis on 'earning' the opportunity for autonomy (Mannion et al, 2007), FTs had to demonstrate their ability to manage themselves 'free' from central oversight. Implementation of the FT programme was slow and many of the 'freedoms' (such as the ability to alter pay rates) were not exercised. This was explained by ongoing forms of centralisation, the ways in which some managers were inured to centralisation and the fear of destabilising relations among local health and care organisations (Exworthy et al, 2011).

The professional and state axis

Here, we focus on the relationship between the state the medical profession. As we have seen earlier in this chapter, the character of the NHS was shaped by this state–profession relationship. In many ways, this has remained largely recognisable 75 years later. Such continuity can be explained by the fundamental nature of the state and the profession, but equally profound differences are also apparent.

The mutual inter-dependency of the state and the profession confers benefits to both parties – for the state, the delivery of an electorally popular service while for the latter, a degree of protected autonomy with adequate resources. Such inter-dependency was termed the 'politics of the double bed' by Klein (1990). The 'irreducible core' (Rueschemeyer, 1983) of the autonomy that clinicians, most notably doctors, enjoy effectively means that the state cannot fully determine the scope and nature of health services delivered locally. Doctors have the freedom to diagnose, treat, refer and prescribe.

For much of the first few decades of the NHS, the state-profession relationship was stable. However, the consensus teams of the 1970s and early 1980s (in which doctors' representatives had a veto over local decisions) was seen by the state as increasingly untenable. With the rise of NPM across the UK public sector (Ferlie, Lynn and Pollitt, 2005), general managers were introduced in the NHS following the 1983 report by the managing director of Sainsbury's supermarket, Sir Roy Griffiths. The established a direct conflict between the competing logics of professionalism and managerialism. The managerial challenge to doctors included the imposition of resource management and performance measurement, among others. Over time, the conflict was lessened somewhat as the medical profession adapted to managerialism by occupying some key managerial positions, as medical-managerial hybrids (McGivern et al, 2015). Indeed, many of the health policy reforms (such as GP fund-holding and Clinical Commissioning Groups) were premised on this basis. As such, conflict gave way, in some cases to collaboration and compromise (Exworthy and Halford, 1999). Arguably, some parts of the medical profession (especially those in managerial/quasi-managerial roles) have inculcated managerialism. This has also involved a shift in language towards leadership (Martin and Learmonth, 2010), as evident in the Faculty of Medical Leadership and Management.

Therefore, the managerial 'turn' of the 1980s highlighted more starkly than ever before the competing logics between state and the medical profession because the newly appointed managers were effectively acting on behalf of the state (Harrison, 1988). However, with greater local decision-making autonomy (since the Foundation Trust policy in England), managers arguably developed their own interests which may diverge from those of the state. That said, the medical profession has, through adapting to the managerial challenge, retained its dominant position among healthcare stakeholders (Alford, 1975). It has managed to deflect or subsume many of the threats from challenging interests whether from political, organisational or managerial interests.

The tension in this profession/state axis is, of course, to the exclusion of patients' interests. Alford (1975) recognised that health reform was contested between dominant and challenging interest groups, to the exclusion of patient interests. Newbigging (2016) comments how patient perspectives have increasingly been individualised in recent years, despite repeated claims of localism. She adds that the formal structures of patient involvement in the NHS have been 'depowered', reducing the influence of 'voice, choice, representation, scrutiny and redress' (Newbigging 2016: 313).

Evaluating policy success in 75 years of the NHS

We now turn to the evaluative dimension, focusing on the evaluation, public management, performance measurement, public service improvement and policy success literatures. There is a long tradition of evaluation in health systems, but this is rooted in examining effectiveness in Randomized Clinical Trials (RCT) (for example, Cochrane, 1972; see Ovretveit, 1978; Mays and Fraser, forthcoming). There have been evaluations of individual policies or programmes, but fewer examples of evaluations of health systems (however, see , Blank, Burau and Kuhlmann, 2017). However, there is limited agreement on the issues of 'what' (criteria) and 'how' (methods).

As suggested earlier, the classic RCT examines the effectiveness of an intervention. The most widely known framework for assessing quality in health services is Donabedian's (1980) model of structure-process-outcome. A number of writers have suggested broad frameworks related to this model that are built on the input-output-outcome (I-O-O) model. These concepts, and the relationships between them, generate a set of criteria of evaluation of effectiveness and efficiency (Powell, 1997: 6–7; see next).

Similarly, the public management and performance management literatures stress the '3E' or the '3E+1' of economy, effectiveness, efficiency and equity (Carter et al, 1992; Boyne et al, 2003). Carter, Klein and Day (1992: 35) state that 'if there is a unifying theme to performance measurement, then it lies in the genuflection to the objectives of economy, efficiency, and effectiveness, and to the production of measures of input, output, and outcome'. They adopt a simple model which regards PIs in terms of inputs, processes, outputs and outcomes. They then go on to discuss the '3Es', before adding the fourth E, as 'equity should be a bottom-line PI for any public service' (1992: 39). They also note that a further criticism of the PIs generated by the 'three Es' model is that they tend to ignore the quality aspect of service delivery (1992: 40).

Finally, the general conclusion of Marsh and McConnell (2010) is that the literature on policy success is thin, with a key problem that many claims or assessments about policy outcomes do not establish any systematic criteria for assessing success or failure. They claim that much of the evaluation literature is produced from within government but rarely, if ever, moves beyond the assumption that success equates with meeting policy objectives or producing 'better' policy. They review two broad sets of literature. First, they explore the 'public service improvement' literature (Boyne, 2003). Second, they outline the work of Bovens, 't Hart and Peters (2001) on policy success, which examines policy success/failure in four areas (including management of institutional reform – health services) in six European countries (the UK, the Netherlands, France, Germany, Sweden and Spain). Bovens, 't Hart and Peters (2001) make a key distinction between programmatic (improvement) and political success. However, Marsh and McConnell (2010) point out that Bovens, 't Hart and Peters (2001) do not discuss the process dimension of policy. They add this category to form three dimensions. They claim that 'programmatic' success is often seen as synonymous with policy success, and has three sub-dimensions: 'Operational': was it implemented as per objectives?; 'Outcome': did it achieve the intended outcomes?; and 'Resource': was it an efficient use of resources? They continue that the 'process' of policy formation is an important, but often unacknowledged, element in any consideration of whether a policy is successful or not. In broad terms, it refers to the stages of policy making in which issues emerge and are framed, options are explored, interests are consulted and decisions made. Finally, 'Political' success is the final benchmark for policy success. From a governmental perspective, a policy may be successful if it assists their electoral prospects, reputation or overall governance project.

They move to discuss a number of complexity factors: 'Whose success?' (linked with distributional issues, outlined next); 'Time, space and culture' (the temporal and spatial issues, outlined next). In terms of methodological problems, they stress that success is not all or nothing, as a policy can be partially successful on a continuum, and may achieve some of its objectives and not others. Finally, they note that policies also have unintended consequences, making it important to examine their impact and importance and to what extent they might undermine the original policy objectives.

An additional lens for evaluating the NHS might be the ways and extent to which it has balanced the competing priorities: improving the individual experience of care (including quality and satisfaction), improving the health of populations and reducing per capita cost of care for populations (Mery et al, 2017). Although the wording of the triple aim varies somewhat, the political choices which are inherent in reconciling (as far as possible) these trade-offs are indicative of the outputs and outcomes which all health systems can and do deliver.

Evaluating the NHS

It has been claimed that performance evaluation in the NHS is both conceptually and organisationally problematic, as it ranks high on a number of dimensions: uncertainty about the relationship between inputs and outputs; heterogeneity of activities and aims; the ambiguity of the available information (Carter, Klein and Day, 1992; Klein, 1982). As Carter, Klein and Day (1992) put it, there is no way of summing up the myriad activities of the NHS or of translating these into a currency of evaluation which will allow the overall performance of the organisation as a whole to be measured from year to year. This view of the problems of evaluation has been shared by a number of politicians and institutions (see Guillebaud, 1956; Royal Commission on the NHS, 1979). For example, former Minister of Health, Enoch Powell stated that the attempts to find satisfactory measurements of yardsticks of performance have been persistently baffled (in Carter, Klein and Day, 1992). Some years later, the House of Commons Social Services Committee (1988: xi) lamented that 'the last major weakness of the National Health Service is that it is not possible to tell whether or not it works'.

Powell (1997) explores temporal, intrinsic and extrinsic evaluation. Temporal evaluation focuses on changes over time: is the NHS improving or deteriorating over time? Intrinsic evaluation compares the NHS to its stated objectives: for example, has it lived up to its founding principles? Extrinsic evaluation compares the NHS to other healthcare systems: for example, how do survival rates after disease diagnosis compare to other nations?

Temporal

This relates to Boyne's notion of public service improvement as a dynamic concept, and Marsh and McConnell's (2010) temporal dimension. It examines temporal changes of criteria such as expenditure (such as when was the highest NHS funding in real terms?), outputs such as waiting lists, and outcomes such as patient satisfaction. It can also explore a simple 'before–after' evaluation design (Ovretveit, 1998: ch 3; Mays and Fraser, forthcoming) to determine whether (say) avoidable mortality reduced after the 2012 Health and Social Care Act, in line with one of its stated objectives (Secretary of State for Health, 2010). Was there a 'golden period' of the NHS at its best?

Intrinsic

This has similarities with the 'goal model' (see Boyne, 2003) in which an organisation is examined on its own terms. There are two broad possible approaches. The first involves examining if the NHS has kept to its principles. While there has been much debate about the principles of the NHS, there is broad agreement that they are related to comprehensiveness and universality; largely funded by taxation; largely free at the point of delivery; and some notion of equity (Powell, 1997). There has been a long and sometimes acrimonious political and academic arguments about whether the NHS has lived up to its principles (Powell, 1997).

   The second approach focuses on aims or objectives, which are arguably as problematic as principles. According to Klein (1982), in so far as there has any clearly stated objectives which might be used as NHS criteria of performance they are 'to secure improvement in the physical and mental health of the people' and 'in the prevention, diagnosis and treatment of illness' in the words of the 1946 Act creating the Service. However, the Royal Commission of the NHS (1979) was forced to conclude that this question was strictly unanswerable. The Royal Commission then set out its own objectives (RCNHS, 1979, para. 2.6) which are arguably equally problematic (see Klein, 1982). Subsequent chapters are likely to show that it is often difficult to point to clear aims and objectives, certainly in the form of 'SMART' (Specific, Measurable, Achievable, Relevant, Timed) targets. For example, many government documents often contain non-SMART and vague goals such as 'culture change' (Mannion and Davies, 2018).

Extrinsic

This can similarly be approached in two rather different senses. First, the NHS may be judged by external third-party views on what it should be trying to achieve, rather than by its own stated criteria (outlined previously). Clearly, different commentators may choose different criteria, but they tend to be rooted in the input-outputs-outcomes and 3Es + 1 literatures (Carter, Klein and Day, 1992) or programmatic' success (Marsh and McConnell, 2010). For example, Powell (1997) discusses inputs (expenditure, staff, beds); outputs (patients treated, waiting lists, patient satisfaction) outcomes; economy; effectiveness; efficiency (operational and allocative). This may be particularly important in some spheres stressing 'patient and public involvement' (PPI) where the idea of the traditional 'Gentleman in Whitehall' or 'Doctor knows best' is being challenged.

Second, the NHS may be judged in terms of Marsh and McConnell's (2010) geographical dimension. It has often been claimed that the NHS is the 'best in the world', but the criteria or evidence to support this assertion is sometimes unclear. Such comparisons have become commonplace in recent years but for much of the period since 1948, evidence of the NHS' performance as a health system has been lacking. It is hard therefore to judge how far it has improved over time, in comparison with similar health systems.

There have been a number of attempts to compare the performance of health systems (Marino and Papanicolos, forthcoming b). However, they have used different criteria with different results. For example, the WHO (2000) used eight criteria of comprising the level and distribution of health, the level and distribution of responsiveness of the health system, fairness in financial contribution, overall goal attainment, health expenditure, and performance on the level of health in order to determinant the 'overall health system performance'. It found France to be the best in the world with the British NHS ranked 18th out of 191 nations. On the other hand, the Commonwealth Fund (2021) compared the performance of healthcare systems of 11 high-income countries by means of 71 performance measures across five domains (access to care, care process, administrative efficiency, equity and healthcare outcomes). After some years as the best performing system, the NHS slipped from first to fourth place overall behind Norway, the Netherlands and Australia, but was ninth in terms of healthcare outcomes.

Conclusion

This anniversary is therefore a moment to reflect analytically on NHS' 75 years. While many of the issues it faced at the outset remain similar, the axes around which it has revolved have pivoted, sometimes significantly, in scale and scope. These axes have implications for how the NHS is evaluated.

Combined, the axes and evaluation dimension provide the basis for the subsequent chapters.

Having outlined the background and broad template for the remainder of the book, each chapter will provide chronological, analytical and evaluative material. First, the NHS narrative will be brought up to date, including the period not covered by other chronological texts. Second, the relevant key analytical 'axes' (markets, hierarchies and networks; centralisation and decentralisation; public and private; professional and managerial) will be explored. The blend of these will vary between chapters, according to the contingencies of topic. Third, an evaluative perspective will explore policy success in terms of temporal, intrinsic and extrinsic evaluation.

References

Alford, R. (1975) *Health Care Politics*. Chicago: University of Chicago Press.

Anand, P., Exworthy, M., Frosini, F. and Jones, L. (2012) 'Autonomy and improved performance: Lessons from an NHS policy reform'. *Public Money and Management*, 32, 3, 209–216.

Anderson, M., Pitchforth, E., Edwards, N., Alderwick, H., McGuire, A. and Mossialos, E. (2022) *United Kingdom: Health System Review 2022*. WHO European Observatory on Health Systems and Policies. https://eurohealthobservatory.who.int/publications/i/united-kingdom-health-system-review-2022

Blank, R., Burau, V. and Kuhlmann, E. (2017) *Comparative Health Policy*. London: Bloomsbury.

Bovens, M., 't Hart, P. and Peters, B.G. (eds) (2001) *Success and Failure in Public Governance: A Comparative Analysis*. Cheltenham: Edward Elgar.

Boyne, G. (2003) 'What is public sector improvement?'. *Public Administration*, 81, 2, 211–227.

Burau, V. and Blank, R. (2006) 'Comparing health policy: An assessment of typologies of health systems'. *Journal of Comparative Policy Analysis: Research and Practice*, 8, 63–76.

Carter, N., Klein, R. and Day, P. (1992) *How Organisations Measure Success*. London: Routledge.

Cochrane, A. (1972) *Effectiveness and Efficiency: Random Reflections on Health Services*. London: Nuffield Provincial Hospitals Trust.

Donabedian, A. (1980) *Explorations in Quality Assessment and Monitoring: The Definition of Quality and Approaches to its Assessment*. Ann Arbor, MI: Health Administration.

Durant, R. and Warber, A. (2001) 'Networking in the shadow of hierarchy: Public policy, the administrative presidency, and the neo-administrative state'. *Presidential Studies Quarterly*, 31, 2, 221–244.

Exworthy, M. and Halford, S. (eds) (1999) *Professionals and the New Managerialism Across the Public Sector*. Buckingham: Open University Press.

Exworthy, M. and Peckham, S. (2006) 'Access, choice and travel: The implications for health policy'. *Social Policy and Administration*, 40, 3, 267–287.

Exworthy, M. and Freeman, R. (2009) 'The United Kingdom: Health policy learning in the NHS', in T.R. Marmor, R. Freeman and K.G.H. Okma (eds) *Comparative Studies and the Politics of Modern Medical Care*. New Haven, CT: Yale University Press, pp 153–179.

Exworthy, M. and Lafond, S. (2021) 'Commercialization of the English National Health Service: A necessity in times of financial austerity?'. *Public Money & Management*, 41, 1, 81–84.

Exworthy, M., Powell, M. and Mohan, J. (1999) 'Markets, bureaucracy and public management: The NHS: quasi-market, quasi-hierarchy and quasi-network?'. *Public Money & Management*, 19, 4, 15–22.

Exworthy, M., Frosini, F., Jones, L., Peckham, S., Powell, M., Greener, I. et al (2010) *Decentralisation and Performance: Autonomy and Incentives in Local Health Economies*. NIHR (SDO) final report, SDO Project (08/1618/125). Southampton: National Institute for Health Research Service Delivery and Organisation Programme.

Exworthy, M., Frosini, F. and Jones, L. (2011) 'NHS Foundation Trusts: You can take a horse to water …'. *Journal of Health Services Research and Policy*, 16, 4, 232–237.

Exworthy, M., Mannion, R. and Powell, M. (2016) *Dismantling the NHS?* Bristol: Policy Press.

Goddard, M. and Mannion, R. (1998) 'From competition to co-operation: New economic relationships in the National Health Service'. *Health Economics*, 7, 105–119.

Ferlie, E., Lynn, L. and Pollitt, C. (eds) (2005) *The Oxford Handbook of Public Management*. Oxford: Oxford University Press.

Frisina Doetter, L., Schmid, A., de Carvalho, G. and Rothgang, H. (2021) 'Comparing apples to oranges? Minimizing typological biases to better classify healthcare systems globally', *Health Policy Open*, 2, December. https://doi.org/10.1016/j.hpopen.2021.100035

Gabbay, J., le May, A., Pope, C. and Robert, G. (2011) *Organisational Innovation in Health Services: Lessons from the NHS Treatment Centres*. Bristol: Policy Press.

Greener, I., Exworthy, M., Peckham, S. and Powell, M. (2009) 'Has Labour decentralised the NHS? Terminological obfuscation and analytical confusion'. *Policy Studies*, 30, 4, 439–454.

Greener, I. (2011) 'The case study as history: "Ideology, class and the National Health Service" by Rudolf Klein', in M. Exworthy, S. Peckham, M. Powell and A. Hann (eds) (2011) *Shaping Health Policy: Case Study Methods and Analysis*. Bristol: Policy Press, pp 77–93.

Guillebaud, C.W. (1956) *Report of the Committee of Enquiry into the Cost of the National Health Service*. London: HM Stationery Office.

Harrison, S.R. (1988) *Managing the National Health Service: Shifting the Frontier?* London: Chapman and Hall.

Haywood, S. and Aleszewski, A. (1980) *Crisis in the NHS*. London: Croom Helm.

Health Foundation. (2022) *NHS Vacancy Rates Point to Deepening Workforce Crisis*. London: Health Foundation, 1 December. https://www.health. org.uk/news-and-comment/news/nhs-vacancy-rates-point-to-deepen ing-workforce-crisis#:~:text=The%20latest%20NHS%20Vacancy%20Sta tistics,the%20quarter%20to%20September%202022.

Heritier, A. and Lehmkuhl, D. (2008) 'The shadow of hierarchy and new modes of governance'. *Journal of Public Policy*, 28, 1–17.

Hodgson, D.E., Bailey, S., Exworthy, M., Hassard, J., Bresnan, M. and Hyde, P. (2021) 'On the character of the new entrepreneurial NHS in England: reforming health care from within?', Public Administration. https://onlinelibrary.wiley.com/doi/abs/10.1111/padm.12797

Hodgson, L., Farrell, C.M. and Connolly, M. (2007) 'Improving UK public services: A review of the evidence'. *Public Administration*, 85, 2, 355–382.

Hogwood, B.W. and Gunn, L.A. (1984) *Policy Analysis for the Real World*. Oxford: Oxford University Press.

House of Commons Social Services Committee. (1988) *The Future of the National Health Service*, HC 613. London: HSMO.

Jenkins, S. (1996) *Accountable to None: The Tory Nationalization of Britain*. Harmondsworth: Penguin.

Johnson, P., Stoye, G., Warner, M. and Zaranko, B. (2022) *NHS Waiting Lists*. London: IFS. https://ifs.org.uk/collections/nhs-waiting-lists

Jones, L. (2017) 'Sedimented governance in the English NHS', in M. Bevir and J. Waring (eds) *De-Centring Health Policy: Learning from British Experiences in Healthcare Governance*. London: Routledge.

King's Fund. (2023) *Social Care 360*. London; King's Fund. 2 March. https:// www.health.org.uk/news-and-comment/news/nhs-vacancy-rates-point- to-deepening-workforce-crisis#:~:text=The%20latest%20NHS%20Vaca ncy%20Statistics,the%20quarter%20to%20September%202022

Klein, R. (1982) 'Performance, evaluation and the NHS'. *Public Administration*, 60, 385–407.

Klein, R. (1990) 'The state and the profession: The politics of the double bed'. *BMJ*, 3, 301(6754), 700–702.

Klein, R. (2003) 'The new localism: Once more through the revolving door?'. *Journal of Health Services Research and Policy*, 8, 4, 195–196.

Klein, R. (2013) *The New Politics of the NHS* (7th ed). Abingdon: Radcliffe Medical.

Mannion, R. and Davies, H. (2018) 'Understanding organisational culture for healthcare quality improvement'. *BMJ*, 363, 4907.

Mannion, R., Goddard, M. and Bate, A. (2007) 'Aligning incentives and motivations in health care: The case of earned autonomy'. *Financial Accountability and Management*, 23, 4, 401–420.

Mannion, R., Harrison, S., Jacobs, R., Konteh, F., Walshe, K. and Davies, H. (2009) 'From cultural cohesion to rules and competition: The trajectory of senior management culture in NHS hospitals, 2001–2008'. *Journal of the Royal Society of Medicine*, 102, 8, 332–336.

Marsh, D. and McConnell, A. (2010) 'Towards a framework for establishing policy success'. *Public Administration*, 88, 2, 564–583.

Marino, A. and Papanicolos, I. (forthcoming) 'The best in the world?', in M. Powell, D. Beland and T. Argatan (eds) *The Elgar Handbook of Health Care Policy*, Cheltenham: Elgar.

Marmot, M.G., Allen, J., Boyce, T., Goldblatt, P. and Morrison, J. (2020) *Health Equity in England: The Marmot Review 10 Years On*. London: Health Foundation.

Martin, G.P. and Learmonth, M. (2010) 'A critical account of the rise and spread of leadership: The case of UK healthcare'. *Social Science and Medicine*, 74, 3, 281–288.

Mays, N. and Fraser, A. (forthcoming) 'Evaluation', in M. Powell, D. Beland, and T. Agartan (eds) *The Elgar Handbook of Health Care Policy*. Cheltenham: Elgar.

McGivern, G., Currie, G., Ferlie, E., Fitzgerald, L. and Waring, J. (2015) 'Hybrid Manager-Professionals' identity work: The maintenance and hybridization of medical professionalism in managerial contexts'. *Public Administration*, 93, 2, 412–432.

Mery, G. Majumder, S., Brown, A. and Dobrow, M.J. (2017) 'What do we mean when we talk about the Triple Aim? A systematic review of evolving definitions and adaptations of the framework at the health system level'. *Health Policy*, 121, 6, 629–636.

Morris, J., Schlepper, L., Dayan, M., Jefferies, D., Maguire, D., Merry, L. and Wellings, D. (2023) 'Public satisfaction with the NHS and social care in 2022 Results from the British Social Attitudes survey'. Research report, March. London: King's Fund. https://www.kingsfund.org.uk/sites/defa ult/files/2023-03/Public%20satisfaction%20with%20the%20NHS%20 and%20social%20care%20in%202022_FINAL%20FOR%20WEB.pdf

Newbigging, K. (2016) 'Blowin' in the wind; the involvement of people who use services, carers and the public in health and social care', in M. Exworthy, S. Peckham, M. Powell and A. Hann (eds) (2011) *Shaping Health Policy: Case Study Methods and Analysis*. Bristol: Policy Press, pp 301–322.

NHS England. (2022) 'Delivery plan for tackling the COVID-19 backlog of elective care'. 8 February. https://www.england.nhs.uk/coronavirus/publication/delivery-plan-for-tackling-the-covid-19-backlog-of-elective-care/

Nuffield Trust. (2023) 'Staff survey and performance figures "stark illustration" of backdrop to strikes'. Press release, 9 March. https://www.nuffieldtrust.org.uk/news-item/staff-survey-and-performance-figures-stark-illustration-of-backdrop-to-strikes

Ovretveit, J. (1998) *Evaluating Health Interventions*. Buckingham: Open University Press.

Peckham, S., Exworthy, M., Greener, I. and Powell, M. (2005) 'Decentralising health services: More local accountability or just more central control?'. *Public Money and Management*, 25, 4, 221–228.

Powell, M. (1997) *Evaluating the National Health Service*. Buckingham: Open University Press.

Powell, M. (1998) 'In what sense a National Health Service?'. *Public Policy and Administration,* 13, 3, 57–69.

Powell, M. (2003) 'Quasi-markets in British health policy: A longue durée perspective'. *Social Policy and Administration*, 37, 7, 725–741.

Powell, M. (2019) 'Parliamentary debates on the anniversaries of the British National Health Service 1958–2008: "plus ça change?"'. *Revue Française de Civilisation Britannique* [Online], XXIV-3. http://journals.openedition.org/rfcb/4133

Powell, M. and Miller, R. (2013) 'Privatizing the English National Health Service: An irregular verb?'. *Journal of Health Politics, Policy and Law*, 38, 5, 1051–1059.

Robinson, R., Evans, D. and Exworthy, M. (1994) *Health and the Economy*. Research paper no. 14. Birmingham: National Association of Health Authorities and Trusts.

Royal Commission on the National Health Service. (1979) *Report*, Cmnd 7615, London: HSMO.

Rueschemeyer, D. (1983) 'Professional autonomy and the social control of expertise', in R. Dingwall and P. Lewis (eds) *The Sociology of Professions*. Basingstoke: Macmillan, pp 38–58.

Secretary of State for Health. (1989) *Working for Patients*, Cm 555. London: HSMO.

Secretary of State for Health. (2010) *Equity and Excellence: Liberating the NHS*. London: The Stationery Office.

Sutaria S., Roderick P. and Pollock, A.M. (2017) 'Are radical changes to health and social care paving the way for fewer services and new user charges?' *BMJ*, 358: j4279. DOI:10.1136/bmj.j4279.

Thompson, G., Frances, J., Levacic, R. and Mitchell, J. (1991) *Markets, Hierarchies, Networks: The Co-ordination of Social Life*. London: Sage.

Timmins, N. (ed) (2008) *Rejuvenate or Retire? Views of the NHS at 60*. London: Nuffield Trust.

Timmins, N. (2017) *The Five Giants* (3rd ed). London: William Collins.

Ungerson, C. (1997) 'Social politics and the commodification of care'. *Social Politics*, 4, 3, 362–381.

Veronesi, G., Kirkpatrick, S.F. and Altanler, A. (2022) 'Corporatization, administrative intensity and the performance of public sector organizations'. *Journal of Public Administration Research and Theory* (early version online). https://academic.oup.com/jpart/advance-article-abstract/doi/10.1093/jopart/muac048/6833649?redirectedFrom=fulltext&login=false

Webster, C. (1988) *The Health Services Since the War. Volume I. Problems of Health Care*. The National Health Service before 1957. London: HMSO.

Webster, C. (1996) *The Health Services Since the War. Volume II. Government and Health Care*. The British National Health Service 1958–1979. London: HMSO.

Webster, C. (1998) *The National Health Service. A Political History*. Oxford: Oxford University Press.

World Health Organization (WHO). (2000) *Health Systems: Improving Performance*. Geneva: WHO.

2

NHS governance: the centre claims authority

Scott Greer

In 1968 Samuel Huntington wrote that the 'most important political distinction among countries concerns not their form of government but their degree of government' (Huntington, 1968: 1). How governance is organised and what governments try to do is not the same thing as the extent to which governments have the tools and information to govern.

The story of NHS governance is most commonly told in terms of its *form*. Outside the UK, the NHS is often taken as the ideal type of a monolithic, centralised, state-run health system. Endless classes in health policy and systems teach it as the original and purest Beveridgean system, with strong political and administrative control over health services. Students or readers are lucky if there is much recognition of the fact that administrative devolution to Northern Ireland, Wales and Scotland existed for decades before political devolution in 1999, let alone the variable degree of central control that existed within the systems at any given time (Klein, 2003). Sometimes it doubles as an ideal-type for neoliberalism or marketisation, a useful story of a country that had a strikingly unified social democratic system and turned away from it to a series of very visible experiments with markets and 'neoliberalism', 'privatization' or 'Americanization' (Powell, Béland and Waddan, 2018).

Inside the UK, the history of the NHS is often written in much more subtle terms, influenced by a long tradition of research into NHS reforms, their politics and their effects. They are often superficially focused on *form*, as seen in the organigrammes of the NHS that decorate their pages. But there is a thread of something else, namely an interest in *degree* of governance. We can see this interest in discussions, reviewed in this volume's introductory chapter, of the tension between central control and local activity (Klein, 2010), the balance of public and private ownership and finance, centralising and decentralising policies, the relationships between professionals and the state, efforts to understand the different kinds of relations at work in it (Exworthy, Powell and Mohan, 1999) and debates about the conditions under which various central policy tools are effective.

This chapter focuses squarely on contestation over the *degree* of government and reading changes in the form of governance as part of that story. Drawing on English debates, I argue that the theme of the evolution of NHS governance over 75 years is the increasing prominence of state claims to authority over the organisation and delivery of healthcare. State claims to authority mean that the government creates policy tools which assert that it can organise and manage healthcare and its delivery rather than somebody else (for example, professions, local notables, hospital boards). They are a claim of authority rather than centralisation because it is not always intended to be centralising; some of the most centralising reforms have been undertaken in the name of decentralisation. They are, more importantly, a claim of authority rather than centralisation because central policy tools frequently fail to centralise or deliver their expected outcomes. These claims to authority come at the expense of somebody else, intermediate bodies – which in England usually means professions and professionals (Harrison and Ahmad, 2000) but can also mean the appointed boards that acted something like the traditional gentry in managing local political and governance problems.

The argument, in brief, is that this rising set of state claims of authority happens because governments, once they have accepted the challenge of providing necessary healthcare to a population, automatically collide with serious fiscal and political challenges. Cost containment becomes their problem, since the healthcare system becomes a powerful rival to every other component of the budget and the destination of much government revenue. But cost containment is politically and practically hard – practically hard because it often does not work in practice, and politically hard because popular and well-regarded interest groups will 'wave the bloody shroud' and make cost containment policies politically costly. In particular, cost containment will often degrade healthcare quality, if nothing else because limited access or long waits are not conducive to good patient experience and outcomes – and there are many interest groups and media actors happy to publicise failings.

Governments, if they cannot limit access, try to escape the cost-quality trade-off – manifesting as pressure on budgets and from the public and interest groups – by adopting policy tools as diverse as electronic health records and management schemes. They also seek to make the system *legible* to them, so they can, as the state, see into it and know what it is doing and what the outcomes are (Scott, 1998). Legibility is a precondition for effective central governance, and one frequently resisted by workers and local leaders of all descriptions who bear costs of reporting and are aware that greater legibility to the centre might tighten and change their accountability.

NHS governance: a schematic history

The broad organisational history of the NHS is well known and forms the core of some of the classic histories, which generally inform this account (Rivett, 1998; Webster, 2002; Ham, 2009; Klein, 2013a; Greener et al, 2014). The account here looks at key moments in the development of state claims to authority and policy tools to match as they accumulated through different reorganisations. Permanent austerity (Pierson, 1998) led to permanent receptiveness to those who promised to find a way that the government could get more and better care, and less blame, for what it did.

1948: the fiduciary model of health policy

The creation of the NHS meant a transformative expansion of state responsibility for healthcare by promising universal access to healthcare and the removal of financial barriers to seeking care. It meant nationalising a set of charity and municipal hospitals and putting primary care on a nationwide basis with, effectively, a government monopsonist. The structure, on paper, was set: a giant organisation accountable to the Secretary of State, financed out of taxes and available to all, and accountable to a government which was then accountable to parliament and the people. It looked rather like the monolith of later comparative caricatures, and there is an apparently unsourced but widely attributed quotation from Aneurin Bevan, saying that the clang of a dropped bedpan in Tredegar should resound through the Palace of Westminster.

Bevan might have uttered the line about the bedpan, but what is striking is how little evidence exists that the bedpan was heard beyond the ward in Tredegar. The removal of financial barriers to access via a dramatic expansion of the central role did not actually mean the creation of a unified central organisation (Ham, 2009: 15–16).

The initial approach to NHS governance was essentially fiduciary, entrusting resources and decisions to the medical profession and to a far lesser extent other self-governing professions, and appointed boards. Governance in practice was through intermediate bodies, notably professions (especially medicine and surgery) (Klein, 1990) and boards of politically connected and sensitive local worthies. The combination of professional 'club government' (Moran, 2003) and boards of what amounted to the twentieth-century version of gentry had many virtues if what governments wanted was a quiet life: it solved government problems in a decentralised and politically sensitive manner and aligned the interests of the professions with policy. At the centre of the system, there was remarkably little administrative capacity to monitor or shape what the appointees did. After Bevan left office, there was no Cabinet-level minister specifically for health until the 1980s (save for two years in the 1960s). The government was content to let the systems get on with their work without a dedicated high-level politician overseeing them in a political backwater (Webster, 2002: 35). Exhort-and-hope was the central approach, rather than the command and control of stylised textbook presentations (Klein, 2010).

Consensus management

The inherited structure, reflecting political compromises made by the Attlee government, looked anachronistic by the 1970s, and therefore a candidate for efficiency measures that would reorganise it to better coordinate with other social services while making decisions in a responsive way. That gave rise to the first major organisational change affecting the whole NHS, in 1974. It was a comprehensive reorganisation that imposed a consistent structure and introduced the novel approach to healthcare services called 'consensus management'.

Consensus management was substantially the intellectual creation of a team surrounding Brunel University social psychologist Elliott Jaques (also known for creating the concept of the midlife crisis) (Jaques, 1978). While it still stands out as an unusually theoretically articulated approach to healthcare management and organisation, it was of a type with other policies to address healthcare costs around the world. The 1970s were a good decade for efforts to rely on professionals, corporatism, and consensus to manage healthcare costs in countries as different as the US and Germany.

The 1974 reforms combined a claim to authority over how the NHS should run with the deliberate creation of a decentralised structure. The NHS was reorganised into consistent local tiers with different sets of responsibilities for different functions and coordinating responsibilities (public health was removed from local government and moved into the NHS, leaving behind work like restaurant inspection and social work that had formerly been under local Medical Officers of Health). Anywhere in England, the governance of any given organisation or person would be consistent. But the governance of that organisation would be remarkably decentralist, run by 'consensus management'. Consensus management meant governance by committees of representatives of key parties, namely doctors, nurses, administrators and variable others. In this model, 'administration' was relatively subordinate, a functional unit responsible for issues like accounting, estates and catering, and was represented on consensus committees on a formally equal footing with medicine or nursing (informally, it seems that catering and estates rarely defeated medicine in conflict). Consensus management was more a form of corporatism than a management structure as conventionally understood, and relied heavily on mobilising professionals' local problem-solving capacities. Regional boards remained, politically appointed with professional representation which continued to absorb, manage, defuse and diffuse conflict and stabilise finances by balancing over- and under-spends across the region.

Management

Consensus management was also about as far as could be from Margaret Thatcher's concept of a viable organisation. Thatcher, early in her career as prime minister, commissioned a supermarket executive, Roy Griffiths, to report on the organisation of the NHS. Griffiths, in a short letter that is often wrongly referred to as a report, suggested a series of changes that would start to make the NHS resemble the well-known organisational form of a firm (NHS Management Inquiry, 1983). His letter suggested that the NHS establish a general management cadre, with executives at every significant level who would be empowered to manage resources and people and make strategic decisions, and who would be accountable for the results of their units (Edwards and Fall, 2005).

The establishment of general management can from one point of view seem unobjectionable, ending the NHS' experiment with professional governance and consensus as a principle and replacing it with the management and hierarchy typical of public and private enterprises at the time. Well-known theories of institutional isomorphism – predicting organisations gain legitimacy if they look like each other – would suggest a truly original organisational model is always in peril (DiMaggio and Powell, 1991). It was also in keeping with the turn away from corporatist policy worldwide, managerialism and the developing New Public Management model (Pollitt, 1993; Ferlie, Fitzgerald and Pettigrew, 1996). New Public Management came to mean many things but its core involved trying to insulate operations from politics, use competition and incentives more effectively and borrow skills from private sector management. Relative to the professional dominance encoded in consensus management, it was striking because of its explicit goals of centring hierarchical, general, management in the NHS. Instead of the essentially fiduciary model of consensus management and its predecessors, in which the governance of the NHS was entrusted to committees and professions, the new NHS would focus on general managers who would be accountable for goals determined further up the managerial hierarchy.

The introduction of general management at the local level was an immense task since merely rebranding 'administrators' (the first thing to happen) was nothing like creating general managers with the skills or authority to do anything much resembling management. Many professionals did not appreciate their formal disempowerment and had the resources to resist it at the local level (Harrison, 2004). Luckily, it was a topic that attracted excellent social science research which still illuminates the complex relations between management and professionals in health systems (Strong and Robinson, 1990; Cox, 1991; Hunter and Williamson, 1991; Harrison et al, 1992; Harrison and Pollitt, 1994; Harrison, 2004). The introduction of general management did nonetheless create something that had heretofore not existed: a clear set of people with formal authority who were accountable to the centre for NHS management as determined by the top of government.

Internal market

The introduction of general management on paper, let alone in reality, was still underway when Thatcher announced a surprise review of NHS funding on television in January 1988. The review was quickly constituted and worked quickly and paid little attention to consensus. Notably, the usual big interest groups such as the doctor's union BMA were excluded from the review; reviving the fiduciary model or corporatism were among few organisational models that the government did not consider.

Their conclusion, loosely based on the 'managed competition' ideas of a Stanford business professor named Alain Enthoven, would become known as the 'internal market' (Enthoven, 1985). The basic idea was that markets could more efficiently (and with less public accountability) allocate resources in a way that reflected the preferences of patients. At its most basic, it created 'trusts', meaning individual hospitals or other service providers, constituted as little publicly owned firms with their own managerial hierarchies and boards. These trusts would sell their services internally within the NHS. The customers were individual GP 'fundholders' who would buy consultant and hospital services for their patients, and district Health Authorities which would purchase services when GPs could not or would not do so (Butler, 1992). District Health Authorities would also be responsible, in ways that were not theoretically or legally clear, for making things work (avoid politically salient failures) in their areas.

Regional boards and the Management Executive would, in similarly unspecified but important ways, manage the overall system – thereby retaining both the politically aware regional level, which could make problems go away, and a management hierarchy accountable not just to the internal market or boards but to the Chief Executive and therefore the Secretary of State. This introduced a theme which would remain in subsequent market-focused NHS reforms: a recognition that the market would produce disequilibria and political problems and would therefore require not just the legal and regulatory structure of a real market but also centrally accountable organisations which would be able to manage problems. Policy documents and law often left it hazy just what these structures would do but looking at the use of phrases such as 'holding the ring' in conversation suggested that avoiding local failures or politically unpleasant consequences of markets, such as provider exits, would be the job of these managerial structures.

A vast amount of ink has been spilled on the subject of the internal market, ranging from subtle studies to simple caricature. Most of them take it at face value and study it as an introduction of market mechanisms. But, like all subsequent forms of the NHS internal market, it was a very strange market, utterly unlike the putatively spontaneous ones in economics textbooks. The government constituted the buyers (GP fundholders and residual Health Authorities), the sellers (trusts) and increasingly both prices and products. The use of transactions between entities created by the government made the system more legible to the government; the stated goal that 'money should follow the patient' had the corollary that a good reporting system would allow government to follow money and patients. As with the 1974 reorganisation, the creation of an entire organisational ecology by law, fleshed out in Management Executive and Department of Health (DH) guidance, was another claim of authority: the government that had created your organisation, its formal environment, its revenue and expenditure systems and your job title, would presumptively know what you did and be able to manipulate your activities.

Department of Health

The Ministry of Health had been downgraded to part of the Department of Health and Social Security, but in July 1988, with the NHS Review that would lead to the internal market underway, it was reinstated as a department on its own with a Secretary of State. This development – one also seen in other countries in the 1980s and 1990s – reflected and enabled a greater political focus on management of healthcare as a specific policy priority (Briatte, 2010; Mätzke, 2010; Sheard, 2010).

On one hand, the case for creating a specific department was obvious: if the government were to be responsible for managing the NHS and making major reforms, it would need focus and expertise at the centre. Getting a politician of enough stature to force through such reforms would be easier if it were a Secretary of State position, and having a department with enough staff and organisational profile to make and implement reforms was easier than trying to do so with a minister inside a larger organisation that had other priorities and accountability. The result, though, was that the government now claimed expertise and a specific managerial role as part of the department it had created, and people within the department, including newly installed senior politicians like Kenneth Clarke, had resources and tools with which to fulfil that claim (Day and Klein, 1997; Greer and Jarman, 2007).

The Blair governments

Twenty-four hours before the 1997 general election, Labour texted voters that they had '24 hours to save the NHS'. From the start of the Labour governments, 'saving' the NHS was a priority. Tony Blair's governments (1997–2007) presided over a dramatic expansion of NHS funding (as well as the creation of elected devolved governments for Northern Ireland, Scotland and Wales) (Greer, 2004). Unlike the Conservatives, Blair and Labour ran and would continue to run as defenders of the NHS. Every Labour manifesto since 1996 has emphasised the NHS, and a few, for example 2005, had surprisingly little else. Labour leadership under Blair were also convinced that if all they managed to do was raise taxes to fund it without making the NHS obviously better, they would damage their own electoral prospects and the fundamental political sustainability of the NHS. The additional funds allocated to the NHS in England from 1997 to 2010 were dramatic, enabling a great deal of investment in workforce, facilities and equipment. So was the investment of money and political energy in making claims to authority over the NHS and developing the policy tools to make them real.

There was nearly constant reorganisation of the NHS in the Blair years, including the merging of regions into the Management Executive and then the merging of the Management Executive with the DH under a person double-hatted as NHS Chief Executive and DH Permanent Secretary. This move effectively turned the Department into the Executive, with the Department largely staffed by NHS managers rather than conventional officials (Greer and Jarman, 2007; Jarman and Greer, 2010; Greer and Jarman, 2010). Legislation in 2003 created Foundation Trusts, a more autonomous kind of trust with more financial discretion and more autonomous boards, outside the NHS lines of authority and instead responsible to its regulators and commissioners. The explicit goal was to decentralise – by centrally creating a new form of regulated NHS body with greater managerial discretion but also legibility to the centre and responsiveness to central regulators. The upshot was fewer and fewer tiers with less and less discretionary authority and real power over the health systems in their areas. On paper, at least, the central authorities had a direct relationship with more and more of the NHS. Foundation Trust hospitals, for example, were not accountable in any hierarchical fashion to the remaining regional tier (Strategic Health Authorities). Rather, they were accountable to regulators (discussed next).

GPs' status as small businesses made them formally harder to manage, but the new contracts, at considerable expense, took away discretion in areas where most businesses owners would prefer to keep it. Central initiatives in detailed areas such as targets for GP performance (appointment times, screening) (Checkland and Harrison, 2010), patient booking (Choose and

Book) and hospital capital investment (Private Finance Initiative (PFI) contracts) likewise eroded discretion at the local level.

The NHS had a long history of professional self-regulation that was a model of club governance (Eckstein, 1960; Moran & Wood, 1993; Moran, 2003; Salter, 2004; McKee and Greer, 2022) as well as a tradition of legalistic professional regulators in other areas. A series of highly public problems, including a serial killer GP and care or ethical scandals dotted around England, led the government to plunge into a global conversation about ways to improve quality and regulate it while also helping to make Labour's case for more funding (Smee, 2005). Increasingly good data on outcomes also alerted government and others to the scale of disparities in outcomes and treatment around the country, making more real the prospect of an NHS that always delivered the outcomes seen in its best performing areas (Walshe, 2003). The quality and regulation area is complex and diffuse, ranging from policies and approaches that emphasise learning to tough inspectors with the power to ask courts to close providers at little notice. Eventually the Care Quality Commission became the key quality regulator for the NHS and care sector, with an elaborate inspection process, grades and authority to ask for closures. Meanwhile, changes to the governance of doctors created 'Responsible Officers' with accountability for their colleague's practice in the eyes of regulators – which is just as much an effort to extend the scope of governance into medical care as the creation of general managers decades earlier (Bryce et al, 2018). Inspections are nothing new in the public sector, but investment in the Care Quality Commission (CQC) was an investment in making facilities more responsive, legible and accountable to the centre for standards it set – and a loss of discretion for local doctors, boards and self-regulating professions.

The next innovation was the introduction of market, rather than quality, regulators. The NHS had a great deal of experience with managers, professional regulation and health and safety. It did not have a great deal of experience with market regulators. Labour began to introduce market regulators. The charge of these regulators was to maintain a market and discipline the participants in the market. Monitor was the NHS one, charged with certifying and overseeing trusts as they graduated to their new and more autonomous Foundation Trust status (Greer, Jarman and Azorsky, 2014; Greer, Rowland and Jarman, 2016). The regulators were designed to be somewhat separate from government and to have clear orders on the theory that this would increase their credibility. Managing the result was a problem for somebody else; leadership's focus on gaining Foundation Trust status led to problems at the Stafford hospital (Francis, 2013: 9).

The centre was also empowered by investment in financial processes and data that would increase the legibility of the system. The 2003–2004 creation of a standard tariff, called payment by results, was quite in keeping with international trends (Busse et al, 2011). It meant that NHS bookkeeping and finances became much more legible, since finance directors lost many of the tools they had once used to balance budgets across organisations or regions. This was emphatically a goal of the central policy-makers.

Payment by Results was not just about financial records and discipline. The incentive effects were clear to all, and so the shape and contents of the tariff were sure to affect clinical care and healthcare planning. Trusts, in particular, would have incentive to focus on the areas where they combined a low cost of delivery with a good price – rudimentary business thinking, but also substantially alien to the NHS where the cost-effectiveness of a given local service was often less important than the importance of the service and the politics surrounding it. Writing the tariff is the job of the department, so it was also nothing like the spontaneous emergence of prices that conventional markets are supposed to have (Street and AbdulHussain, 2004; Allen, 2013). Rather, it was a central tool for deciding what should be valued.

Health Technology Assessment (HTA) is a complex and internationally varied area, one that the UK also entered with gusto. HTA involves, broadly, government payers employing economists and health services researchers to evaluate the comparative effectiveness of different technologies and treatments. It more or less automatically intrudes on the autonomy of pharmaceutical companies, doctors, devices makers and various local decision-makers, which has led to many overt campaigns against it and subtle campaigns to make it ineffective (Löblová, 2018; Löblová et al, 2020). The National Institute for Clinical Excellence (NICE), the UK's HTA agency, is internationally known for its sophistication and apparent policy influence – which we can read as a state claim of authority. HTA in general (and perhaps the whole of health services research) might be best read as an effort by governments to build up the analytical capacity to argue with professions about the best way to deliver care; a claim of competency to match a claim of authority.

Electronic health records (EHRs) are, globally, a fine tool for monitoring, evaluation, and financial planning of care (their impact on quality of care, workforce morale and patients is rather less clear). Labour governments invested a great deal of money in building out nationally interconnected EHR systems connected to every local NHS installation. The claim of authority was tremendous, even if often normalised by the global ubiquity of ambitious EHR programs. In the name of efficiency and quality, the government would create a single national system with data on the problems and treatments of effectively every citizen and be able to identify, for example, practice variations and outcomes. The claim of authority is even bigger when we remember the well-documented ways in which EHRs, intentionally and unintentionally, shape healthcare through their suggestions, questions, reporting and other components. Whomever designs an EHR is going to necessarily shape care at least as much as they reflect it. The claim of authority in this case was clearly not substantiated; the centralising potential of the national EHR strategy remains theoretical because the contractors simply failed to build out most of what was promised (Robertson, Bates and Sheikh, 2011). Not all claims of authority work; the policy tools can be inadequate or fail.

The Blair-Brown years will rightly be remembered as a time of enormous new NHS investment coupled with constant change in the *form* of governance (Kay, 2019). They should also be remembered as years of a great deal of investment – of political, bureaucratic, creative and financial resources – in increasing the *degree* of governance. One can easily get lost in the organisational story, distinguishing the 'NHS Plan' from 'Shifting the Balance of Power' or parsing the family trees of quangos, but they can perhaps all be best viewed as part of a project of increasing not just resources for the NHS, but also the degree of governance in the NHS. Statements by key participants can be read as saying so, explicitly (Stevens, 2004; Barber, 2007; Crisp, 2011).

The Lansley reforms

After the 2010 election, a coalition government led by David Cameron took office. In a frankly inexplicable decision whose contingency testifies to the centralisation of political power in the UK, Cameron and the Liberal Democrats let Secretary of State Andrew Lansley enact a major reorganisation of the entire NHS in the shape of the 2012 Health and Social Care Act (Timmins, 2012; Klein, 2013b; Exworthy, Mannion and Powell, 2016; Greer, 2016). The Health and Social Care Act (HSCA) fell into the great tradition of putatively decentralising reforms whose process of enactment and actual operation were amounted to centralising claims of authority. The core idea of Lansley was to revisit Thatcher's reforms by eliminating the geographic bodies that had commissioned healthcare and to replace them with doctors, namely groups of GPs organised as 'Clinical Commissioning Groups' (CCGs). The full range of NHS territorial organisations would be eliminated; organisations would either be local (CCGs and trusts) or central. The regional levels which had used their discretion largely to avoid politically salient problems, would no longer be available to cushion local services from central policy – or central politicians from local problems. Public health was transferred to local government (never a formula for increased status in English public life) and a national agency, Public Health England.

Predictably enough, the actual results were centralising (Greer, 2013). The CCGs were subscale for most purposes including needs analysis and bargaining with large trusts. Even in the policy documents leading up to the enactment of the HSCA, it was clear that the organisation which came to be called 'NHS England' (NHSE) would be absolutely crucial as the body that would be responsive to ministers and responsible for the overall stability of the system should the new internal market fail to produce the desired results (Greer, 2016). Monitor, the economic regulator, was in charge of ensuring that individual organisations were financially stable and conformed to norms of financial management, but Monitor had no overall authority to shape the market or focus on its overall outcomes and resilience. Given that no government could let the market alone shape healthcare (for example by forcing less efficient hospitals out of business), the result was a key role for NHSE as a tool for central intervention. Unsurprisingly, it was to NHSE that the DH staff mostly moved when the DH itself shrank; NHSE looked a lot like the Management Executive reborn (Greer, Jarman and Azorsky, 2014).

Implementing the reforms at the same time as a major effort to shrink public expenditure increased the pressure on health services, so the emphasis under NHS England quickly shifted from competition to care integration. Reading some of the highest quality reports on, for example, relational contracting, it can seem a lot like 1991 over again (Checkland et al, 2012; Porter et al, 2013).

NHSE's focus on integration, combined with the government's distraction and deep reluctance to legislate on healthcare after the bruising HSCA experience, produced some curious effects. Monitor was increasingly sidelined, reorganised and renamed since the market it was supposed to regulate no longer had the political support it required. The dismantling of the Lansley scheme was largely orchestrated by NHSE, while the Department of Health became increasingly the preserve of Whitehall officials and a few NHS managers (Greer, Jarman and Azorsky, 2015). The government, having concluded that major healthcare reform was unwise, was happy to let NHSE, under the politically astute Simon Stevens, quietly redesign the system (Jarman, 2023). Sustainability and Transformation Plans (STPs), for example, grouped CCGs with NHSE support to plan services and manage austerity. They had neither a legal framework nor their own staff, and while CCGs had to formally pass their decisions, it was clear the STPs, working primarily for NHSE, were orchestrating local service planning and reconfigurations. Over time STPs became Accountable Care Systems, then Integrated Care Systems, and slowly became a key policy tool (Hammond et al, 2017; Jarman, 2023). While there was a clear policy case for some larger commissioning unit than the CCGs if there was to be any strategic thinking about services, it was also clear that creating an entire tier of regional management accountable to the centre and nobody else was anything but decentralising.

COVID-19

The Conservative governments after Cameron's resignation were preoccupied with Brexit, COVID-19 and their own internal political difficulties (Jarman, 2023). Health, a topic on which Conservatives have had to play defence since

1945, was an especially unpromising use of their scant political capital. Brexit created challenges for the NHS in a variety of areas, from medicines supply chains to workforce, but pro-Brexit Conservative governments focused on other issues and generally refused to admit the problems or develop structural solutions such as a post-Brexit workforce strategy (McCarey et al, 2022; Greer Löblová, 2020).

The government obviously could not ignore COVID-19, and its erratic public health response coupled with pre-existing inequalities and the legacy of austerity since 2010 led to a UK response that could clearly have been better (Williams, Rajan and Cylus, 2021). The governance story was perhaps not surprising. As in most high-income countries (Greer et al, 2022; Schmidt et al, 2022; Waitzberg et al, 2022) the UK responded with a high degree of centralisation within government. Complex purchasing systems, financial formulas and even reporting requirements were brushed aside in the scramble to keep services supplied and operational. Local NHS managers scrambled to run their services and handle the huge redistribution of work from elective and preventative to emergency services, with the government quite directly paying them and telling them what to do. Key COVID-19 response functions, including PPE acquisition, testing and tracing and vaccines acquisition and distribution were essentially run directly from the centre, with widely varying and sometimes scandalous results. The apparatus of the normal health system was, for a while, swept aside (Montás et al, 2022).

At the time of writing in late 2022 it is not entirely clear what the next stage will be, since the NHS remained under enormous pressure from COVID-19, other contagious diseases, the long-awaited implosion of the social and long-term care sector, the long-awaited workforce crisis and a giant backlog of every other kind of care as well as the potential threat from long COVID, while the government remained distracted and rudderless. What COVID-19 showed, though, was that in a big enough crisis, the government could claim essentially unlimited authority over the NHS, regardless of the laws that supposedly bound it.

Conclusion: rising claims of authority

Each of these episodes had the same basic characteristic. The UK government had accepted effectively universal access to services (in 1948 with the removal of financial barriers, and since then, in the efforts to remove geographic and other barriers to access). While subsequent governments successfully reintroduced financial barriers to access, notably in dentistry, it has been politically difficult to reintroduce them in core healthcare services. It therefore took on the burden of balancing cost and quality, and quickly learned that resolving those trade-offs by reinstating financial barriers to access to core healthcare services was bad politics (Cutler, 2006). Bearing that burden gave its politicians an appetite for managerial, organisational or other policy ideas which promised to reduce the trade-offs by creating more efficiency, better quality or at least less blame for the Secretary of State when things went wrong. The combination of Westminster's flexible policy making and the major formal role of the central government in the NHS meant that they could choose from possibly the widest range of options of any rich democracy, from data systems to massive organisational reforms. Whether the policies produced quality or efficiency, or even effective legibility and accountability to the centre, is a complex empirical question. But in each case, the result was the government making more and more claims of detailed, discretionary authority over the practice of medicine, at the expense of professionals and boards whose problem-solving role was increasingly eroded in favour of centrally chosen tools and policies that made the operation of the system more legible and putatively responsive to the centre.

This happened when austerity was clearly the policy agenda of the broader government, as with Thatcher and Cameron. It also happened when the opposite of austerity happened in the NHS under Blair. In times of famine, each claim of authority was a way to avoid blame for any quality effects of reduced funding; in times of feast, each claim of authority was a way to justify expenditure by arguing that organisational changes would ensure that the money would not be wasted.

This chapter has argued that the story of NHS governance is one of governments, trapped by their own commitments, making more and more detailed and discretionary claims of authority over the organisation of healthcare and practice of medicine. For all that many of these policies failed on their own terms, or were never really implemented as intended, they have contributed to the creation of a huge regulatory, managerial and financial apparatus intended to allow the government to govern the NHS more and more. The form of NHS governance changes constantly – in large part because of a decades-long campaign by politicians to increase its degree.

References

Allen, P. (2013) 'An economic analysis of the limits of market based reforms in the English NHS'. *BMC Health Services Research*, 13, 1, 1–10.

Barber, M. (2007) *Instruction to Deliver: Tony Blair, the Public Services, and the Challenge of Delivery*. London: Politico's.

Briatte, F. (2010) 'A case of weak architecture: The French Ministry of Health'. *Social Policy and Administration*, 44, 2, 155–170.

Bryce, M., Luscombe, K., Boyd, A., Tazzyman, A., Tredinnick-Rowe, J., Walshe, K. et al (2018) 'Policing the profession? Regulatory reform, restratification and the emergence of Responsible Officers as a new locus of power in UK medicine'. *Social Science & Medicine*, 213, 98–105. DOI:10.1016/j.socscimed.2018.07.042

Busse, R., Geissler, A., Quentin, W. and Wiley, M. (eds) (2011) *Diagnosis-Related Groups in Europe: Moving Towards Transparency, Efficiency and Quality in Hospitals*. Basingstoke: Open University Press.

Butler, J. (1992) *Patients, Policies and Politics: Before and After Working for Patients*. Buckingham: Open University Press.

Checkland, K. and Harrison, S. (2010) 'The impact of the Quality and Outcomes Framework on practice organisation and service delivery: Summary of evidence from two qualitative studies'. *Quality in Primary Care*, 18, 2, 139–146.

Checkland, K., Snow, S., McDermott, I., Harrison, S. and Coleman, A. (2012) '"Animateurs" and animation: What makes a good commissioning manager?'. *Journal of Health Services Research and Policy*, 17, 1, 11–17. DOI:10.1258/jhsrp.2011.011010

Cox, D. (1991) 'Health service management: A sociological view: Griffiths and the non-negotiated order of the hospital', in J. Gabe, M. Calnan and M. Bury (eds) *The Sociology of the Health Service*. London: Routledge, pp 89–114.

Crisp, N. (2011) *24 Hours to Save the NHS: The Chief Executive's Account of Reform 2000–2006*. Oxford: Oxford University Press.

Cutler, T. (2006) 'A double irony? The politics of National Health Service Expenditure in the 1950s', in M. Gorsky and S. Sheard (eds) *Financing Medicine: The British Experience since 1750*. Abingdon: Routledge, pp 201–220.

Day, P. and Klein, R. (1997) *Steering but Not Rowing? The Transformation of the Department of Health: A Case Study*. Bristol: Policy Press.

DiMaggio, P.J. and Powell, W.W. (1991) 'The iron cage revisited: Institutional isomorphism and collective rationality in organization fields', in W.W. Powell and P.J. DiMaggio (eds) *The New Institutionalism in Organizational Analysis*. Chicago: University of Chicago Press, pp 63–82.

Eckstein, H. (1960) *Pressure Group Politics: The Case of the British Medical Association*. London: Allen & Unwin.

Edwards, B. and Fall, M. (2005) *The Executive Years of the NHS: The England Account 1985–2003*. London: The Nuffield Trust/Radcliffe.

Enthoven, A.C. (1985) *Reflections on the Management of the National Health Service*. London: Nuffield Provincial Hospitals Trust.

Exworthy, M., Mannion, R. and Powell, M. (eds) (2016) *Dismantling the NHS? Evaluating the Impact of Health Reforms*. Bristol: Policy Press.

Exworthy, M., Powell, M. and Mohan, J. (1999) 'The NHS: Quasi-market, quasi-hierarchy and quasi-network?'. *Public Money and Management*, 19, 4, 15–22.

Ferlie, E., Fitzgerald, L. and Pettigrew, A. (1996) *The New Public Management in Action*. Oxford: Oxford University Press.

Francis, R.Q.C. (2013) *Report of the Mid Staffordship NHS Foundation Trust Public Inquiry*. London: Stationery Office.

Greener, I., Harrington, B., Hunter, D.J., Mannion, R. and Powell, M. (2014) *Reforming Healthcare: What's the Evidence?* Bristol: Policy Press.

Greer, S.L. (2004) *Territorial Politics and Health Policy: UK Health Policy in Comparative Perspective*. Manchester: Manchester University Press.

Greer, S.L. (2013) 'The rise and fall of territory in United Kingdom health services', in J. Costa-Font and S. L. Greer (eds) *Federalism and Decentralization in European Health and Social Care*. Basingstoke: Palgrave Macmillan, pp 81–100.

Greer, S.L. (2016) 'Claiming authority over the NHS', in M. Bevir and R.A.W. Rhodes (eds) *Rethinking Governance: Ruling, Rationalities and Resistance*. Abingdon: Routledge, pp 87–104.

Greer, S.L. and Jarman, H. (2007) *The Department of Health and the Civil Service: From Whitehall to Department of Delivery to Where?* London: Nuffield Trust.

Greer, S.L. and Jarman, H. (2010) 'What Whitehall? Definitions, demographics and the changing home civil service'. *Public Policy and Administration*, 25, 3, 251–270.

Greer, S.L., Jarman, H. and Azorsky, A. (2014) *A Reorganisation You Can See from Space: The Architecture of Power in the New NHS*. London: Centre for Health and the Public Interest.

Greer, S.L., Jarman, H. and Azorsky, A. (2015) 'Devolution and the civil service: A biographical study'. *Public Policy and Administration*, 30, 1, 31–50.

Greer, S.L. and Löblová, O. (2020) 'Networks after Brexit', in S.L. Greer and J. Laible (eds) *The European Union after Brexit*. Manchester: Manchester University Press, pp 146–161.

Greer, S.L., Rozenblum, S., Falkenbach, M., Löblová, O., Jarman, H., Williams, N. et al (2022) 'Centralizing and decentralizing governance in the COVID-19 pandemic: The politics of credit and blame'. *Health Policy*, 126, 5, 408–417.

Greer, S.L., Rowland, D. and Jarman, H. (2016) 'The central management of the English NHS,' in M. Exworthy , R. Mannion and M. Powell (eds) *Dismantling the NHS? Evaluating the Impact of Health Reforms*. Bristol: Policy Press, pp 87–104.

Ham, C. (2009) *Health Policy in Britain* (6th ed). Basingstoke: Palgrave Macmillan.

Hammond, J., Lorne, C., Coleman, A., Allen, P., Mays, N., Dam, R. et al (2017) 'The spatial politics of place and health policy: Exploring Sustainability and Transformation Plans in the English NHS'. *Social Science & Medicine*, 190, 217–226. DOI:10.1016/j.socscimed.2017.08.007

Harrison, S. (2004) 'Medicine and management: Autonomy and authority in the National Health Service', in A. Gray and S. Harrison (eds) *Governing Medicine: Theory and Practice*. Maidenhead: Open University Press, pp 51–60.

Harrison, S. and Ahmad, W.U. (2000) 'Medical autonomy and the UK state 1975 to 2025'. *Sociology*, 34, 5, 129–246.

Harrison, S., Hunter, D., Marnoch, G. and Pollitt, C. (1992) *Just Managing: Power and Culture in the National Health Service*. Basingstoke: Macmillan.

Harrison, S. and Pollitt, C. (1994) *Controlling Health Professionals: The Future of Work and Organization in the NHS*. Buckingham: Open University Press.

Hunter, D. and Williamson, P. (1991) 'General management in the NHS: Comparisons and contrasts between Scotland and England'. *Health Services Management*, 87, 4.

Huntington, S.P. (1968) *Political Order in Changing Societies*. New Haven: Yale University Press.

Jaques, E. (1978) *Health Services: Their Nature and Organization and the Role of Patients, Doctors, Nurses, and the Complementary Professions*. London: Heinemann.

Jarman, H. (2023) 'The submerged welfare state: Health and social care policy in England from 2015 to 2020', in M. Beech (ed), *Conservative Governments in the Age of Brexit*. New York: Springer, pp 147–170.

Jarman, H. and Greer, S.L. (2010) 'In the eye of the storm: Civil servants and managers in the department of health'. *Social Policy and Administration*, 44, 2, 172–192.

Kay, A. (2019) 'Cutting the wait – at least for a while: The NHS's assault on waiting times'. *Great Policy Successes*, 0. DOI:10.1093/oso/9780198843719.003.0004.

Klein, R. (1990) 'The state and the profession: The politics of the double bed'. *British Medical Journal*, 301, 700–702.

Klein, R. (2003) '"The new localism": Once more through the revolving door'. *Journal of Health Services Research & Policy*, 8, 4, 195–196.

Klein, R. (2010) 'The eternal triangle: Sixty years of the centre-periphery relationship in the National Health Service'. *Social Policy & Administration*, 44, 3, 285–304. DOI:10.1111/j.1467-9515.2010.00714.x

Klein, R. (2013a) *The New Politics of the NHS* (7th ed.). Boca Raton, FL: CRC Press.

Klein, R. (2013b) 'The twenty-year war over England's National Health Service: A report from the battlefield'. *Journal of Health Politics, Policy and Law*, 38, 4, 849–869.

Löblová, O. (2018) 'What has health technology assessment ever done for us'. *Journal of Health Services Research & Policy*, 23, 2, 134–136.

Löblová, O., Trayanov, T., Csanádi, M. and Ozierański, P. (2020) 'The emerging social science literature on health technology assessment: A narrative review'. *Value in Health*, 23, 1, 3–9.

Mätzke, M. (2010) 'The organization of health policy functions in the German Federal Government'. *Social Policy & Administration*, 44, 2, 120–141.

McCarey, M., Dayan, M., Jarman, H., Hervey, T., Fahy, N., Bristow, D. et al (2022) *Health and Brexit: Six Years On*. London: Nuffield Trust.

McKee, M. and Greer, S.L. (2022) 'Doctors are accountable to the GMC, but who is the GMC accountable to'. *BMJ*, 379, o2676.

Montás, M.C., Klasa, K., van Ginneken, E. and Greer, S.L. (2022) 'Strategic purchasing and health systems resilience: Lessons from COVID-19 in selected European countries'. *Health Policy*, 126, 9, 853–864.

Moran, M. (2003) *The British Regulatory State*. Oxford: Oxford University Press.

Moran, M. and Wood, B. (1993) *States, Regulation, and the Medical Profession*. Maidenhead: Open University Press.

NHS Management Inquiry. (1983) *Letter to the Rt. Hon Norman Fowler MP, Secretary of State for Social Services*. London: Department of Health and Social Services.

Pierson, P. (1998) 'Irresistible forces, immovable objects: Post-industrial welfare states confront permanent austerity'. *Journal of European Public Policy*, 5, 4, 539–560.

Pollitt, C. (1993) *Managerialism and the Public Services* (2nd ed). Oxford: Blackwell.

Porter, A., Mays, N., Shaw, S.E., Rosen, R. and Smith, J. (2013) 'Commissioning healthcare for people with long term conditions: The persistence of relational contracting in England's NHS quasi-market'. *BMC Health Services Research*, 13, 1, S2. DOI:10.1186/1472-6963-13-S1-S2

Powell, M., Béland, D. and Waddan, A. (2018) 'The Americanization of the British National Health Service: A typological approach'. *Health Policy*, 122, 7, 775–782.

Rivett, G. (1998) *From Cradle to Grave: Fifty Years of the NHS*. London: King's Fund.

Robertson, A., Bates, D.W. and Sheikh, A. (2011) 'The rise and fall of England's National Programme for IT'. *Journal of the Royal Society of Medicine*, 104, 11, 434–435. DOI:10.1258/jrsm.2011.11k039

Salter, B. (2004) *The New Politics of Medicine*. Basingstoke: Palgrave Macmillan.

Schmidt, A.E., Merkur, S., Haindl, A., Gerkens, S., Gandré, C., Or, Z. et al (2022) 'Tackling the COVID-19 pandemic: Initial responses in 2020 in selected social health insurance countries in Europe'. *Health Policy*, 126, 5, 476–484. DOI:10.1016/j.healthpol.2021.09.011

Scott, J.C. (1998) *Seeing Like a State: How Certain Schemes to Improve the Human Condition Have Failed*. New Haven: Yale University Press.

Sheard, S. (2010) 'Quacks and clerks: Historical and contemporary perspectives on the structure and function of the British Medical Civil Service'. *Social Policy & Administration*, 44, 2, 193–207.

Smee, C. (2005) *Speaking Truth to Power: Two Decades of Analysis in the Department of Health*. London: The Nuffield Trust/Radcliffe.

Stevens, S. (2004) 'Reform Strategies for the English NHS'. *Health Affairs*, 23, 3, 37–44. Retrieved from http://content.healthaffairs.org/content/23/3/37.full.pdf

Street, A. and Abdul Hussain, S. (2004) 'Would Roman soldiers fight for the financial flows regime? The re-issue of Diocletian's edict in the English NHS'. *Public Money and Management*, 25, 5, 301–308.

Strong, P. and Robinson, J. (1990) *The NHS Under New Management*. Buckingham: Open University Press.

Timmins, N. (2012) *Never Again? The Story of the Health and Social Care Act 2012: A Study in Coalition Government and Policymaking*. London: Nuffield Trust.

Waitzberg, R., Gerkens, S., Dimova, A., Bryndová, L., Vrangbæk, K., Jervelund, S.S. et al (2022) 'Balancing financial incentives during COVID-19: A comparison of provider payment adjustments across 20 countries'. *Health Policy*, 126, 5, 398–407. DOI:10.1016/j.healthpol.2021.09.015

Walshe, K. (2003) *Regulating Healthcare: A Prescription for Improvement?* Maidenhead: Open University Press.

Webster, C. (2002) *The National Health Service: A Political History*. Oxford: Oxford University Press.

Williams, G.A., Rajan, S. and Cylus, J.D. (2021) 'COVID-19 in the United Kingdom: How austerity and a loss of state capacity undermined the crisis response', in S.L. Greer, E.J. King, E. Massard da Fonseca and A. Peralta-Santos (eds) *Coronavirus Politics: The Comparative Politics and Policy of COVID-19*. Ann Arbor: University of Michigan Press, pp 215–234.

3

Health and care funding at 75

Anita Charlesworth, Nihar Shembavnekar and George Stevenson

Introduction

Public spending on health has increased substantially over the past 75 years. In 1949–1950, the first financial year after the founding of the National Health Service (NHS), UK public spending on health was £16 billion (2022–2023 prices; HM Treasury, 2022b). This was 3.5 per cent of national income and accounted for 9.2 per cent of total public spending. By 2019–2020, just before the COVID-19 pandemic, publicly funded health spending had increased more than tenfold to almost £180 billion (2022–2023 prices), accounting for 18.6 per cent of overall public spending, 7.3 per cent of GDP.

Throughout the last 75 years, funding for the NHS has risen by more than inflation and by more than GDP, and, on average, healthcare spending has increased by 3.6 per cent in real terms (Figure 3.1).

Reductions in real spending have been rare. Spending fell in the early 1950s as budgets fluctuated sharply in the early years of the NHS and prescription charges were introduced. In the late 1970s health spending fell as part of widespread cuts to public spending under the terms of a loan from the International Monetary Fund.

As the NHS marks its 75th anniversary, health service funding is under pressure and the outlook is hugely challenging. The health service has experienced comparatively low funding growth for more than a decade, and now faces the pandemic's legacy of major backlogs, questions over the service's resilience to future health shocks and the pressures of an ageing population with rising multi-morbidity and inequality.

The pressures on NHS funding are not happening in isolation: Office for Budget Responsibility and OECD forecasts for the UK economy and public finances for 2023 are bleak (Office for Budget Responsibility, 2022b). The performance of the economy is very important for healthcare. In 2019 before the pandemic health spending as a share of GDP was broadly in line with that of the 14 major European countries (9.9 per cent compared to the EU14 average of 9.8 per cent). But when we look at spending per head over the decade 2010 to 2019, UK spending was almost a fifth lower than the EU14. The decade preceding the COVID-19 pandemic was one of relative economic decline for the UK economy, with low productivity growth

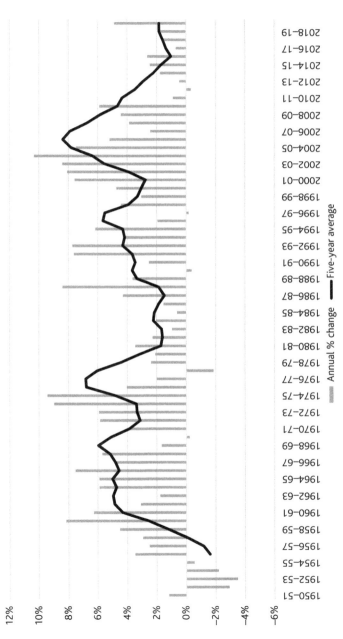

Figure 3.1: Annual change in real UK publicly funded health spending, 1950/51–2019/20

Annual % change ▬▬▬ Five-year average

Note: Real spending refers to 2022/3 prices, using the GDP deflator from the Office for Budget Responsibility (OBR) in March 2022.

Source: Nominal health spending data from the Office of Health Economics (1949/50 to 1992/93) and HM Treasury Public Expenditure Statistical Analyses (1993/94 to 2019/20)

affecting earnings and GDP per head. Analysis by the National Institute of Economic and Social Research (NIESR) shows that GDP would have been almost £10,000 higher per person in 2023 if the pre-2008 recession trend rate of growth had continued (Figure 3.2) (Chadha and Samiri, 2022). Before the great recession in 2008, GDP per head in the UK was 6 per cent below Germany, by 2019 the gap had increased to 11 per cent (Resolution Foundation, 2022).

The former Secretary of State for Health and Social Care Sajid Javid questioned whether the health service can continue to grow as a share of public spending and GDP (Javid, 2022). Questions about the balance of public and private funding and the possibility of reform to the funding model are beginning to re-emerge after two decades of broad consensus (Andrews, 2022).

In this chapter we examine the current financial settlement for the NHS, including the role of public and private funding and the pressures and outlook for future funding. This analysis is primarily for England as healthcare is a devolved responsibility for Scotland, Wales, and Northern Ireland. Some data is UK wide, notably spending as a share of GDP and spending by funding source (public, private and out of pocket). We provide some international comparisons and where this is the case these are for the UK as a whole. The analysis is for the NHS but over the last decade the interdependencies between the health and care system have become increasingly apparent. We therefore include a short section on the current settlement and outlook for the English adult social care system. We present funding in real terms – allowing for inflation. We use the GDP deflator measure of economy wide inflation in 2022–2023 prices.

The funding settlement for health in England

COVID-19 has resulted in significant changes to the pattern of health spending in England. Overall health spending (public and private) has increased from almost 10 per cent of GDP in the year before the pandemic to 12 per cent of GDP in 2020 and 2021 (Office for National Statistics, 2021a) (Figure 3.3). As the Office for Budget Responsibility (the UK's independent official economic forecasting body) notes, this is one of the largest increases among OECD countries (Office for Budget Responsibility, 2021). It's a reflection of the fall in GDP that occurred in 2020 but also the scale of additional healthcare spending required for COVID-19 – spending per head of population in 2021 was more than a fifth higher in than in 2019.

The pandemic resulted in government spending accounting for a greater share of overall health spending – up from 79 per cent of total health spending in 2019 to 83 per cent in 2021 (Office for National Statistics, 2022a). The big areas of increased spending during COVID-19 were for

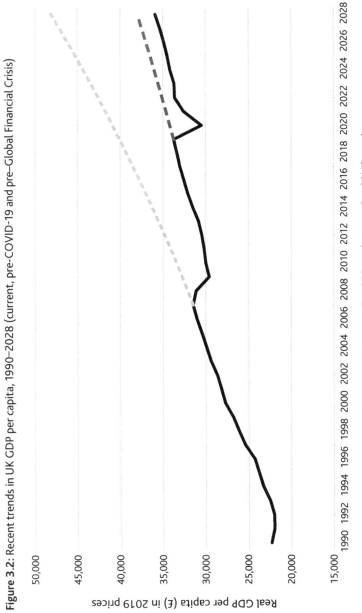

Figure 3.2: Recent trends in UK GDP per capita, 1990–2028 (current, pre-COVID-19 and pre-Global Financial Crisis)

Note: Real GDP per capita expressed in 2019 prices. GDP per capita data for 2022 onwards are based on NIESR forecasts.

Source: Chadha and Samiri (2022)

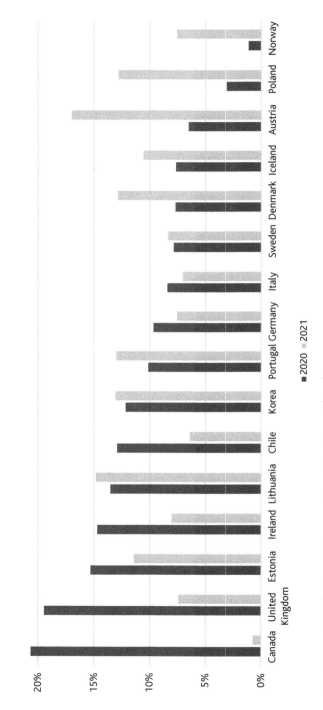

Figure 3.3: Annual growth (per cent) in health spending per head of population, 2019–2020 and 2020–2021

Source: Organisation for Economic Co-operation and Development (2023)

the test-and-trace system (£16 billion in 2021) and personal protective equipment (£2.4 billion), there was also additional spending on vaccination (£2.7 billion). Funding for the core of NHS services increased in real terms (£8.5 billion) but accounted for less than half of COVID-19-related health spending through the pandemic.

Much of the COVID-related spending is one-off, in 2022–2023 COVID-related spending is expected to fall to £6.6 billion. But it is increasingly apparent that while the impact on health services has reduced since the peak of the pandemic, it is likely to become endemic, putting additional pressure on the system.

Out-of-pocket and private spending

Prior to COVID just over a fifth of health spending was non-government funded. Non-governmental spending includes private voluntary insurance (for international travel and care domestically), charitable funding, occupational health provided by employers and individual's out-of-pocket payments.

Non-governmental spending is a smaller share of overall health spending in most countries, reflecting the comprehensive coverage within the NHS and low level of co-payments. The average across European countries is 23 per cent and it's significantly less than the OECD average (27 per cent).

The main areas of out-of-pocket spending are for pharmaceuticals (prescription charges and over the counter medicines), outpatient care (including dentistry and opticians) and long-term care (Table 3.1). Out-of-pocket payments are more than a quarter of long-term care spending, reflecting the limited provision of publicly funded adult social care support in England. Out-of-pocket spending on healthcare services is higher in households with the most disposable income. However, as a proportion of disposable income, those in more well-off households spend roughly an equal amount to that seen in the least well-off households (Holmes, 2023).

However, levels of out-of-pocket spending have increased substantially over recent years, with spending rising from 1 per cent to 1.8 per cent of GDP between 1990 and 2020. Within that, hospital costs have risen at the fastest rate for households in the lowest income groups (Figure 3.4).

While the average amount of out-of-pocket payments is important, the distribution also matters. Health and care costs are often 'lumpy', involving potentially very large levels of expenditure concentrated on certain individuals or at certain points in people's lives (those with lifelong severe health problems or at the end of life). Since 2015 the UN has tracked two measures as part of the Sustainable Development Goal (SDG) 3.8 – coverage of essential health services and catastrophic spending on health. The World Bank and the WHO, the custodian agencies for SDG 3.8, calculate health and care costs to be catastrophic if they are 10 per cent or more of overall

Table 3.1: UK out-of-pocket, private insurance and general government health expenditure shares 2020

	Inpatient care	Outpatient care	Long-term care	Ancillary services	Pharmaceuticals	Public health	Administration	Other services	Total
General government	22.9	22.5	11.5	1.9	7.1	5.5	1.1	3.7	82.9
Private insurance	1.0	0.9	0.9	0.1	0.2	0.4	0.8	0.0	4.8
Out-of-pocket	0.2	1.5	4.5		6.1	0.2			12.3
Total expenditure	24.1	24.9	16.9	2.0	13.3	6.1	1.9	3.7	100.0

Source: Organisation for Economic Co-operation and Development (2023)

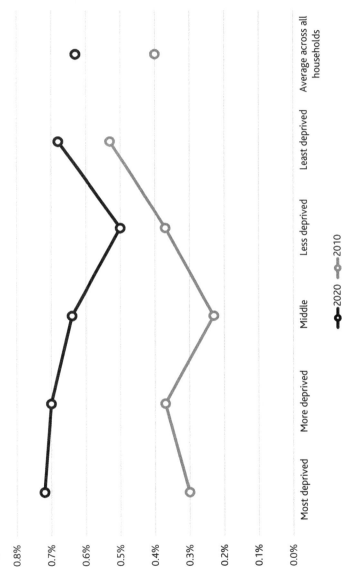

Figure 3.4: Hospital costs as a share of total household spending (per cent), by year and level of household income

Note: The ONS includes private and NHS medical, optical, dental and medical auxiliary services as a part of their definition of hospital costs.

Source: Office for National Statistics (2022b)

income (United Nations, 2022). Overall, the NHS performs well in terms of protecting people from high costs (Rice et al, 2018) or out-of-pocket payments, while increases are low by international standards as are the number of people reporting cost as a barrier to using services (Dilnot, 2011). But the same is not true for social care where costs aren't capped.

It's important to note that the international definition of health spending includes spending on long-term care (Office for National Statistics, 2021b). Long-term care is provided by a mixture of NHS and social care services and these international comparisons of health spending include a considerable proportion of adult social care expenditure. Since 2008 real terms funding and access to social care has fallen.

In 2018, 6.8 million people in the UK had private medical insurance cover, below the peak of 7.6 million covered in 2008. Coverage has fallen to around 10 per cent of the population from that peak of around 12 per cent the UK population. Coverage failed to bounce back following the 2008 great recession. While employers have continued to increase their spending in real terms, individual paid private medical insurance has been on a downward trend since 1996. This trend has continued in recent years despite the increases in average waiting times in the NHS since 2010. While private medical insurance has declined the self-pay market for healthcare has increased (LaingBuisson, 2022).

The average annual price of private medical cover in 2020 was £1,223 per subscriber/enrolee; with big differences between employer paid cover (£1,010 per enrolee) and individual paid policies (£2,036 per enrolee). Historically, prices have increased at a faster rate for individual paid rather than company paid private medical cover. As a result, since the 1990s, the differential between employer and individual insurance premiums has increased. The late 1990s saw rapid real terms inflation for individual paid private medical insurance (PMI) and this continued, albeit at a slower pace, in the 2000s. Since the great recession of 2008 individually paid PMI inflation has continued to outpace price increases for employer paid insurance, but at a lower rate than previously (LaingBuisson, 2022) (Figure 3.5).

Government funding for the NHS in England

The seven years from 2010 to 2017, alongside the late 1970s and early 1980s, saw one of the longest periods of below average real terms funding growth in the history of the NHS (Rocks et al, 2021). Funding increases were below demand pressures (Roberts et al, 2012). NHS wages fell in real terms (NHS Pay Review Body, 2018), and capital investment, health prevention and workforce training budgets all declined.

However, even with these measures, the NHS couldn't bridge the gap between demand pressures and constrained funding growth. Pay is the largest

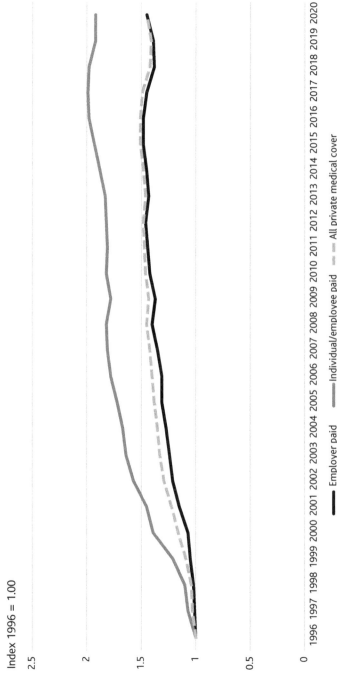

Figure 3.5: Private medical cover, real terms price index by source 1995–2000

Index 1996 = 1.00

Source: LaingBuisson (2022) surveys of health cover provider

single cost for the NHS (Department of Health and Social Care, 2016) accounting for 46.6 per cent of the total budget in 2019–2020. Over the long term NHS pay has increased by an average of 2 per cent a year in real terms, but between 2010 and 2017 real earnings fell reducing pressure on the wage bill (Charlesworth et al, 2018).

However, wage restraint was not sufficient to bridge the gap between funding growth and pressures on the services. In response, providers limited workforce growth to attempt to avoid overspending and to drive productivity improvements in an attempt to meet challenging efficiency targets set nationally (Exworthy et al, 2016). Over the period 2010 to 2017 NHS productivity increased by 1 per cent a year, above the past trend and faster than whole economy productivity. This was the result of a significant slowdown in input growth. Growth in healthcare inputs slowed from an average of 5.3 per cent annually in the 2000s to an average of 1.9 per cent between 2010 and 2017. Healthcare output growth also fell but by much less, from an average of 5.6 per cent a year in the 2000s to 3.8 per cent between 2010 and 2017 (Office for National Statistics, 2017).

While workforce data time series are patchy, the number of full-time equivalent staff employed in the NHS (including general practices) increased by only around 0.1 per cent a year (NHS Digital, 2019) through these seven years, a sharp decline on the previous decade (3 per cent a year; NHS, 2011) and below the number required to keep pace with demand. Data on staff vacancies are also difficult to compare over time, but vacancy numbers increased substantially over this period from around 2,000 in March 2010 to around 31,000 in March 2017 (NHS Digital, 2017) and spending on temporary staff grew rapidly, with the cost of agency staff in trusts in England alone increasing by 40 per cent from £2.6 billion in 2013–2014 to a peak of £3.6 billion in 2015–2016 (DHSC, 2022). Alongside this, the period between 2010 and 2016 saw an increase in the reliance of the NHS on international recruitment, perhaps most visibly through a surge in the number of nurses trained in EEA countries (Buchan and Shembavnekar, 2022). The post-2016 period, following the Brexit vote and new English language test requirements being introduced for nurses, saw a 'switch' in nurse recruitment away from EEA countries, with a marked increase in the number of nurse recruits trained in non-EEA countries between 2017 and 2022 (Nursing and Midwifery Council, 2019).

By 2017 the NHS was falling to meet the main NHS constitution standards for A&E, elective waiting, and cancer care (Morris and Reed, 2022). Hospitals were in deficit, peaking at £2.5 billion in 2015–2016 when two-thirds of NHS trusts overspent their budget. In 2016–2017 the government ring-fenced part of the health settlement to reduce deficits with the sustainability and transformation fund (STF). But even with the targeted additional support, more than 4 in 10 NHS providers were in deficit with a combined overspend of more than £800 million (Charlesworth, 2018).

A new financial settlement for NHS England

In 2018, the year of the 70th anniversary of the founding of the NHS, Prime Minister Theresa May announced a five-year funding settlement that would increase NHS England's budget by £20.5 billion per year, in 2018–2019 prices, by 2023–2024. This represented a 3.4 per cent real terms annual increase in day-to-day funding of the NHS in England, more than double the rate of funding growth since 2010 but below the average rate of increase over the NHS first 70 years (see Table 3.2).

While a significant increase compared to the recent past, the new funding settlement was only just in line with the core funding pressures from a growing and ageing population with multi-morbidity and to allow pay to keep up with future projected earnings growth across the economy (Charlesworth et al, 2018). Improvements in care would have required funding growth of around 4 per cent a year.

Alongside the funding commitment, the government announced that the NHS would develop a 10-year plan later that year. The plan's priorities would include delivering agreed performance standards that had been missed in recent years, improving cancer outcomes in line with other European countries, improving access to mental health services, greater integration of health and social care, and a focus on prevention. This led in 2019 to the publication of the NHS Long Term Plan, which included a range of ambitions for further improvements in quality and outcomes and to introduce new models of care investing in primary, community and mental health services. With funding only increasing in line with core pressures, this meant that once again the NHS was falling back on ambitious targets to improve

Table 3.2: Real terms England and UK publicly funded healthcare spending

Government	Time period	Annual growth
Whole period	1949–50 to 2024–25	3.6%
Pre 1979 (various governments)	1949–50 to 1978–79	3.5%
Thatcher and Major Conservative governments	1978–79 to 1996–97	3.3%
Blair and Brown Labour governments	1996–97 to 2009–10	6.0%
Coalition government	2009–10 to 2014–15	1.1%
Cameron and May Conservative governments	2014–15 to 2018–19	1.6%
NHS Long Term Plan	2019–20 to 2023–24	3.4%

Note: The long-term average is taken from all UK health spending, not just the NHS.
Source: PESA tables, HM Treasury (2022b)

efficiency and productivity. The reasury set five tests for financial stability, eliminating deficits, achieving cash-releasing productivity growth of 1.1 per cent a year, reducing growth in demand, reducing variation across the system, and using capital investment to drive transformation (NHS, 2019).

Theresa May's government funding settlement did not cover other areas of the Department of Health and Social Care budget, such as public health, medical training or capital spending on important resources such as buildings, equipment and technology. Investment in these areas is important for the long-term efficiency and effectiveness of the health service.

Public health spending

Spending on the services covered by the public health grant is up to four times more productive than spending on treatment services funded within the NHS England budget. Each additional year of good health achieved in the population by public health interventions, measured using Quality Adjusted Life Years (QALYs), costs £3,800 compared to £13,500 for NHS interventions (Martin et al, 2019). As spending from the grant tends to be more preventative – taking place before the full consequences become apparent rather than meeting acute need to treat ill-health – short-term decision-making has led to it being underfunded. In contrast, the NHS, where the demand is more visible, has been continually prioritised for additional spend.

The failure to match the increased spending on NHS England services with additional real terms increases for public health meant that spending on the public health grant per head of population fell by a quarter in the period 2015–2016 to 2019–2020. While funding has now stabilised in 2022–2023, it was still a fifth lower per person than in 2015–2016 (Figure 3.6).

Workforce

Established in 2012, Health Education England (HEE) has held the remit for national and regional workforce planning in England, with a focus on central funding for education and training. Between 2013–2014 and 2018–2019, the HEE budget fell by around £1 billion in real terms, from £5.3 billion to £4.3 billion (Beech et al, 2019).

On the back of the real terms fall in the HEE budget, the NHS tuition bursary for nursing and allied health professional course students was closed in 2016 (Buchan et al, 2020). This was followed by a significant drop in the number of applicants to nursing degrees living in England, from around 51,400 to 40,000 between 2016 and 2017. This did not, however, go hand in hand with a similar drop in university acceptance numbers, which fell only marginally in 2017 after having increased gradually between 2010 and 2016 (Buchan et al, 2020).

Figure 3.6: Real terms historic spending on the public health grant

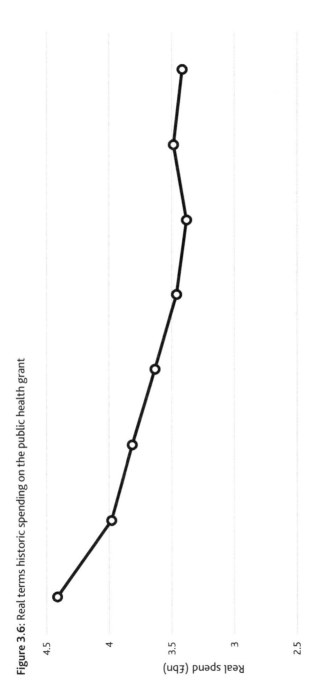
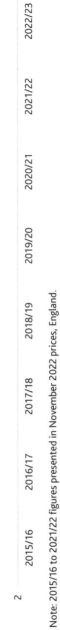

Note: 2015/16 to 2021/22 figures presented in November 2022 prices, England.

Source: Ministry of Housing, Communities and Local Government: Local authority revenue expenditure data, OBR Economic and Fiscal Outlook November 2022

Subsequently, acceptances to nursing degrees – arguably a better indicator of long-term nurse supply than application numbers – did not change substantially in 2018 and 2019, before registering a 25 per cent increase in 2020 (Shembavnekar et al, 2022). Whether, and how much, this was attributable to the unusual circumstances engendered by the COVID-19 pandemic remains to be seen.

Capital spending

The capital budget is used to finance long-term investments in the NHS in England. This includes spending on new buildings, equipment and IT, improvements to and maintenance of NHS trusts and research and development. Between 2010 and 2017, capital spending by NHS trusts fell by a fifth in real terms (Charlesworth, 2019). The Treasury allocates separate funding for capital and resource spending for public services. While the NHS struggled to balance is budget, there were repeated transfers from the capital to the revenue budget, to focus more funding on day-to-day running costs. This meant that the share of health spending devoted to longer-term capital investment fell between 2010 and 2017.

The fall in capital spending contributed to the UK having a low level of capital investment in healthcare by international standards. When the government announced the additional funding to mark the NHS' 70th birthday, and the UK spent about half the share of GDP on capital in healthcare compared with similar countries, it was far behind other countries in the number of MRI and CT scanners per capita. With constrained capital budgets, the maintenance backlog in NHS trusts increased, from £4.9 billion in 2010 to over £6.78 billion by 2017, around double the amount of annual capital spending in NHS trusts. Over £3.49 billion of this backlog was 'high' and 'significant' risk, the two highest risk categories (NHS Digital, 2022).

Social care

The key principle of the NHS – free at the point of use, based on need not ability, to pain – continues to command huge popular support. While this principle has remained at the core of the NHS for 75 years, the mismatch between comprehensive financial protection for health and a means-tested social care system has become increasingly stark.

Adult social care services cover both residential and home based (domiciliary care) for people who need support with the activities of daily living (washing, dressing, cooking, and eating, working and social interaction). The system is run by local government funded by a mix of locally raised revenue (council tax and business rates) and national government grants.

Care home residents with capital (including the value of their home) below £23,250 are eligible for publicly funded social care. They have to contribute their income (and some of their capital if in excess of £14,250) towards the cost on an ongoing basis without limit (Foster, 2021). For those receiving social care at home, local government establish their own frameworks for charging but the support must be at least as generous as the care home means-test. The value of a person's home is excluded from the domiciliary care means-test. There is no limit to the amount an individual can spend on social care. In 2011, the independent Dilnot Commission estimated that around one in ten adults aged 65 face lifetime costs of more than £100,000. With rising care costs, that estimate is now one in seven (Cabinet Office, 2022). In England, councils' spending on social care per adult resident fell by 11 per cent in real terms between 2009–2010 and 2015–2016 (Bottery et al, 2018), the initial years of 'austerity', and the number of people in receipt of publicly funded care correspondingly fell by 400,000 – a 26 per cent drop – between 2009–2010 and 2013–2014 (Watt and Charlesworth, 2018). Although there was a big focus on cost saving, productivity growth in a highly people-intensive sector was largely static.

In 2010 the coalition government had established a commission on the future funding of social care led by Sir Andrew Dilnot (Dilnot, 2011). His proposals to raise the capital threshold for the means-test and introduce a cap on lifetime care costs to pool catastrophic risks were included in the 2014 Care Act (DHSC, 2016). However, in 2015 the government announced the cap would be delayed until 2020 as local authority leaders requested that implementation be delayed largely for affordability reasons (Jarret, 2018).

The government looked for alternative options and Theresa May included revised proposals in the Conservative Party 2017 Manifesto. Unusually, social care became a focus on the election as the proposals were dubbed the 'dementia tax'. In 2019 her successor, Boris Johnson, in his first speech as prime minister stated that the government would 'fix the crisis in social care once and for all with a clear plan we have prepared to give every older person the dignity and security they deserve'. But in practice there was little detail on what fixing social care would involve. Adult social care had three main issues that required fixing; the pressures on the existing means-tested publicly funded system, workforce shortages and poor pay, terms and conditions and the fairness of the funding system that left people facing catastrophic care costs with limited state support and no workable private insurance options.

The government did put some funding into the adult social care system after 2015, and social care funding recovered somewhat and grew by around 2 per cent a year, amounting to nearly £20 billion in 2019–2020 (Rocks et al, 2021) – very close in real terms to 2009–2010 levels. On a per adult basis, however, 2019–2020 spending was still around 7 per cent below 2009–2010 (Rocks et al, 2021). To compound this underfunding, adult social care has also long faced glaring workforce challenges (Allen and Tallack, 2022). The median care worker in the independent sector in social care – which accounts for a lion's share of providers – earned £8.50 an hour in 2019–2020, just 29 pence more than the prevailing National Living Wage (£8.21 an hour in 2019–2020) (Skills for Care, 2021b). Staff turnover rates in both the local authority and independent sectors increased by 10.2 percentage points between 2012–2013 and 2019–2020 and stood at nearly 32 per cent on the eve of the pandemic. Over the same period, nearly 1 in 4 (around 24 per cent) of the social care workforce were employed on zero-hours contracts (Skills for Care, 2022), as opposed to just 3 per cent of all UK employees in October-December 2019 (Office for National Statistics, 2022c). Skills for Care have repeatedly emphasised the need to improve not only pay rates but also working conditions in the sector, with a focus on investing in staff training, providing better development and career growth opportunities, and tackling discrimination and racism (NHS Employers, 2017).

On funding reform, the Johnson government announced a package of reform in September 2021 which recommitted to the Dilnot Commission's cap on care costs from October 2023 – albeit at a higher level – and raised capital allowance threshold. With HM Treasury concerned about the affordability of the NHS and social care, the government announced the introduction of a new NHS and social care levy. The main component of the levy was an increase in employer and employee national insurance of 1.25 percentage points. Levy funding was due to address the cost of the waiting list backlog in its first three years and then shift to funding social care reform. Following Johnson's resignation as prime minister and opposition the levy in the subsequent contest for party leader and economic turmoil, the levy was abolished and in the 2022 Autumn Statement the Chancellor Jeremy Hunt confirmed that once again the reforms to social care funding would be delayed.

NHS funding after the pandemic

The NHS Long Term Plan proposed to achieve better outcomes by focusing the additional funding on the key areas of mental health, primary and community services. Around a third of the additional funding provided for the NHS between 2018–2019 and 2023–2024 was earmarked for investment in mental health, primary and community health services (NHS, 2019). Funding for these areas was planned to grow at a faster rate than the overall NHS budget.

This would have been a major change from the pattern between 2010 and 2017 when acute hospital services took an increasing share of the NHS budget. International comparisons show that the NHS devotes a greater share of its budget to acute care services than many other countries and that has been increasing while in many other countries it has fallen (see Figure 3.7).

Prioritising spending on mental health, primary and community services is widely supported and may improve the allocative efficiency of the NHS as a whole in the long term. However, while one of the five Treasury tests for the long-term plan was to reduce activity through more integrated care, there is little evidence that integrated care can significantly reduce efficiency and that where it does hold the potential to do so the impact takes many years to realise. In the short term, earmarking a larger share of the funding growth for mental health, primary and community services reduces the funding growth for acute and specialist hospital.

Between 2010 and 2017 the amount of care provided by acute hospitals increased by 3.0 per cent per year on average (Charlesworth and Watt, 2019). This covers all care provided in acute settings, including inpatient and outpatient care. Over the five years covered by the May government's funding plan, without any improvements in the quality or range of services, projections suggest that acute and specialist hospital activity would need to rise by at least 2.7 per cent per year just to keep pace with demand. The additional funding available for acute and specialist care under the NHS Long Term Plan would have been sufficient for activity growth of up to 2.3 per cent per year. This implies a requirement for the NHS to significantly moderate growth in demand for hospital services over the five years or make difficult trade-offs in how the investment is allocated or to see standards fall (Figure 3.8) (Charlesworth and Watt, 2019).

COVID-19 was an unanticipated health shock and required the NHS to put the long-term plan on hold. Spending rose by much more than planned but funding was devoted to the one-off costs of COVID-19 not underlying demand and cost pressures.

As the NHS emerges from COVID-19, the budget has been reset and it is tasked with service recovery and reform to implement the broad vision of a service more focused on primary, community and mental health services with greater emphasis on integrated care, prevention and earlier diagnosis.

The period 2023–2024 was to have been the final year of Theresa May's funding boost. Core NHS England funding is £9 billion greater than was planned under the 2018 spending settlement. This £9 billion reflects the continuing impact of COVID-19 on hospital productivity (for example with greater staff absence and lower throughput). Although much has changed, despite COVID-19, the government has held core NHS England funding to an annual average increase of 2 per cent in real terms for 2023–2024 and 2024–2025.

Pressures on the system in the near term are very significant. The NHS England budget for the next few years was based on assumptions about pay

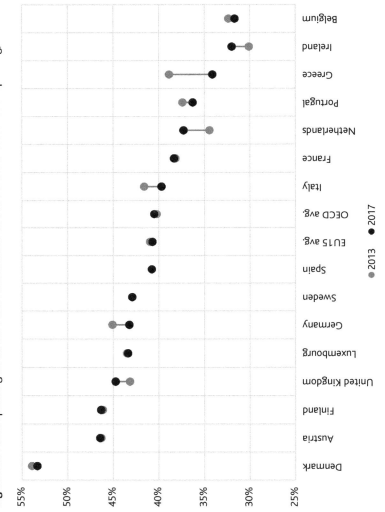

Figure 3.7: Public spending on curative and rehabilitative care as a share of total health spending, 2013–2017

Source: Organisation for Economic Co-operation and Development (2023)

Figure 3.8: Estimated acute activity growth and recent growth rates from the NHS Long Term Plan

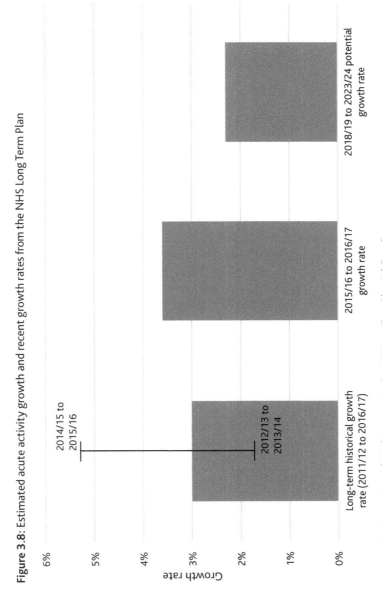

Source: Charlesworth et al (2019), *Investing in the NHS Long Term Plan: Job Done?*

and inflation that predates the significant increase in energy costs and cost of living in 2022.

To tackle the backlog of waiting, the NHS is aiming to increase activity so that it is 30 per cent higher by end of 2024–2025 than pre-pandemic. This is 10 percentage points higher than the activity growth anticipated under the NHS Long Term Plan, an extra 3 million completed pathways (NHS, 2023). However, increasing activity at this rate is still likely to mean that more people are on the waiting list for NHS care in March 2025 than at the start of the elective recovery plan. Additional funding will therefore be required beyond March 2025 to reduce waiting lists and improve waiting times. But the backlog of elective care is not the only pressure facing the NHS over the medium term. The NHS wasn't meeting performance standards in cancer and emergency and urgent care before the pandemic. In part this reflects a progressive slowdown in the amount of care that could be provided with the spending settlement (Figure 3.9).

Over the medium term the ageing of the population and rising levels of morbidity, particularly multi-morbidity, will lead to continuing demand pressures. By 2030 the population over 85 will be a third greater than pre-pandemic. The number of people in the last year of life – important as this is a period of intensive healthcare utilisation – is expected to be a fifth higher. To meet rising demand without significant changes in the way care is provided, activity growth would need to increase closer to the long-term averages. Current funding plans for the NHS are around £2 billion a year less that would be required to support underlying activity growth of around 3 per cent a year (Boccarini, 2023).

Demand is one half of the coin of pressures on healthcare spending. The other major long-term driver of healthcare spending is what happens to pay and how much pay growth can be offset by productivity improvements. This is known as the Baumol effect. The Baumol effect occurs as it is assumed that in order to recruit and retain staff, average wages in the medium to long-term must keep pace with earnings in the wider economy. Real earnings across the economy are linked to productivity growth. In the UK the Office for Budget Responsibility assumes that the long-term trend rate of productivity is 1.5 per cent a year on average (Office for Budget Responsibility, 2022a). The OBR project wages will increase by inflation (2.3 per cent a year on average over the long-term) plus productivity, giving a headline rate of earnings growth of 3.8 per cent a year, over coming decades. If this sets the benchmark for earnings growth in the NHS over the medium to long-term, the issue is how much of the earnings growth can be offset by productivity. Baumol argued that services such as healthcare couldn't sustain rates of productivity growth that matched the whole economy as there is less opportunity to substitute workers for capital as so much of quality depends on human interaction. This is not unique to the English NHS, it's a feature of all health systems

Figure 3.9: NHS output growth, 1995/1996 to 2019/2020

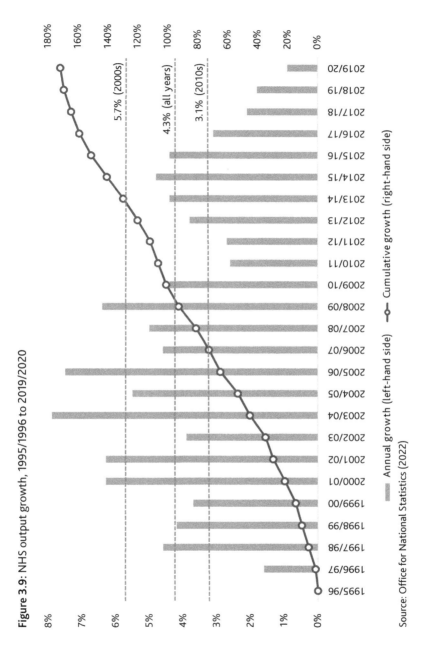

Source: Office for National Statistics (2022)

however organised and funded. If NHS productivity grows over the medium to long term at a rate similar to the long-run average of around 1 per cent a year, not all of wage pressures will be offset by productivity and so the cost of delivering care will rise in real terms.

The OBR project that the combined impact of the Baumol effect and rising demand, over the medium to long-term, will be for health spending to continue to increase by more than inflation and GDP. It projects that health spending will continue to grow as a share of GDP over time. This assessment is common among high-income countries. The OECD project that on average the share of GDP devoted to health will increase from 8.8 per cent of GDP in 2015 to 10.2 per cent in 2030 (Lorenzoni et al, 2019).

The Lancet/LSE commission on the future of the NHS after COVID-19 argued for an ongoing increase in funding for the NHS, social care and public health is essential to ensure that the health and care system can meet demand, rebuild after the pandemic and develop resilience against further acute shocks and major threats to health. This funding should be targeted towards increased investment in capital, workforce, preparedness, prevention, diagnosis, health information technology (HIT) and research and development. It argued that in the long term, health spending should increase by at least 4 per cent per year in real terms to maintain and improve the quality of services (Anderson et al, 2021).

Increasing capacity

Without further increases in productivity the NHS would need almost half a million more staff by 2030 and a workforce growth of 2.8 per cent a year. This increase in workforce would be mirrored by increased hospital beds. If care in 2030/31 was delivered in the same way as pre-pandemic (in terms of length of stay and mix of inpatient and day cases), the NHS in England would need 70,000 extra beds relative to its pre-pandemic bed capacity: 70,000 beds would be a 63 per cent increase on the current level of general and acute beds in England.

Productivity improvements in the past have mitigated the need for workforce and bed growth to match activity growth. In part this is the result of reductions in the average length of stay in hospital and an increasing number of patients that can be treated on a day case rate. Falling length of stay and increasing day case rates reflect technological advances in surgery and anaesthetics but also improvement in the management of patient flow and understanding of how to manage patients pre- and post-operatively. On average, admitted patients spent 4.5 days in hospital in England before the pandemic – lower that the OECD average. Average length of stay has fallen by a day over the last decade (22 per cent). The proportion of planned care delivered on a day case basis is now around 70 per cent, an increase of 84 per cent over the last decade (Rocks, and Rachet-Jacquet, 2022).

But the other factor which has allowed capacity and workforce to increase at a much slower rate than activity since 2010 has been the level of bed occupancy across the NHS. Bed occupancy rates have increased from 87 per cent in 2011–2012 to 90 per cent in 2018–2019. Higher bed occupancy has been associated with a decline in performance and is above NICE guidance (85 per cent). There is also some evidence that higher bed occupancy is associated with some aspects of poorer quality of care and outcomes (Kaier et al, 2012; Bosque-Mercader and Siciliani, 2022). Hospital bed occupancy was at around 87 per cent when the NHS last met the A&E 4-hour standard.

If the NHS were to reduce bed occupancy back to 87 per cent and average length of stay continued to fall, but at a slower rate than the decade pre-pandemic, the NHS would need between 23,000 and 39,000 extra general and acute beds, an increase of 20–35 per cent (NHS Digital, 2011). For the workforce this would reduce by a third the number of additional staff required across the NHS (around 314,000 full-time equivalents projected to be needed by 2030/31 compared to around 488,000 if average length of stay (ALOS) and day case rates were held constant). This would mean workforce growth of around 2 per cent a year, much higher than in the period 2010 to 2019 but below the levels seen in the 2000s.

Productivity improvements can mitigate some of the pressure for more staff and capacity but if the NHS wants to be more resilient to health shocks and improve performance, capacity would need to increase over the next decade. This would require investment in capital. Ballpark estimates suggest a one-off capital cost of £17 to £29 billion. Increasing the workforce would require sustained investment in workforce training and education budgets.

Social care funding after the pandemic

Government spending on adult social care in England barely increased in real terms in the decade to 2019–2020, but this changed with the onset of the pandemic. Between 2019–2020 and 2020–2021, real terms spending on social care increased by 7.4 per cent, with central government grants to local authorities driving the majority of this increase. The additional spending amounted to £3.2 billion of the £20.7 billion (Institute for Government, 2022) spent on adult social care in 2020–2021 and represented an overestimate of the additional care costs incurred by local authorities during the pandemic. Despite this, the evidence points to current levels of funding not being sufficient (NHS Digital, 2011) to meet existing pressures facing social care (Levelling Up, Housing and Communities Committee, 2022). The 2022 Autumn Statement announced some additional funding over the subsequent two years (to 2024–2025) for core adult social care spending, particularly focused on aiding discharge from hospital (Institute for Government, 2022). However, this failed to address the need for a long-term solution to the social care funding gap. The additional funds are partly due to the government delaying a long overdue promise to cap care costs and extend the means-test (HM Treasury, 2022a). It also relies on local governments raising more council tax, and even assuming that a significant chunk of this can be ring-fenced for social care – a tall order given the many competing pressures on councils' budgets – this is a regressive policy.

As with the NHS, workforce shortages are a huge challenge for adult social care. Skills for Care recently highlighted that vacancies in the sector (Skills for Care, 2021a) increased by 52 per cent between 2020–2021 and 2021–2022 to reach 165,000 – the highest level on record. This occurred alongside a fall of around 3 per cent (50,000) in the number of filled posts, highlighting the severe recruitment and retention challenges faced by providers. Alongside this, vacancies in NHS trusts are also on the rise and stood at around 133,400 FTE in the quarter to September 2022 (NHS Digital, 2010) – well above pre-pandemic highs and highlighting growing workforce gaps, a huge concern against a backdrop of record care backlogs (British Medical Association, 2022) and delayed hospital discharges (The Nuffield Trust, 2022).

Further, at 29 per cent, the social care staff turnover rate (Skills for Care, 2021a) is much higher than for the overall economy, and the starter rate fell from around 37 per cent to 31 per cent between 2018–2019 and 2021–2022. Low pay and poor working conditions are endemic problems facing adult social care – the largely female care workforce has consistently been underpaid and undervalued. Recent research points to over a quarter (Allen et al, 2022) of residential care workers in the UK living in or on the brink of poverty. With high inflation and a cost of living crisis dominating the headlines in 2022, grave concerns remain around how the adult social care workforce will fare, with question marks around the long-term sustainability of quality care provision in the aftermath of the pandemic. A comprehensive long-term care workforce strategy, backed by full funding, has never been more urgently needed.

Conclusion

The NHS at 70 was a moment of cautious optimism about the future. At the end of a decade of austerity, the health service had a five-year funding settlement close to the historic average rate of growth. The five-year financial settlement was accompanied by a long-term plan charting priorities for improvement. Although there were major areas of unfinished business; workforce, capital investment, social care funding and reform and prevention, action was promised to address each of these.

Five years later, cautious optimism looks much harder to sustain. The pandemic exposed major fault lines in the NHS and social care that have at their heart the common problems of a lack of capacity and short-termist leadership. In 2023 the government have come up with a much delayed long-term NHS workforce plan, but there continues to be no social care plan and no capital plan. The population is ageing and multi-morbidity increasing. The funding pressures facing the NHS and care system mean spending will have to increase by more than inflation and more than GDP. With the abolition of the proposals for the NHS and social care levy there is no plan for how to meet rising costs into the future. At 75, while public support for the principle of universal health coverage free at the point of use remains as strong as ever, the uncertainty about how to sustain that has never been greater.

References

Allen, L. and Tallack, C. (2022) *A Short-term Drive on International Recruitment Is No Quick Fix for Social Care.* The Health Foundation, 25 August. https://www.health.org.uk/news-and-comment/blogs/a-short-term-drive-on-international-recruitment-is-no-quick-fix-for-social

Allen, L., Williamson, S., Berry, E. and Alderwick, H. (2022) *The Cost of Caring: Poverty and Deprivation Among Residential Care Workers in the UK.* The Health Foundation, 11 October. https://www.health.org.uk/publications/long-reads/the-cost-of-caring

Anderson, M., Pitchforth, E., Asaria, M., Brayne, C., Casadei, B. and Charlesworth, A. (2021) *Lancet Commission on the Future of the NHS: Re-Laying the Foundations for an Equitable and Efficient Health and Care Service after COVID-19.* https://doi.org/10.1016/S0140-6736(21)00232-4

Andrews, K. (2022) 'Patients are getting nothing for extra NHS spending.' *The Telegraph*, 9 December. https://www.telegraph.co.uk/business/2022/12/09/patients-getting-nothing-extra-nhs-spending/

Beech, J., Bottery, S., Charlesworth, A., Evans, H., Gershlick, B., Hemmings, N. et al (2019) *Closing the Gap: Key Areas for Action on the Health and Care Workforce.* Health Foundation. https://www.health.org.uk/publications/reports/closing-the-gap

Boccarini, G. (2023) *What is the Outlook for Health Funding?* The Health Foundation. https://www.health.org.uk/publications/long-reads/what-is-the-outlook-for-health-funding

Bosque-Mercader, L. and Siciliani, L. (2022) 'The association between bed occupancy rates and hospital quality in the English National Health Service.' *The European Journal of Health Economics.* https://link.springer.com/article/10.1007/s10198-022-01464-8

Bottery, S., Varrow, M., Thorlby, R. and Wellings, D. (2018) *A Fork in the Road: Next Steps for Social Care Funding Reform.* The Health Foundation and the King's Fund. https://www.health.org.uk/publications/a-fork-in-the-road-next-steps-for-social-care-funding-reform

British Medical Association. (2022) *NHS Backlog Data Analysis*. [Online] The British Medical Association. https://www.bma.org.uk/advice-and-support/nhs-delivery-and-workforce/pressures/nhs-backlog-data-analysis

Buchan, J., Ball, J., Shembavnekar, N. and Charlesworth, A. (2020) *Building the NHS Nursing Workforce in England: Workforce Pressure Points*. The Health Foundation. https://doi.org/10.37829/HF-2020-RC14

Buchan, J. and Shembavnekar N. (2022) *How Reliant is the NHS in England on International Nurse Recruitment*. https://www.health.org.uk/news-and-comment/charts-and-infographics/how-reliant-is-the-nhs-in-england-on-international-nurse-recruitment

Cabinet Office. (2022) *Build Back Better: Our Plan for Health and Social Care*. https://www.gov.uk/government/publications/build-back-better-our-plan-for-health-and-social-care/build-back-better-our-plan-for-health-and-social-care

Chadha, J.S. and Samiri, I. (2022) *Macroeconomic Perspectives on Productivity, Working Paper No. 030*. The Productivity Institute. https://www.productivity.ac.uk/research/macroeconomic-perspectives-on-productivity/

Charlesworth, A. (2018) *False Economy: An Analysis of NHS Funding Pressures*. https://www.health.org.uk/publications/false-economy

Charlesworth, A. (2019) *Failing to Capitalise: Capital Spending in the NHS*. https://www.health.org.uk/publications/reports/failing-to-capitalise

Charlesworth, A., Firth, Z., Gerschlick, B., Johnson, P., Kelly, E., Lee, T. et al (2018) *Securing the Future: Funding Health and Social Care to the 2030s*. https://www.health.org.uk/publications/reports/securing-the-future-funding-health-and-social-care-to-the-2030s

Charlesworth, A., Gershlick, B., Firth, Z., Kraindler, J., Watt, T. (2019) *Investing in the NHS Long Term Plan: Job Done?* https://www.health.org.uk/publications/reports/investing-in-the-nhs-long-term-plan

Department of Health and Social Care (DHSC). (2016) *Guidance: Care Act Factsheets*. Updated 19 April 2016. https://www.gov.uk/government/publications/care-act-2014-part-1-factsheets/care-act-factsheets#factsheet-6-reforming-how-people-pay-for-their-care-and-support

DHSC. (2021) *DHSC Evidence for the NHSPRB: Pay Round 2021 to 2022*. https://www.gov.uk/government/publications/dhsc-evidence-for-the-nhsprb-pay-round-2021-to-2022

DHSC. (2022) *DHSC Evidence for the NHSPRB: Pay Round 2022 to 2023*. https://www.gov.uk/government/publications/dhsc-evidence-for-the-nhsprb-pay-round-2022-to-2023

Dilnot, A. (2011) 'Fairer care funding.' The Report of the Commission on Funding of Care and Support. Vol. 1. *HMSO*. https://webarchive.nationalarchives.gov.uk/ukgwa/20130221130239/https://www.wp.dh.gov.uk/carecommission/files/2011/07/Fairer-Care-Funding-Report.pdf

Exworthy, M., Mannion, R. and Powell, M. (2016) *Dismantling the NHS? Evaluating the Impact of Health Reforms.* Policy Press Scholarship Online, 18 May. https://doi.org/10.1332/policypress/9781447330226.001.0001

Foster, D. (2021) *Reform of Adult Social Care Funding: Developments Since July 2019 (England)*, House of Commons Library. https://commonslibrary.par liament.uk/research-briefings/cbp-8001/

HM Treasury. (2022a) *Autumn Statement 2022.* https://www.gov.uk/gov ernment/publications/autumn-statement-2022-documents

HM Treasury. (2022b) *Public Expenditure Statistical Analyses 2022.* https:// www.gov.uk/government/statistics/public-expenditure-statistical-analyses-2022

Holmes, J. (2023) *Independent health care and the NHS.* https://www.kingsf und.org.uk/sites/default/files/2023-01/Independent%20health%20c are%20and%20the%20NHS%20online%20version%202.pdf

Institute for Government. (2022) *Performance Tracker 2022: Adult Social Care.* https://www.instituteforgovernment.org.uk/performance-tracker-2022/ adult-social-care

Jarret, T. (2018) *Social care: Announcements Delaying the Introduction of Funding Reforms (Including the Cap) (England).* House of Commons Library. https:// researchbriefings.files.parliament.uk/documents/CBP-7265/CBP-7265.pdf

Javid, S. (2022) *Health and Social Care Secretary speech on Health Reform 8th March 2022.* https://www.gov.uk/government/speeches/health-and-soc ial-care-secretary-speech-on-health-reform

Kaier, K., Mutters, N.T. and Frank, U. (2012) 'Bed occupancy rates and hospital-acquired infections: Should beds be kept empty?' *Clinical Microbiology and Infection.* https://pubmed.ncbi.nlm.nih.gov/22757765/

LaingBuisson. (2022) *Private Healthcare Self-Pay Statistics & Analysis: LaingBuisson UK Report.* https://www.laingbuisson.com/shop/private-healthcare-self-pay-uk-market-report-4ed/

Levelling Up, Housing and Communities Committee. (2022) *Long-term Funding of Adult Social Care.* House of Commons. https://committees.par liament.uk/publications/23319/documents/170008/default

Lorenzoni, L., Marinoi, A., Morgani, D. and Jamesi, C. (2019) *Health Spending Projections to 2030: New results Based on a Revised OECD Methodology.* OECD Health Working Papers, No. 110, OECD Publishing, Paris. https://doi.org/10.1787/5667f23d-en

Martin, S., Lomas, J.R.S. and Grant, U.O.Y. (2019) *Is an Ounce of Prevention Worth a Pound of Cure? A Cross-sectional Study of the Impact of English Public Health Grant on Mortality and Morbidity.* (CHE Research Paper; No. 166). Centre for Health Economics, University of York. https://www. york.ac.uk/media/che/documents/papers/researchpapers/CHERP166_ Impact_Public_Health_Mortality_Morbidity.pdf

Ministry of Housing, Communities and Local Government. (2022) *Local Authority Revenue Expenditure and Financing*. https://www.gov.uk/government/collections/local-authority-revenue-expenditure-and-financing

Morris, J. and Reed, S. (2022) *How Much is COVID-19 to Blame for Growing NHS Waiting Times?* QualityWatch. Nuffield Trust and Health Foundation. https://www.nuffieldtrust.org.uk/resource/how-much-is-covid-19-to-blame-for-growing-nhs-waiting-times

NHS. (2011) *NHS Workforce, Summary of staff in the NHS Results from September 2010 Census*. The Information Centre. https://digital.nhs.uk/data-and-information/publications/statistical/nhs-workforce-statistics

NHS. (2019) *The NHS Long Term Plan*. NHS Long Term Plan. https://www.longtermplan.nhs.uk/publication/nhs-long-term-plan/

NHS. (2023) *Delivery Plan for Tackling the COVID-19 Backlog of Elective Care*. https://www.england.nhs.uk/coronavirus/publication/delivery-plan-for-tackling-the-covid-19-backlog-of-elective-care/

NHS Digital. (2010) *NHS Vacancies Survey – England, 31 March 2010*. https://digital.nhs.uk/data-and-information/publications/statistical/nhs-vacancies-survey/nhs-vacancies-survey-england-31-march-2010

NHS Digital. (2011) *Hospital Episode Statistics, Admitted Patient Care – England, 2010-11*. https://digital.nhs.uk/data-and-information/publications/statistical/hospital-admitted-patient-care-activity/hospital-episode-statistics-admitted-patient-care-england-2010-11

NHS Digital. (2017) *NHS Vacancy Statistics England, February 2015 – March 2017*. Provisional Experimental Statistics. https://digital.nhs.uk/data-and-information/publications/statistical/nhs-vacancies-survey/nhs-vacancy-statistics-england-february-2015-march-2017-provisional-experimental-statistics

NHS Digital. (2019) *NHS Workforce Statistics & NHS Digital. (2023). General Practice Workforce*. https://digital.nhs.uk/data-and-information/publications/statistical/nhs-workforce-statistics and https://digital.nhs.uk/data-and-information/publications/statistical/general-and-personal-medical-services

NHS Digital. (2022) *Estates Returns Information Collection*. https://digital.nhs.uk/data-and-information/publications/statistical/estates-returns-information-collection

NHS Employers. (2017) *Social care roles added to the Shortage Occupation List*. https://www.nhsemployers.org/news/social-care-roles-added-shortage-occupation-list

NHS Pay Review Body. (2018) *Thirty First Report on Agenda for Change pay 2018*. https://www.gov.uk/government/publications/national-health-service-pay-review-body-31st-report-2018

Nuffield Trust, The. (2022) *Hospitals at Capacity: Understanding Delays in Patient Discharge.* https://www.nuffieldtrust.org.uk/news-item/hospitals-at-capacity-understanding-delays-in-patient-discharge

Nursing and Midwifery Council. (2019) *Registration Data Reports.* Nmc.org.uk. https://www.nmc.org.uk/about-us/reports-and-accounts/registration-statistics/

Office for Budget Responsibility. (2021) *Fiscal Risks Report July 2021.* https://obr.uk/frs/fiscal-risks-report-july-2021

Office for Budget Responsibility. (2022a) *Fiscal Risks Report July 2022.* https://obr.uk/frs/fiscal-risks-and-sustainability-july-2022/

Office for Budget Responsibility. (2022b) *Economic and Fiscal Outlook – November 2022.* https://obr.uk/efo/economic-and-fiscal-outlook-november-2022/

Office for National Statistics. (2017) *Public Service Productivity: Healthcare, England.* https://www.ons.gov.uk/economy/economicoutputandproductivity/publicservicesproductivity/articles/publicservicesproductivityestimateshealthcare/financialyearending2017

Office for National Statistics. (2021a) *Healthcare Expenditure, UK Health Accounts.* https://www.ons.gov.uk/peoplepopulationandcommunity/healthandsocialcare/healthcaresystem/bulletins/ukhealthaccounts/2019

Office for National Statistics. (2021b) *UK Health Accounts: Methodological Guidance.* https://www.ons.gov.uk/peoplepopulationandcommunity/healthandsocialcare/healthcaresystem/methodologies/ukhealthaccountsmethodologicalguidance

Office for National Statistics. (2022a) *Healthcare Expenditure, UK Health Accounts Provisional Estimates.* https://www.ons.gov.uk/peoplepopulationandcommunity/healthandsocialcare/healthcaresystem/bulletins/healthcareexpenditureukhealthaccountsprovisionalestimates/2021

Office for National Statistics. (2022b) *Family Spending in the UK.* https://www.ons.gov.uk/peoplepopulationandcommunity/personalandhouseholdfinances/expenditure/bulletins/familyspendingintheuk/latest#related-links

Office for National Statistics. (2022c) *People in Employment on Zero-hour Contracts.* https://www.ons.gov.uk/employmentandlabourmarket/peopleinwork/employmentandemployeetypes/datasets/emp17peopleinemploymentonzerohourscontracts/current

Office for National Statistics (2022d) *Public Service Productivity: Healthcare, England* https://www.ons.gov.uk/economy/economicoutputandproductivity/publicservicesproductivity/articles/publicservicesproductivityestimateshealthcare/financialyearending2020

Organisation for Economic Co-operation and Development. (2023) *OECD statistics: Health Expenditure and Financing.*

Resolution Foundation. (2022) *Stagnation Nation, Navigating a Route to a Fairer and More Prosperous Britain.* https://economy2030.resolutionfoundat ion.org/reports/stagnation-nation/

Rice, T., Quentin, W., Anell, A., Barnes, A.J., Rosenau, P., Unruh, L.Y. et al (2018) 'Revisiting out-of-pocket requirements: Trends in spending, financial access barriers, and policy in ten high-income countries.' *BMC Health Services Research*, 18, 1. https://doi.org/10.1186/s12913-018-3185-8

Roberts, A., Marshall, L. and Charlesworth, A. (2012) *A Decade of Austerity? The Funding Pressures Facing the NHS from 2010/11 to 2021/22.* Research report. Nuffield Trust. https://www.nuffieldtr ust.org.uk/research/a-decade-of-austerity-the-funding-pressures-fac ing-the-nhs-from-2010-11-to-2021-22

Rocks, S., Boccarini, G., Charlesworth, A., Idriss, O., McConkey, R. and Rachet-Jacquet, L. (2021) *Health and Social Care Funding Projections 2021.* The Health Foundation. https://doi.org/10.37829/HF-2021-RC18

Rocks, S. and Rachet-Jacquet, L. (2022) *How Many Hospital Beds Will the NHS Need Over the Coming Decade? Projections: General and Acute Hospital Beds in England (2018–2030).* https://www.health.org.uk/publications/ reports/how-many-beds-will-the-nhs-need-over-the-coming-decade

Shembavnekar, N., Buchan, J., Bazeer, N., Kelly, E., Beech, J., Charlesworth, A. et al (2022) *NHS Workforce Projections 2022.* The Health Foundation. https://doi.org/10.37829/HF-2022-RC01

Skills for Care. (2021a) *The State of the Adult Social Care Sector and Workforce in England.* https://www.skillsforcare.org.uk/adult-social-care-work force-data/Workforce-intelligence/publications/national-information/ The-state-of-the-adult-social-care-sector-and-workforce-in-England.aspx

Skills for Care. (2021b) *Pay Rates.* https://www.skillsforcare.org.uk/Adult-Social-Care-Workforce-Data/Workforce-intelligence/publications/Top ics/Pay-rates.aspx

Skills for Care. (2022) *The Size and Structure of The Adult Social Care Sector and Workforce in England.* https://www.skillsforcare.org.uk/Adult-Social-Care-Workforce-Data/Workforce-intelligence/publications/national-informat ion/The-size-and-structure-of-the-adult-social-care-sector-and-workfo rce-in-England.aspx

United Nations. (2022) *Goal 3: Ensure Healthy Lives and Promote Well-being for All at All Ages.* https://sdgs.un.org/goals/goal3

Watt, T. and Charlesworth, A. (2018) *Social Care Funding Options: How Much and Where From?* The Health Foundation. https://www.health.org. uk/publications/social-care-funding-options

4

The devolved nations

John Stewart

When ... established 70 years ago, inspired by Aneurin Bevan and the model of the Tredegar Medical Aid Society, the NHS was visionary, bold and radical. ... But we no longer live in the world the NHS was originally designed for. ... We acknowledge the level of challenge to meet the aspirations of this plan, but ... this can be met if we can rediscover the confidence and bold ambition that made Wales the birthplace of the greatest National Health Service in the world. (Welsh Government, 2021)

The government decides the policy for the NHS, it decides the funding for the NHS, we fund the NHS to a higher level proportionately than other governments across the UK and we'll continue to do that. We'll continue to have the difficult discussions with those who run the NHS ... about how we ensure the sustainability of the service. But the founding principles on which that service is based are not up for discussion by government and will not change. (Scottish First Minister, 2022)

The World Health Organization defines health as 'a state of complete physical, mental and social wellbeing and not merely the absence of disease or infirmity'. That is the health outcome I want to deliver for our people. ... We are facing a time of change for our health system but it is change that must happen. This document sets out a direction of travel that I hope all of our society can embrace and support in the challenging but exciting time ahead. (Northern Ireland Executive, 2016)

Introduction

The first of these revealing statements, by the Welsh Labour Secretary for Health and Social Care, gives a partial account of the origins of the National Health Service (NHS). The second, by the then Scottish National Party (SNP) first minister, emphasises her government's commitment to NHS 'founding principles'. The third ignores NHS history, with the Sinn Féin minister citing a post-war World Health Organization aspiration. None mentions the UK or NHS England. We are thus alerted to healthcare's highly politicised nature, the relevance of its history, the significance of devolution, and that its treatment in many social policy and historical texts notwithstanding, the 'NHS' is not monolithic. Greer found it 'no surprise' that Welsh, Scottish and Northern Irish politics differed from those in England. Devolution was 'poorly thought out' while reflecting longstanding 'distinctive policy communities, different debates, and … a different "feel"' (Greer, 2008: 117). A Nuffield Trust report, meanwhile, found the NHS in all four UK nations 'subject to extensive politicisation' (Dayan and Heenan, 2019: 25). These observations should be located, too, in perceptions of 'crisis' embracing the NHS throughout its history.

This chapter examines the devolved nations' health policies under the headings 'Devolved Health Policy', 'Divergence' and 'Brexit and COVID-19'. Brief analyses of Northern Irish, Scottish and Welsh health policies come next, before concluding with a 'Summary/Discussion' which engages with issues raised in Chapter 1. The following points inform the argument:

- The histories of Northern Ireland, Wales and Scotland have shaped their health policies, pre- and post-devolution.
- These nations see themselves, now and historically, as distinct – politically, socially and culturally – from the UK/England. Relatively poorer socio-economic circumstances, and health outcomes, exemplify such distinctions.
- Political devolution (the usual meaning of 'devolution' here) was achieved by Northern Ireland in 1921 (the 1998 Belfast/Good Friday Agreement modified this arrangement[1]), and Wales and Scotland in 1999. These changes followed the Labour Party's 1997 UK general election victory. Devolution is, though, a process, not an event, while its meaning varies across the three nations.
- Prior to political devolution, Wales and Scotland enjoyed a degree of administrative devolution, which included health policy.
- Devolution is 'asymmetrical'. The UK government 'reserves' key policy areas, crucially macroeconomic affairs and constitutional matters. The devolved administrations' responsibilities rest primarily with social policy, especially health and education. Devolution is also asymmetrical in that the combined population (and hence political clout) of the devolved nations is less than one fifth of England's.
- Funding mostly comes from the UK Treasury, although devolved administrations can, in principle, spend allocations as they choose.
- Devolution's first decade saw, at UK level, Labour administrations which, if half-heartedly, nonetheless bought into the project. Since 2010, UK government has been dominated by the Conservative Party, at best indifferent to devolution and to the devolved administrations. The latter's politics, furthermore, have generally differed from those of the UK, a situation pre-dating 1999.

- The devolved administrations' health services retain much in common with NHS England (they share familial origins in the 1940s). Nonetheless, differences have emerged.

Devolved health policy

Historically, there has never been a UK-wide budget for the NHS. A 2012 official report observed that devolved administrations had been empowered to 'choose how much money to spend on health services, what their policy priorities should be, and how services should be delivered, as the UK Government does for England' (National Audit Office, 2012: 5). Recent data show Scotland spending £13,700 million on health, Wales £8,000 million and Northern Ireland £5,000 million – in each case roughly 25 per cent of total expenditure on all public services (HM Treasury, 2021: table 9.21). England has spent less per capita, and more as a proportion of total public expenditure. Health indicators, though, tend to be more favourable there than elsewhere in the UK (for example, National Audit Office, 2012: 12). Health services are economically important to the devolved nations. A 2021 Institute of Welsh Affairs piece observed that while it had been well documented that health expenditure consumed about 50 per cent of the Welsh government's budget, the NHS' contribution to local and national economies was less well understood. Health, wellbeing and the economy were 'tightly bound together' with health gains producing positive economic benefits. NHS Wales supported around 145,000 jobs, roughly 11 per cent of the workforce, and so had a 'unique opportunity' to, for instance, reduce health inequalities (Institute of Welsh Affairs, 2021). The Barnett Formula, initially devised as a 'short-term fix', determines the volume of resources for the devolved nations. It has lasted over 40 years and remains intact, if only because of potential difficulties in change. In particular, any replacement would almost certainly 'disadvantage Scotland', creating 'substantial political headaches' for the UK government, given its recurrent current struggle with the SNP administration 'over the future of the union' (Paun, Cheung and Nicholson, 2021: 8–9, 33–34 – although see Birrell and Gray later).

Within this financial context, what can we say about Northern Irish, Welsh and Scottish health policy? A health warning – the expression 'devolved nations' is descriptively accurate while raising complex issues, including interpretations of the UK as a unitary state. Whether this accurately describes the United Kingdom is, and long has been, contestable, while its future is not unconditionally guaranteed. A case can certainly be made for uniformity and continuity. Mackinnon notes devolution as a global trend, with the UK a latecomer. While devolved powers change over time, parallel pressures seek to ensure that no measures are adopted conflicting with 'those of the central state', so encouraging 'policy convergence'. Political devolution built on a 'substantial legacy of administrative devolution', making its introduction '*deceptively* straightforward' (Mackinnon 2015: 47–48, 53 – my emphasis). Simpson identifies 'subnational differences of approach' as a longstanding feature of UK social policy, but within 'an *apparently* unassailable consensus round core principles', for example healthcare free at point of use (Simpson 2022: 4 – my emphasis). Kaehne and his colleagues remark that integrating health and social care services has 'now been placed on a statutory basis in England, Wales, Scotland and Northern Ireland', reflecting a 'global interest in responses to common factors' including demographic change, expenditure cuts and more 'holistic approaches' to health and wellbeing (Kaehne et al 2017: 84). Smith and Hellowell, meanwhile, stress the UK's health services' commonalities, including mode of financing. Comparable economic circumstances, and fiscal policy mostly in London's hands, means that healthcare throughout the UK is likely to remain largely uniform. So, debates about the constitutional settlement and greater devolved fiscal powers notwithstanding, differences can be construed as 'rhetorical' (Smith and Hellowell, 2017: 193). As to outcomes, a 2014 Health Foundation/ Nuffield Trust report noted that 'despite hotly contested policy differences' since devolution over, for instance, competition, no evidence linked these 'to a matching divergence of performance' (Bevan et al, 2014: 2).

The terms 'political headaches', 'deceptively', 'apparently' and 'hotly contested' nonetheless give pause for thought. A former civil servant closely involved in the process proposes that Scottish devolution involved 'no overarching plan' while, more broadly, the three settlements were distinct, 'each adapted to the particular circumstances of its own territory' (Rycroft, 2022: 6). This raises the question what is 'national' about the 'National Health Service'? The English and Welsh service was created by the National Health Service Act 1946, those in Scotland and Northern Ireland by Acts of 1947 and 1948 respectively. The Scottish Act, like that for England and Wales, was welcomed but, nonetheless, acknowledged Scotland's 'relative autonomy' in welfare matters. The Northern Ireland legislation, though, was imposed on a unionist-dominated administration with equivocal views about welfare reform.

Separate legislation notwithstanding, healthcare in the post-war 'welfare state' also incorporated UK-wide, familial, dimensions. For Scotland, but more generally applicable, the 'Anglo-Scottish Union was renewed by the arrival of the welfare state' (Jackson, 2020b: 90) – hence the 'social union'. For service users, access and expectations throughout the UK were virtually identical. In mental health, for instance, all four UK nations 'have well-developed, complex systems of mental health care with shared roots in the era of the asylum'. Nonetheless, Hannigan also identifies Welsh policy difference in the face of the 'dominant, Anglocentric narrative' generally prevalent 'in the health policy, mental health and nursing fields' in a context wherein health policy 'reflects prevailing ideologies and power' (Hannigan, 2022: 200–201).

From the 1970s the 'post-war consensus' – the 'welfare state' and the pursuit of full employment – crumbled, hurried along by the 1979–1997 Conservative governments, with profound implications for UK unity. In Scotland the 'decomposition of the British social democratic settlement' correlated with nationalism's emergence as a popular political movement. By 1974 the SNP was describing itself as 'social democratic', indicating commitment to 'full employment and the welfare state' (Jackson, 2020b: 90–91, 94). In the early 1990s Labour sought to use devolution to outmanoeuvre 'Celtic nationalists', whose emergence manifested heightening tensions between national identities within the UK at a time when the Welsh and Scottish electorates were already pursuing different paths (Jackson, 2020a: 499). Northern Ireland, meanwhile, remained politically distinct from the mainland, alarmingly so with the onset of 'The Troubles'.

Since 1999, the devolved administrations too have taken different political paths from the UK/England. In Scotland, a Labour-Liberal Democrat coalition was followed, from 2007, by SNP governments, majority and minority. In Wales, Labour has dominated, sometimes in conjunction with the Liberal Democrats and Plaid Cymru. Northern Ireland has, again, followed its own course. From the 1920s to the 1970s it was governed by political unionism. This was followed by, variously, direct rule from London and then, from 2007, a form of power-sharing between the Democratic Unionist Party (DUP) and Sinn Féin.[2] The situation now (2022) is different again, power-sharing having run into trouble while Sinn Féin dominates the Executive. More broadly, devolution itself has been subject to change, with further powers gained by Scotland in 2012 and 2016, and Wales in 2007 and 2011 (Greer, 2019: 554).

Pro-union politicians, though, insist on the need for a 'larger unit … to sustain welfare and social solidarity' (Keating, 2021: 10). During the 2014 independence referendum campaign Gordon Brown, former Labour prime minister, claimed Scotland as a 'natural leader' within a United Kingdom pooling and sharing resources 'to deliver the objectives of full employment, free healthcare and a welfare state' (Brown, 2017: 401). In 2019, the Conservative PM, Theresa May, laid claim to a social union underpinned by 'shared institutions, including the armed forces, the BBC and the NHS'. As Keating comments, in a remark illuminating healthcare's role in national identities, while the NHS is frequently portrayed as exemplifying UK unity, seeing universal credit in the same manner is more difficult (Keating, 2021: 153, 169). For Simpson, the 2014 referendum highlighted 'competing claims of the social benefits of the union' alongside 'irreconcilable differences between UK and Scottish visions of social citizenship'. Devolution has thus foregrounded the nature and future of the social union and, thereby, the political union (Simpson, 2022: 2 and passim).

The opportunity nonetheless exists for policy learning between UK administrations. Discussions around greater integration of health and social care in England noted its presence in Northern Ireland since 1973 (with further reform under the terms of the Health and Social Care [Reform] [NI] Act 2009). In the event, this has been problematic, but at least offered an evidence base for English policy-makers (Donnelly and O'Neill, 2018: 1–3). It has also had notable achievements, for example in integrated practice and hospital patient discharge (Heenan and Birrell, 2009: 7–8). NHS Scotland's trajectory, it has likewise been suggested, offers lessons for other administrations (Dayan and Edwards, 2017: 3).

Given their asymmetrical relationship, though, UK governments do not see devolved administrations as equal partners. In 2015 Wales was described as 'this small polity ... still too often buffeted about', with 'eternal vigilance' the 'price of devolution' (Rawlings, 2015: 497). Rycroft claims that London 'barely adjusted' to political devolution. Accustomed to administrative devolution, Whitehall 'saw no need to invest in a refreshed understanding of territorial governance'. Scotland and Northern Ireland's Brexit results 'counted for nothing in the eventual outcome', while the Welsh and Scottish governments' commitments 'made no dent in the UK's negotiating position' (Rycroft, 2022: 6–7).

This raises interpretative issues about small polities on the 'periphery' of larger welfare formations. It has been argued, first, that peripheral entities often embrace difficult physical terrain with consequent implications for welfare delivery. Second, that social provision 'can clearly act as a unifying force within society', and may help shape 'national identity or even nationalism'. And, third, that small nations' governments may be more responsive to non-governmental pressures (King and Stewart, 2007: 25, 33–34). Such ideas have purchase given, for example, healthcare delivery challenges in remote Scottish regions, Welsh claims regarding the NHS' origins, civic society's apparently greater role in the devolved nations, and their simpler (than England's) organisational structures.[3] The last are attributable to history, smaller populations, and the centrality of social policy responsibilities. Stewart and her colleagues remark that devolved nations' health services have 'broadly converged on a simple and flat organisational structure', and that while a local hospital problem 'can easily become a national political debate' it would not attract such attention in England, especially if outside London (Stewart et al, 2020: 291).

Divergence

The devolved administrations may pursue health policies potentially divergent from, essentially, England, distinguished by its 'far larger political system and NHS', 'much stronger Conservative Party with a weaker attachment to public services including the NHS' and 'long-standing set of assertive advocates' of expanded management and competition. Consequently, Greer concludes, NHS England's standing is less solid, with even political supporters 'constantly seeking ways to make it show its usefulness through high customer satisfaction' (Greer, 2016: 20). The National Audit Office commented in 2012 that the preceding decade had witnessed 'notable divergence in policy and performance management between the nations, particularly in the use of competition between healthcare providers'. Health service commissioners and providers had been 'reintegrated in Scotland and Wales, thus removing the internal market' (National Audit Office, 2012: 8). The Health and Social Care Act 2012 was a crucial piece of English legislation introducing, by one account, the 'most wide-ranging reforms of the NHS' since its inception (King's Fund, 2012). Pollock argued that the service was erected on moral foundations, so providing a 'political and legal contract for citizens'. This survived in the devolved nations, but the Act effectively abolished England's NHS, notably by removing restraints on the 'complete marketisation of funding and break up of delivery' (Pollock, 2015: 399). Klein was more circumspect, while agreeing that since devolution 'Scotland, Wales, and Northern Ireland have increasingly diverged' from England's healthcare model (Klein, 2013: 849 n1).

Surveying the post-2012 situation, Hawkes argued that, from London, the devolved administrations' policies seemed 'timid and complacent'. They, however, saw NHS England pursuing 'a chimera of market driven improvement' owing 'more to doctrine than to evidence', hence their 'distinctive policies' – for instance Scotland's stress on public health, Wales' provision of free prescriptions and hospital parking, and Northern Ireland's implementation of 'a major change in health and social care' aimed at providing more care in the community, and less in hospitals (Hawkes, 2013: 18–20). Reviewing Scotland's position, also in 2013, Fox commented that its recent health policy history had 'already started to inform conversations between Scottish policy makers and their peers in other jurisdictions' while crucially illustrating 'that a political party can accord high priority to reducing health inequality and win the next election' (Fox, 2013: 511). In 2014, meanwhile, it was suggested that, unlike England, Northern Ireland had 'no role for the market' (McGregor and O'Neill, 2014: 409).

The Community Care and Health Act (Scotland) 2002, which sought to integrate health and social care and provided free care for the elderly, was an early instance of post-devolution divergence (Stewart, 2004: 126–30 – for what integration might involve, Elliott, Sinclair and Hesselgreaves, 2020). Provision for the elderly was expanded in 2019 but has no English, Welsh or Northern Irish equivalents. One policy common to the devolved administrations, but not England, is free prescriptions (The

Lancet Commissions, 2021, 1924). The promotion of 'social partnerships', meanwhile, has characterised NHS Wales and NHS Scotland. Bacon and Samuel argue that this arose post-devolution with the transfer of power to governments 'opposed to the marketization of public services'. In Scotland 'extensive cooperation developed to dismantle the internal health market, improve services and enhance staff terms and conditions' while NHS Wales, following a slightly more cautious path, nonetheless 'dismantled' the internal market. Discussions between various actors reflected the 'broadly social democratic approach to industrial relations' in the Welsh and Scottish health services (Bacon and Samuel, 2017: 125, 137–38).

Brexit and COVID-19

Scotland and Northern Ireland voted to remain in the European Union (EU). Wales voted 'leave', although this did not align with its government's position. EU withdrawal was, Keating suggests, predicated on returning to 'a unitary nation-state that had never fully existed and from which the devolution settlements had further deviated' (Keating, 2021: 1). Costa-Font observes that the NHS was 'intrinsically associated with the Brexit referendum narrative'. The impact on healthcare of withdrawal would probably vary across the UK, and 'especially in Scotland and Northern Ireland' *if* they remained in the union. Existing health policy differences would, in any event, be amplified (Costa-Font, 2017: 783–785, 793 – my emphasis). Birrell and Gray claim that Brexit might provoke changes to the Barnett Formula, with obvious implications for health expenditure, and, dispiritingly if predictably, that the devolved administrations' concerns were neither sympathetically received nor well understood 'in the UK cabinet or in Whitehall' (Birrell and Gray, 2017: 766, 776–778). McHale and her colleagues note further post-Brexit healthcare concerns for devolved administrations. Access to sparsely populated, inaccessible, locations, for instance, 'poses particular challenges' for staff recruitment and retention. And while devolved governments are responsible for their populations' health, and consequently obliged to 'secure adequate supplies of medicines within those separate systems', their jurisdictions 'have no powers in trade agreements or medicines regulations' (McHale et al, 2021: 1567, 1562).

As to COVID-19, for Jackson early responses highlighted 'the tension inherent within the devolution settlement', especially the London government's 'curious double role' – responsible for the UK 'across certain policy areas' while functioning in others, notably health, 'as an unacknowledged government of England alone' (Jackson, 2020a: 499). Rycroft sees an initially unified UK response giving way 'to a more disjointed approach'. This included failing to distinguish properly the respective roles of UK and devolved governments, allowing the latter to establish their own ways of dealing with the virus. Outcomes may not have been markedly different, but perceptions 'certainly were', to the advantage of the Welsh and Scottish political leaderships (Rycroft, 2022: 8–9). The 'significant journalistic attention' enjoyed by Welsh first minister Drakeford, for example, led to a high UK profile (Andrews, 2022: 131).

The 'historically destabilising' pandemic, Bone claims, has apparently 'deepened the growing schism' between England and Scotland. The impression created was that Scotland's government, like those of Wales and of Northern Ireland but unlike that of the UK, placed 'more weight on public health than private wealth', and that then first minister Nicola Sturgeon had handled the emergency more assertively, while being more cautious in relaxing restrictive measures. This conformed to Scotland's 'key tropes' of self-identity, 'reason, egalitarianism, collectivism, empathy and solidarity', irrespective of their actual prevalence (Bone, 2021). Audit Scotland, however, notes that Scotland's NHS 'was not financially sustainable before the pandemic', a situation exacerbated by the necessary response to it. The 'considerable impact on mental health', for instance, meant that both adult and child referrals now exceeded pre-pandemic levels (Audit Scotland, 2022: 3, 19).

Post-2016 events added to the devolved administrations' challenges, and to perceptions that their health policies diverge from England's. Much of this is understood in terms of a recurring theme, that divergence derives from political and cultural differences. We now turn briefly to each devolved nation further to illustrate this approach.

Northern Ireland

Northern Ireland's health services operate, as they always have, in their 'unique context' (Dayan and Heenan, 2019: 3). The post-1921 government had limited powers, relied on Treasury support, and pursued a unionist-driven 'politics of culture-war'. There was a limited attitudinal shift in the 1940s in that the 'welfare state' was embraced, so 'allowing the import of Labourism at no political cost to the Unionist united front' (Mulholland, 2020: 14, 18). Crucial, though, is Northern Ireland's inherent political instability, most obviously manifested by 'The Troubles'. The *Ulster Medical Journal* reported in 2015 that before 1969 most of its doctors had 'rarely seen a gunshot wound'. But in the following three decades there were 'over 3,600 deaths and 47,000 people injured' (McGarry, 2015: 121). Among the consequences are that, more than 20 years after the 1994 ceasefire, paramilitary attacks remain a 'significant burden' on health services, affecting both physical and mental wellbeing (Napier, Gallagher and Wilson, 2017: 101). In 2008 Greer noted the 'glacial nature of Northern Ireland's health services'. Health policy, 'intense interest' notwithstanding, tended to be submerged by sectarian politics and, when government was suspended, the Northern Ireland Office's limitations (Greer, 2008: 127). Following the 2011 Assembly elections, one analysis described devolution as a 'lost opportunity'. The administration had, from the outset, been dominated by 'neo-liberal economics and populist rhetoric', with several hospital accident and emergency departments already closed. An 'agenda set in London', which had failed to take into account Northern Ireland's 'laggard position in relation to social policy and provision', still prevailed (Horgan and Gray, 2012: 474–475).

Unsurprisingly, prognoses for NHS Northern Ireland have generally been downbeat. McGregor and O'Neill suggested in 2014 that in the coming decade 'the public health and social care service ... faces considerable challenges', but the outlook for any 'radical reshaping of services' was 'not optimistic' (McGregor and O'Neill, 2014: 415–416). A few years later, during a suspension of the Executive, a UK-wide nurses pay rise was agreed but could not be implemented in the absence of a Northern Irish health minister. Shortly afterwards, significant cuts in nursing education were proposed. Both decisions encountered considerable protest, and were duly reversed. Drawing on such examples, Heenan and Birrell propose that government suspensions have meant 'that major policy changes in health and education', including the implementation of 'long overdue' reforms necessitated by growing hospital waiting lists, have stalled (Heenan and Birrell, 2018: 308–309).

By 2019 a 'political vacuum' was 'exacerbating chronic problems in making difficult decisions', including in health policy (Dayan and Heenan, 2019: 2). A (temporary) return to power-sharing was attributable less to political manoeuvring than to the 'real tipping point', health workers taking 'unprecedented industrial action' over pay and a 'spiralling' NHS crisis (Haughey, 2020: 134). And as McHale and her colleagues note, Brexit and COVID-19 have contributed to 'increasingly integrated healthcare provision on the island of Ireland', encouraged by 'mutual recognition of professional qualifications, and shared standards, including for data sharing' (McHale et al, 2021: 1566). Brexit was another example of 'British political considerations' delivering an 'exogenous shock' (Mulholland, 2020: 114–115). It fuelled debates about future Irish unity, highlighting Northern Ireland's particular position within the UK. Medical supplies, and staff commuting across the NI/Republic border, are especially problematic. Dayan and Hervey observed in summer 2022 that the current political standoff had come at the worst time for the health and care services. While broad political agreement on reform had existed since 2016, progress had been stymied by periods without a government. Waiting times, 'already appalling before covid', were 'reaching the point where planned care simply is not available in practice, even for critical illnesses' (Dayan and Hervey, 2022). Shortly afterwards, the Royal College of Physicians charged that 'lack of a functioning government' was 'damaging patient care and undermining staff in the health sector', problems manifested by '(e)xcessively long waiting lists, vacant posts, and a deteriorating quality of care' (Baraniuk, 2022).

Scotland

Scotland's pre-NHS healthcare saw notable innovations, for example the Highlands and Islands Medical Service. This involved state financial support for medical staff, the provision of more comprehensive patient care, and addressing the problem, still current, of healthcare for geographically remote areas. During debates over the NHS' creation, much was made of Scotland's history of state intervention in healthcare. The 1947 Act put the Scottish Secretary firmly in charge, administratively and politically, with the result that NHS Scotland has been more centrally controlled than its English counterpart. Scottish doctors, meanwhile, were more committed to post-war healthcare reconstruction than those in England, a situation repeated in late twentieth-century public sector resistance to market-led healthcare initiatives. Post-1940s Scottish health policy continued to enjoy its own legislation and administration. However, the National Health Service and Community Care Act 1990, an expression of Thatcherite zeal for the internal market, was UK-wide. Given Scotland's previous legislative autonomy, and its electoral rejection of Conservatism, this was badly received. Health and health policy became powerful weapons for political devolution's proponents, focusing on Scotland's historically poor health record and, especially after the 1979 UK general election, hostility to London's proposed reforms (Stewart, 2004: 103–112).

Scottish 'distinctiveness' is much discussed, although with necessary attention drawn to 'universal' as well as 'territorial' trends (for example, Cairney, Russell and St Denny, 2016). Nor was NHS Scotland immune to funding mechanisms such PFIs, albeit adopted more reluctantly than in England (Stewart, 2004: 125). Nonetheless, Greer and his colleagues noted in 2016 the SNP government's prioritising of health policy, with improved outcomes part of its 'strategy for independence'. Since devolution both SNP and Labour/Liberal Democrat governments had been 'associated with a consistent and generally enlightened health policy'. The SNP was, therefore, 'effectively pursuing and building on themes in Scottish health policy' both pre-dating, and benefitting from, devolution (Greer, Wilson and Donnelly, 2016: 28, 41). Wiggan likewise argues that since the 1970s the SNP has pursued 'territorial interests with an anti-Conservative Party, pro-welfare state message', an approach heightened with the advent of Coalition/Conservative UK administrations pursuing 'austerity' and 'welfare reform'. New political opportunities had thus arisen for a distinctive 'vision and practice of welfare' (Wiggan, 2017: 651, 639–640).

A 2017 Nuffield Trust report noted Scotland's 'unique system of improving the quality of health care' through engaging frontline staff's 'altruistic professional motivations' and 'building their skills to improve'. Scotland's smaller size (relative to England) enabled 'a more personalised, less formal approach' with healthcare 'overseen by a single organisation' monitoring care quality while helping staff improve it. There were, though, 'particular issues of unequal health outcomes, and very remote areas'. NHS Scotland faced a 'serious financial predicament' with constraints on 'national planning' and a 'polarised, hostile political context' making 'an honest national debate difficult' (Dayan and Edwards, 2017: 3–4). Audit Scotland, meanwhile, records the country's drug-related death rates as Europe's worst, and death rates from alcohol abuse as among the worst in the UK, with deprived areas especially vulnerable (Audit Scotland, 2022: 23). Illustrating the salience of the long-term view, Campbell and his colleagues observed the 'widening gap' between Scottish and English and Welsh mortality rates, exacerbated in the 1980s but established at least a decade previously (Campbell et al, 2013: 184). In a thought-provoking overview, Scotland's post-devolution 'research and healthcare systems' are argued to 'have undergone profound structural and organisational change', while their further evolution in the event of independence has 'animated debates'. More broadly, the 'existence of multiple and competing narratives about the past and future' had implications for viewing Scotland 'as a set of imagined communities/identities', both 'sick' and 'innovative', these being 'problematised within a broader health and wealth policy agenda' (Mittra et al, 2019: 69).

Wales

Wales came late to administrative devolution, the Welsh Office being set up in 1964. Five years later, with the NHS consuming two-thirds of his department's expenditure, the Secretary of State assumed full executive responsibility for health and welfare services, a 'major victory for the devolutionists' (Webster, 2006: 240, 264). Drakeford comments that before political devolution Welsh Office health initiatives were not unknown and that while the NHS remained the 'iconic achievement of the British Labour movement', for Wales 'its ownership has always been a matter of fierce national pride'. Nonetheless, pre-1999 policy making was 'extensively integrated into Whitehall networks', with potential for independent action limited. Political devolution was thus crucial for health policy, becoming a 'major player in the Assembly's roster of responsibilities' with important political dimensions (Drakeford, 2006: 545–547, 558).

Unlike Scotland, debates over health and health policy were minimal in 1990s Wales. Even post-devolution, emerging policy differences in health and education did not fundamentally alter 'the experience of going to school or being treated in hospital' when compared with England. And, it has been argued, such differences were not especially profound (Johnes, 2012: 413, 420, 432). Nonetheless, neither Scotland nor Wales electorally bought into post-1979 Thatcherism. Welsh pro-devolutionists, notably Peter Hain (later Secretary of State for Northern Ireland, then Secretary of State for Wales), argued that 'historical evidence' showed a 'greater willingness to embrace socialist and communitarian values' in Wales than in England. And the Welsh Assembly was, Chaney and Drakeford conclude, from its inception 'a *social policy body*' with one of the 'most significant post-devolution developments' the proposed restructuring of NHS Wales, and a strategic emphasis on primary care and public health (Chaney and Drakeford, 2004: 124, 136, 121, 134 – original emphasis). Riley describes Welsh health ambitions as threefold: 'systems and policies better attuned to Welsh needs; better health for all; and improved service quality' (Riley, 2016, 40). Wales has thus seen 'emerging cultural practices', some diverging significantly from those in England, including a nationwide focus on public service collaboration and partnership (Andrews, 2022, 144). As elsewhere in the UK, integrating health and social care has been much discussed. The Social Services and Wellbeing (Wales) Act 2014 and the Well-Being of Future Generations (Wales) Act 2015, concerned in the first instance with social care, are nonetheless seen as crucial to the NHS, giving the health service and local government the opportunity 'to be equal partners in making a difference to the people and communities they serve'. The 2015 Act, especially, aspired to a healthier and more equal Wales (Greenwell and Antebi, 2017: 265–267).

However, a 2016 official report concluded that existing health and social care provision was 'not fit for the future' (quoted in Willson and Davies, 2021: 295). A further major review, in 2018, repeated the claim about the NHS' origins ('born in Wales, based on … the Tredegar Workmen's Medical Aid Society') before observing that increased demand for health and care was unforeseen. The 'key challenge' now was anticipating and addressing new circumstances. A growing proportion of Wales' budget was allocated to health and social care, at the expense of other public services (a problem admittedly faced by other advanced societies). Although a small country, Wales had 'tremendous assets in its people', especially health and social care users, supporters and staff. The question therefore arose, if 'the case for change is compelling, then why hasn't it compelled?'. A system of 'seamless health and care' should be the aim but this would require a 'revolution from within' (Welsh Government, 2018: 4–7).

Surveying the situation in 2016 Riley found 'significant if unspectacular progress' in adapting healthcare to Welsh circumstances. More might have been achieved, though, with hindrances to change including restricted governmental powers and Welsh Labour's limitations. While NHS Wales sought to be distinct from the rest of the UK, this 'preferred philosophy has not been successfully communicated to the public or the NHS' (Riley, 2016: 41–42). Willson and Davies too identify political shortcomings. NHS Wales simultaneously struggled with pressures to perform and to reform. Slow progress could not, though, be attributed to a 'political vacuum', given Labour's dominance for 20 years (Willson and Davies, 2021: 295).

Conclusion

Political devolution is a messy, dynamic and fluid process wherein the devolved nations' histories have played, and continue to play, a crucial part. Each nation has 'particularities' – Northern Ireland's constitutional distinctiveness and political instability; Scottish nationalism's strength in a society both 'sick' and 'innovative'; Welsh Labour's dominance in a 'communitarian' culture; and, across the board, political trajectories and self-identities separate, partially at least, from those of UK/England. Pre-1999 Scottish and Welsh administrative devolution and Northern Ireland's decades old political settlement further testify to these particularities. Health policy 'divergences' must be seen in such contexts.

One shared characteristic of the devolved nations' healthcare strategies is the need to confront challenges, in delivery and outcomes, in difficult economic and political circumstances (and, implicitly if more contentiously, in common historical experiences of socio-economic disadvantage). Another is resistance to 'the market' and the private sector, sometimes openly contrasted to NHS England's perceived trajectory dating from the 1979–1997 Conservative administrations (although this has not, for instance, precluded post-devolution Scottish engagement with PFI). Their smaller size is likewise significant in that devolved administrations are – or claim to be – more engaged with civic society and healthcare professionals. This is further enabled by political inclination and culture, and by relatively straightforward administrative structures. The latter may in themselves be 'centralised', but the devolved health services' very existence confirms that the 'NHS' is not monolithic, and that devolution accelerated pre-existing, albeit qualified, administrative autonomy.

On the other hand, their constitutional positions and reliance on Treasury funding means that healthcare provision in these small polities operates in the shadows of the UK state and NHS England, and potentially inhibits truly radical divergence. Patient experience and outcomes, meanwhile, are broadly similar throughout the United Kingdom. Taken together, all this suggests values, aims, practices and challenges commonly shared by English, Welsh, Northern Irish and Scottish health services.

Does this mean that health policy divergences are not, ultimately, of real substance? A case can be made for such interpretation. Nonetheless, divergences do exist, and attention has been drawn to their deep historical, political, and cultural roots. Given the UK polity's current (2023) fragility, and the devolved nations' aspirations and propensities, it seems probable that health policy will remain a major input to Scottish, Welsh and Northern Irish attempts further to confirm identities distinct from that of UK/England. To put it another way, this chapter began by emphasising health policy's highly politicised nature. This is unlikely to change any time soon, as commentary on NHS Scotland's alleged shortcomings at the time of the first minister's resignation in 2023 amply illustrated.

Notes

1   Elections shortly followed to the Northern Ireland Assembly, with the period since dominated, politically, by Sinn Féin (SF) and the Democratic Unionist Party (DUP).
2   Generally, 'direct rule' is carried out by the Northern Ireland Office, rather than 'London/ Whitehall' per se.
3   For organisational guides, Dayan and Edwards (2017), Appendix 1; Stewart et al (2020) Table 3; The Lancet Commissions (2021), 1925.

References

Andrews, L. (2022) 'Performing Welsh government 1999–2016: How insider narratives illuminate the hidden wiring and emergent cultural practices'. *Contemporary British History*, 36, 1, 124–156.

Audit Scotland. (2022) *NHS in Scotland 2021*. Edinburgh: Audit Scotland.

Bacon, S. and Samuel, P. (2017) 'Social partnership and political devolution in the National Health Service: Emergence, operation and outcomes'. *Work, Employment and Society*, 31, 1, 123–141.

Baraniuk, C. (2022) 'Northern Ireland: Political turmoil spells "disaster" for healthcare, warn doctors'. *BMJ Online* 379, o2581, 27 October.

Bevan, G., Karanikolos, M., Exley, J., Nolte, E., Connolly, S. and Mays, N. (2014) *The Four Health Care Systems of the United Kingdom: How Do They Compare?* London: Health Foundation/Nuffield Trust.

Birrell, D. and Gray, A.M. (2017) 'Devolution: The social, political and policy implications of Brexit for Scotland, Wales and Northern Ireland'. *Journal of Social Policy*, 46, 4, 765–782.

Bone, J. (2021) 'Scotland and England's colliding nationalisms: Neoliberalism and the fracturing of the United Kingdom', *British Politics*, published online 29 September.

Brown, G. (2017) *My Life, Our Times*. London: The Bodley Head.

Cairney, P., Russell, S. and St Denny, E. (2016) 'The "Scottish approach" to policy and policymaking: What issues are territorial and what are universal?'. *Policy and Politics*, 44, 3, 333–350.

Campbell, M., Ballas, D., Dorling, D. and Mitchell, R. (2013) 'Mortality inequalities: Scotland versus England and Wales'. *Health and Place*, 23, 179–186.

Chaney, P. and Drakeford, M. (2004) 'The primacy of ideology: Social policy and the first term of the National Assembly for Wales', in N. Ellison, L. Bauld and M. Powell (eds) *Social Policy Review 16*. Bristol: Policy Press, pp 121–142.

Costa-Font, J. (2017) 'The National Health Service at a critical moment: When Brexit means hectic'. *Journal of Social Policy*, 46, 4, 783–795.

Dayan, M. and Edwards, N. (2017) *Learning from Scotland's NHS*. London: Nuffield Trust.

Dayan, M. and Heenan, D. (2019) *Change or Collapse: Lessons from the Drive to Reform Health and Social Care in Northern Ireland*. London: Nuffield Trust.

Dayan, M. and Hervey, T. (2022) 'Breaking the Northern Ireland Protocol would create problems for health and care'. *BMJ Online*, 378, o1673.

Donnelly, M. and O'Neill, C. (2018) 'Editorial: integration – reflections from Northern Ireland'. *Journal of Health Services Research and Policy*, 23, 1, 1–3.

Drakeford, M. (2006) 'Health policy in Wales: Making a difference in conditions of difficulty'. *Critical Social Policy*, 26, 3, 543–561.

Elliott, I.C., Sinclair, C. and Hesselgreaves, H. (2020) 'Leadership of integrated health and social care services'. *Scottish Affairs*, 29, 2, 198–222.

Fox, D.M. (2013) 'Health inequality and governance in Scotland since 2007'. *Public Health*, 127, 6, 503–513.

Greenwell, S. and Antebi, D. (2017) 'A new health and social care context in Wales: Promoting resilience through a shift in perspective and different relationships'. *Journal of Integrated Care*, 25, 4, 265–270.

Greer, A. (2019) 'Reflections on devolution: Twenty years on'. *The Political Quarterly*, 90, 3, 553–558.

Greer, S.L. (2008) 'Options and lack of options: Healthcare politics and policy'. *The Political Quarterly*, 79, s1, 117–132.

Greer, S.L. (2016) 'Devolution and health in the UK: Policy and its lessons since 1998'. *British Medical Bulletin*, 118, 1, 17–25.

Greer, S.L., Wilson, I. and Donnelly, P.D. (2016) 'The wages of continuity: Health policy under the SNP'. *Scottish Affairs*, 25, 1, 28–44.

Hannigan, B. (2022) 'Observations from a small country: Mental health policy, services and nursing in Wales'. *Health Economics, Policy and Law*, 17, 2, 200–211.

Haughey, S. (2020) 'Back to Stormont: The *New Decade, New Approach* Agreement and what it means for Northern Ireland'. *The Political Quarterly*, 91, 1, 134–140.

Hawkes, N. (2013) 'How different are the NHS systems across the UK since devolution?' *British Medical Journal*, 346, 7908, 18–20.

Heenan, D. and Birrell, D. (2009) 'Organisational integration in health and social care: Some reflections on the Northern Ireland experience'. *Journal of Integrated Care*, 17, 5, 3–12.

Heenan, D. and Birrell, D. (2018) 'Between devolution and direct rule: Implications of a political vacuum in Northern Ireland'. *The Political Quarterly*, 89, 2, 306–312.

HM Treasury. (2021) *Public Expenditure: Statistical Analyses 2021*. London: HM Treasury.

Horgan, G. and Gray, A.M. (2012) 'Devolution in Northern Ireland: A lost opportunity?'. *Critical Social Policy*, 32, 3, 467–478.

Institute of Welsh Affairs (2021) *Why the NHS Is Fundamental to Economic and Social Recovery*. Cardiff: Cardiff University – iwa.wales, Politics and Policy, 16 November.

Jackson, B. (2020a) 'Commentary: A crisis for devolution?' *The Political Quarterly* 91, 3, 499–501.

Jackson, B. (2020b) *The Case for Scottish Independence: A History of Nationalist Political Thought in Modern Scotland*. Oxford: Oxford University Press.

Johnes, M. (2012) *Wales since 1939*. Manchester: Manchester University Press.

Kaehne, A., Birrell, D., Miller, R. and Petch, A. (2017) 'Bringing integration home: Policy on health and social care integration in the four nations of the UK'. *Journal of Integrated Care*, 25, 2, 84–98.

Keating, M. (2021) *United Kingdom: The Fractured Union*. Oxford: Oxford University Press.

King, S. and Stewart, J. (2007) 'Welfare peripheries in modern Europe', in S. King and J. Stewart (eds) *Welfare Peripheries: The Development of Welfare States in Nineteenth and Twentieth Century Europe*. Bern: Peter Lang, pp 9–38.

King's Fund (2012) 'The NHS after the Health and Social Care Act'. London: The King's Fund. www.kingsfund.org.uk/projects/new-nhs

Klein, R. (2013) 'The twenty-year war over England's National Health Service: A report from the battlefield'. *Journal of Health Politics, Policy and Law*, 38, 4, 849–869.

The Lancet Commissions. (2021) 'LSE-Lancet Commission on the future of the NHS'. *The Lancet* 397, 22 May, 1915–1978.

Mackinnon, D. (2015) 'Devolution, state restructuring and policy divergence in the UK'. *The Geographical Journal*, 181, 1, 47–56.

McGarry, P. (2015) 'The fortunes of the legal and medical professions during the "Troubles"'. *Ulster Medical Journal*, 84, 2, 119–123.

McGregor, P. and O'Neill, C. (2014) 'Resource allocation in the Northern Ireland health service: Consensus or challenge?'. *Public Money and Management*, 34, 6, 409–416.

McHale, J., Speakman, E., Hervey, T. and Flear, M. (2021) 'Health law and policy, devolution and Brexit'. *Regional Studies*, 55, 9, 1561–1570.

Mittra, J., Mastroeni, M., Haddow, G., Wield, D. and Barlow, E. (2019) 'Re-imagining healthcare and medical research systems in post-devolution Scotland'. *Sociological Research Online*, 24, 1, 55–72.

Mulholland, M. (2020) *Northern Ireland: A Very Short Introduction.* 2nd ed. Oxford: Oxford University Press.

Napier, P., Gallagher, B.J. and Wilson, D.S. (2017) 'An imperfect peace: Trends in paramilitary related violence 20 years after the Northern Ireland ceasefires'. *Ulster Medical Journal*, 86, 2, 99–102.

National Audit Office. (2012) *Healthcare Across the UK: A Comparison of the NHS in England, Scotland, Wales and Northern Ireland.* London: The Stationery Office.

Northern Ireland Executive (2016) *Health and Wellbeing 2026. Delivering Together.* Belfast: The Northern Ireland Executive

Paun, A., Cheung, A. and Nicholson, E. (2021) *Funding Devolution: The Barnett Formula in Theory and Practice.* London: Institute for Government.

Pollock, A.M. (2015) 'Morality and values in support of universal healthcare must be enshrined in law'. *International Journal of Health Policy Management*, 4, 6, 399–402.

Rawlings, R. (2015) 'Riders on the storm: Wales, the union, and territorial constitutional crisis'. *Journal of Law and Society*, 42, 4, 471–498.

Riley, C. (2016) 'The challenge of creating a "Welsh NHS"'. *Journal of Health Services Research and Policy*, 21, 1, 40–42.

Rycroft, P. (2022) 'After Brexit: The state of the UK union'. *Revue Française de Civilisation Britannique*, XXVII, 2, 1–13.

Scottish First Minister. (2022) 'Nicola Sturgeon says NHS principles "not up for discussion"'. www.bbc.co.uk/news/uk-scotland-63701717

Simpson, M. (2022) *Social Citizenship in an Age of Welfare Regionalism: The State of the Social Union.* Oxford: Hart.

Smith, K. and Hellowell, M. (2017) 'Beyond rhetorical differences: A cohesive account of post-devolution developments in UK health policy'. *Social Policy and Administration*, 46, 2, 178–198.

Stewart, E., Greer, S.L., Ercia, A. and Donnelly, P.D. (2020) 'Transforming health care: The policy and politics of service reconfiguration in the UK's four health systems'. *Health Economics, Policy and Law*, 15, 3, 289–307.

Stewart, J. (2004) *Taking Stock: Scottish Social Welfare After Devolution.* Bristol: Policy Press.

Webster, C. (2006) 'Devolution and the health services in Wales, 1919–1969', in P. Michael and C. Webster (eds) *Health and Society in Twentieth Century Wales.* Cardiff: University of Wales Press, pp 240–269.

Welsh Government. (2018) *The Parliamentary Review of Health and Social Care in Wales: A Revolution from within: Transforming Health and Care in Wales.* Cardiff: Welsh Government.

Welsh Government. (2021) *A Healthier Wales: Our Plan for Health and Social Care.* Cardiff: Welsh Government.

Wiggan, J. (2017) 'Contesting the austerity and "welfare reform" narrative of the UK government'. *International Journal of Sociology and Social Policy*, 37, 11/12, 639–654.

Willson, A. and Davies, A. (2021) 'Rhetoric or reform? Changing health and social care in Wales'. *International Journal of Health Policy Management*, 10, 6, 295–298.

5

NHS at 75: general practice through the lens of access

*Kath Checkland, Jennifer Voorhees, Jonathan Hammond and
Sharon Spooner*

As the NHS reaches its 75th birthday, general practice represents something of a policy paradox: it is both highly visible, dominating headlines with perceived shortcomings and failings (Mroz, Papoutsi and Greenhalgh, 2022), and yet strangely invisible, with the most recent NHS reorganisation in England barely touching on its role. For example, in the latest Health and Care Act (Department of Health and Social Care, 2021) mention of general practice is confined to a few references to how it might be commissioned, with nothing at all about its form or function. Most strikingly, the most visible aspect of current primary care policy – an additional contract which provides funding for groups of GP practices to work together in networks – is not mentioned at all in the Act.

In part this dichotomy arises from the historical position of general practice in the NHS. In 1948, general practice was established not as an integral function of the hierarchical new NHS, but as a separate service, provided to the NHS by independent contractors (Peckham and Exworthy, 2003). This independent status has been both a strength and a weakness of general practice ever since (Lewis, 1998). Lauded for the fact that it may support innovation, and usefully allowing the central NHS to avoid providing premises, it has also been identified as problematic, generating unwarranted variation and difficulties in integrating primary care with other sectors (Chapman and Groom, 1999; Jones et al, 2015).

In terms of the themes set up in Chapter 1, general practice is perhaps an outlier, insulated by its independent status from the more significant NHS policy switches around competition or managerialism. Nevertheless, general practice policy since 1948 has seen a shift towards a more atomised approach (Norman, Russell and Merli, 2016), with the professional ideal of providing person-centred relationship-based care in ongoing tension with an approach which seeks to identify and manage biomedical problems in the most efficient way possible (Checkland et al, 2008).

In this chapter we consider general practice in the context of its history, and offer some thoughts about the future which take account of the unique status of primary care as both the entry-point to other services and as a semi-detached quasi-independent service. Focusing upon a longstanding area of public and policy concern – access to services – we use this as a case study topic to illuminate a number of persistent policy issues: the aspiration to deliver holistic person-centred care in the context of managerialism; workforce availability and the tensions between patient expectations and service provision in resource-constrained environments; and the tensions between national negotiation and contracting and local assessment of needs and appropriate service adaptation. We then draw these together to consider how they speak to the issues addressed throughout this volume, including persistent inequalities, the ongoing tension between the centralisation and decentralisation of services and the ability of the primary care sector to adapt and be sustainable for the future.

The GP contract

As noted before, GP practices are independent businesses commissioned to provide generalist medical services to a particular patient population. Practices are commonly partnerships between GPs that take on legal responsibility for care provision. The General Medical Services (GMS) contract accounts for the majority of practices in England (approximately 70 per cent).[1] This is negotiated each year between NHS England and the British Medical Association's (BMA) General Practice Committee. The remaining GP practices either hold a Personal Medical Services (PMS) contract or an Alternative Personal Medical Service (APMS) contract, which are more flexible in terms of requirements and allow non-GP partnership providers to deliver services (in the case of APMS (Coleman et al, 2013)). Beyond the core contract, all GP practices have the option of taking up additional nationally negotiated Directed Enhanced Service contracts, or locally commissioned Local Enhanced Services, to provide certain services (for example, vaccination programmes) or engage in defined activities (for example, becoming a Primary Care Network member). Practices receive global sum payments for delivering the core contract, but then receive bespoke levels of income according to, among other things, additional contracts they sign up to or incentive scheme framework indicators that they choose to address. All of this creates a complex mix in terms of the nature of GP practices as care providers, policy levers for affecting change and the political dynamic between government and GP representatives.

This description of the current contractual situation applies to England only. In Scotland, Wales and Northern Ireland, healthcare provision has been a devolved responsibility since 1998, and as such is subject to separate contract negotiations (Greer, 2016). In Scotland, for example, the quality incentive aspects of the contract have been curtailed (Stewart et al, 2022). These differences are addressed elsewhere in this volume.

Access as a lens through which to understand primary care

You do not have to look far to find evidence of a current crisis in access to primary care. Throughout 2021 and into 2022, newspaper headlines have highlighted urgent problems (Oliver, 2021). A combination of increased demand, ongoing problems associated with COVID-19, recruitment and retention challenges, and backlogs elsewhere in the system (Haynes, 2022) have resulted in delays in obtaining care at crisis levels.[2] However, while recent issues such as COVID-19 have undoubtedly exacerbated the problem, access to primary care services has long been a contentious and charged issue. In the early years of the NHS, 'access' was largely thought of as being a population-level issue. The so-called 'inverse care law' (Tudor Hart, 1971) highlighted a perceived mismatch between population health need and service provision, with policy remedies largely confined to the use of local Medical Practices Committees to determine whether and where new practices should be allowed to open (Powell and Exworthy, 2003). During the New Labour years (1997–2010), however, a more consumerist approach was taken, with concern that the public would withdraw their consent from a taxation-funded NHS if access did not improve (Newman and Vidler, 2006). This perceived crisis led to a regime of access targets and mystery shopper exercises (Campbell et al, 2010). A managerial solution known as 'Advanced Access' swept the sector, focusing upon same-day access for anyone who felt they needed it (Salisbury et al, 2007).

These current and past crises have foregrounded access as the most salient problem affecting primary care. Throughout, the focus has been upon *timely* access, in which the length of time taken to obtain an appointment is seen as the most important issue (Simpson et al, 2015). However, there is a richer literature addressing the concept of access to primary care which may be of value in considering where we are now and how the system might need to change (Voorhees et al, 2022). Drawing upon theories related to individual help-seeking and candidacy, practice organisation and management and system design, authors such as Levesque (2013) have sought to understand the complex interactions and individual behaviours which come together to determine who gets an appointment to see whom. From this perspective, access becomes a lens which can illuminate not only straightforward issues of appointment systems and availability, but also more complex questions of who seeks access, what type of primary care is valued and how the wider system is configured, managed and paid for. Moreover, in keeping with the focus of this volume, access to a service might be said to be the most fundamental test of policy success or failure.

In the rest of this chapter we use this more nuanced and complex conception of access to consider three contemporary policy topics: remote access to services; skill mix change and the substitution of nurses and other clinical workers for doctors; and care outside of usual office hours, often referred to as 'extended access'. We then look across these three topics to draw more general lessons about the nature of primary care services in the NHS as it turns 75 and to consider how policy might usefully be targeted in the future.

Access theory: a new model

While this model of access is recently published, the ideas synthesised within it are not new. They are not, however, how access has historically or is currently conceptualised in English health policy. This has several implications for the three areas of tension outlined earlier in this chapter. Here we explain the model of access in terms of 'human fit' (see Figure 5.1).

Scholarship on the complexities of accessing healthcare dates back to at least the 1970s when American sociologists Andersen and Aday (1974) published their initial model of patient factors affecting healthcare utilisation. Around the same time, epidemiologist Donabedian (1973) brought together concepts of needs assessment and care supply to define 'accessibility' as 'characteristics of the resource that facilitate or obstruct use'. Penchansky and Thomas (1981) built on this work to describe access as 'a concept representing the degree of fit between the clients and the system'. More recent models have built on this work and also embraced the dynamic and contingent aspects of access, which is 'constantly … redefined through interactions between individuals and professionals' (Dixon-Woods et al, 2006a). Levesque's conceptualisation of patient-centred access visually depicted much of the aforementioned scholarship (Levesque, Harris and Russell, 2013). Our application of that model in the context of English general practice and the resulting modifications are shown next.

Several features of this model are important for our discussion within this chapter:

1. The definition of access as the fit between the needs, abilities, and capacity of the humans on both the patient/population and the health system sides of ongoing interactions.
2. The people can be thought of as individuals, that is, a patient or carer interacting with a staff member or clinician, or they can be a practice population and practice staff, or the national population and the national workforce.

Figure 5.1: Access conceptualised as 'human fit'

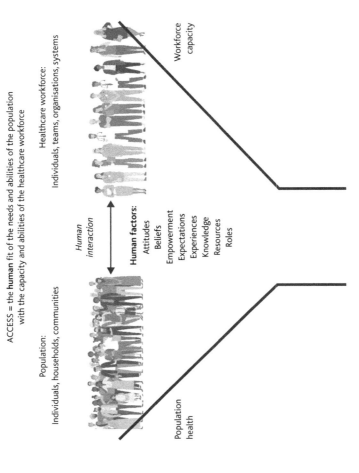

ACCESS = the **human** fit of the needs and abilities of the population
with the capacity and abilities of the healthcare workforce

Population:
Individuals, households, communities

Healthcare workforce:
Individuals, teams, organisations, systems

*Human
interaction*

Human factors:
Attitudes
Beliefs
Empowerment
Expectations
Experiences
Knowledge
Resources
Roles

Population
health

Workforce
capacity

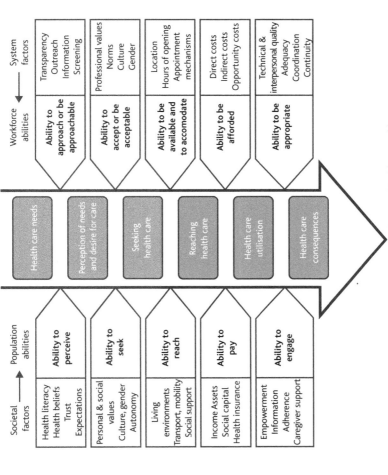

Better fit between abilities of population and healthcare workforce: population needs met/health improved, workforce optimised

Source: Adapted from Voorhees et al (2022)

3. Human interactions, particularly at the individual level, are affected by factors such as each person (or the collective group's) attitudes, beliefs, empowerment, expectations, experiences, knowledge, resources and roles.
4. The overall context of the health of the population and the size/capacity of the workforce affects these ongoing interactions.
5. Along the steps involved in seeking and obtaining care, different abilities within the population and the workforce affect the fit between the needs and the capacity.
6. Various societal factors and system factors on each side affect the interaction of these abilities.
7. When access is conceptualised in this way, improving access does not mean simply more of something, but a better fit between the two sides.
8. Continuity is very much a part of appropriate access and not something that is at odds with access. Indeed, relational and information continuity are relevant throughout the model and depicted in various ways, including having knowledge of the other person to know what to expect from an interaction.
9. Specific aspects of access such as appointment mechanisms and hours of opening, which have received a lot of attention in policy, are included but put into context.
10. Factors on the patient population side, such as health literacy, are potential targets for improving the fit of access.

Finally, this more nuanced approach allows the 'problem' to be contextualised and considered at multiple levels. 'Better access' no longer simply means more or quicker, but 'more appropriate', which may mean different things to different people at different times. It raises significant questions about 'one size' solutions, and brings to the foreground the need for local adaptation and negotiation.

Contemporary policy issues using an access lens

Introduction

In this section we use the theory elucidated earlier to consider three contemporary policy issues. First, we consider remote access to services. Long a policy aspiration, uptake of technology-assisted appointment modalities was initially slow and inconsistent. COVID-19 transformed this, with rapid and complete uptake of a remote-first model of care across general practice (Murphy et al, 2021). However, many questions remain, and public discourse around this topic is often highly critical, including a national newspaper for 'more face-to-face consultations'.[3] Second, we address skill mix change in primary care. Again, this is something which has a long history in general practice, with the rapid development of the practice nurse role attributed to the policy of reimbursing GPs for nurse salaries introduced in the 1980/90s (Smith and Donovan, 1970). Subsequent expansion of their roles included management of minor illness (Shum et al, 2000) and monitoring of long-term conditions (Griffiths et al, 2010). However, skill mix change has been given fresh impetus in the context of a perceived workforce crisis, with successive governments failing in their stated aim to recruit an additional 6000 GPs.[4] Current policy suggests that the recruitment of a wide range of new types of clinical practitioners will alleviate pressures on GPs, thereby improving access, and provide a better service for patients (NHS England, 2019). Finally, we consider extended access to primary care. Historically, routine GP hours have been deemed to be from 8 am to 6 pm. However, successive governments have considered this problematic, with particular emphasis upon those who work. Policy has therefore focused upon providing routine services outside these core hours, with additional contractual payments for the provision of appointments during the evening and at weekends.

Remote-first primary care

Prior to the COVID-19 pandemic, there was considerable policy push to 'modernise' access to primary care via technological solutions such as video and online consultations (Cook, 2018). However, uptake was slow (Mold et al, 2019). The pandemic in 2020 provided an exogenous shock necessitating rapid change. As national lockdowns started, practices restricted access to face-to-face appointments to minimise the risk of infection, with the then health secretary arguing for 'remote by default' access to primary care (Walker, 2020). As a result, accessing care quickly shifted from the historical model by which patients would phone their practice or call in to book a face-to-face appointment, to one by which initial contact was via an online form or a triage phone call, after which the practice would decide what form of appointment to offer. An early mixed-methods evaluation found that the transition had been near complete, with 90 per cent of GP-patient contacts occurring remotely by July 2020. However, it was striking that the legacy technology of the telephone remained the most frequent mode of consultation, with a very small minority of consultations using video or online consultations.

As the vaccination programme rolled out in early 2021, face-to-face appointments gradually restarted, but there had clearly been a shift in how access to primary care was experienced by patients. In autumn 2021, the *Daily Mail* ran a campaign critical of general practice, alleging that general practices had used the pandemic to remove valued access to face-to-face appointments (Oliver, 2021), with other newspapers joining in (Mroz, Papoutsi and Greenhalgh, 2022). The appointments data evidence is

Figure 5.2: Changes in GP and nurse consultations 2019–2020

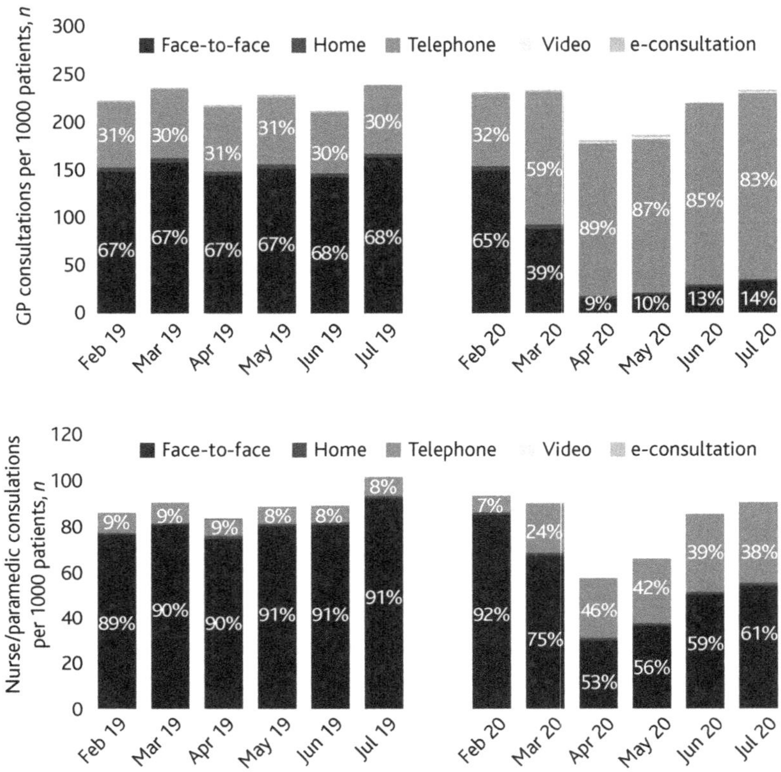

Source: From Murphy et al (2021)

somewhat different to the headlines, with 70 per cent of appointments in October 2022 taking place face to face, compared with 80 per cent pre-pandemic (Potter, 2022); a decline in face-to-face activity, certainly, but not a catastrophic one. However, concealed within this statistic is the fact that triage – the pre-appointment assessment of patient needs to support allocation to an appropriate appointment/practitioner – has become the norm in primary care. Thus, seeing a GP no longer simply involves calling in or phoning up for an appointment. Rather, a patient must contact the practice, either by telephone or by filling in an online form, and someone will then assess the information provided and make a decision about what appointment is warranted and when. Arguments in favour of this approach highlight the fact that not all patients or problems need to be seen, with many problems amenable to an administrative response or a telephone call (Campbell et al, 2014). However, patient satisfaction with GP services has declined sharply,[5] suggesting that something is not working well (see Figure 5.2).

Our extended theory of access may be helpful here. Thinking of access as 'human fit' between the needs and abilities of patients and the capacity and capabilities of staff, potential issues become clear. For patients, ability to engage with triage systems requires access to relevant technology. This might be a phone, or it might be a computer. Time is also required, particularly for phone access – ringing the practice early in the morning is often the only way to get a triage appointment, but many people will be travelling to work at that time and receiving a call-back may not be feasible. For those experiencing homelessness, all of this may be insurmountable, with phone credit and phone charging all potential problems. Many practices no longer engage with people walking in, as this doesn't fit with triage processes – one study documented patients who attended a practice in person being required to stand in the waiting room using their phone to speak to a clinician to be triaged (MacKichan et al, 2017). For practices, triage represents an attempt to manage demand, and to match patients with appropriate appointments, but the blanket requirement for triage represents a one size fits all approach, which doesn't take account of the human characteristics of the person seeking help. Perhaps more troublingly, it is also an approach which requires a patient to be able to articulate a discrete problem. Online forms require the person seeking help to state their problem, and this is then used to decide what response is necessary. A triage phone call requires a person to be able to hear and speak clearly, and to define and articulate their problem. All of this is a long way from an ideal of generalist, holistic and person-centred care (Roberts, 2004; Hasegawa et al, 2005; Rudebeck, 2019). From the perspective of what is sometimes called 'relationship-based care' (Royal College of General Practitioners, 2022), an encounter in primary care is not merely about solving a specific and immediate problem. Rather, it is an opportunity to share concerns, discuss symptoms and seek help with managing their health. Sometimes this might involve a specific and immediate problem, but these very often occur in the context of other health issues and may well not be amenable to simple solutions which do not take account of that context. Moreover, what seems to be the problem to the patient may not be so, and it is within the context of an ongoing relationship between a doctor and a patient that the subtle art of problem definition and elucidation can take place.

We do not argue that triage and associated remote access has no place in general practice, nor that it is not sometimes useful. However, applying our chosen lens of access to care as 'human fit' illuminates a number of potential problems, from practical concerns about how the triage process works, to a more philosophical concern about the nature of care in general practice. The concept of triage requires a vision of care based around the identification and articulation of discrete problems. In the next section we explore this in more detail via an examination of skill mix change in primary care.

Skill mix change in primary care

The notion of 'skill mix' in primary care – that is, that care could and should be provided by a wider range of professionals beyond just medically qualified general practitioners – has a long history. The 1967 Charter for General Practice (Anonymous, 1965; Gillam, 2017) introduced reimbursement for 70 per cent of the salary of up to two nursing or 'ancillary' staff per GP partner. In the early 1970s such roles were seen as support roles, providing delegated care under GP supervision, but by the later part of that decade enthusiasm was growing for multidisciplinary team management, with district nurses and health visitors working alongside nurses and GPs in general practice to provide care in the community (Bramwell et al, 2022). However, multidisciplinary team working, while remaining an ongoing policy aspiration (Goldzahl, Stokes and Sutton, 2022; NHS England, 2022), has proved difficult to operationalise and promised benefits remain elusive (Roland and Abel, 2012; Bramwell et al, 2014; Stokes et al, 2016).

Alongside this aspiration towards team-based working, policy and practice in the UK and elsewhere has evidenced a parallel trend towards skill mix change. Beyond questions of how different professionals might work effectively together in teams (Saint-Pierre, Herskovic and Sepúlveda, 2018), skill mix change rather focuses upon the skills of the different professionals within teams and the extent to which particular types of professionals can substitute for or complement one another (Sibbald, Shen and McBride, 2004). In the UK NHS, problems with recruitment and retention of doctors has driven a renewed focus on this approach (Roland et al, 2015), with a recent add-on to the standard GP contract seeking to explicitly mimic the perceived success of the practice nurse role by providing reimbursement for the employment of a wide range of practitioners (NHS England & BMA, 2019). The range of professionals who can be employed under this new contract has expanded, and now encompasses various different practitioners, including paramedics, pharmacists, mental health workers, advanced nurse and other clinical practitioners, physician associates and physiotherapists. The avowed intention is to provide support for GPs by substitution, with these new practitioners seeing patients who would, in the past, have been seen by GPs (NHS England, 2020).

Applying our access lens to this development, it is clear that there may be some issues which overlap with those identified with regards to remote-first access. Considering access as 'human fit' between patients and the services on offer brings to the fore the processes by which that 'fit' might be achieved. In the past, 'access' to services in primary care generally meant an appointment with either a nurse or a GP, with a relatively clear demarcation between the two roles. Patients knew what was available, and could request an appropriate appointment. Of course, this was not always straightforward, with longstanding problems with appointment availability as well as issues for those with specific needs related to physical access to buildings (Joseph and Bantock, 1982), personal perceptions of entitlement or need for care (Dixon-Woods et al, 2006b) or communication problems including language, hearing and vision. All of these issues are important in considering how appropriate 'human fit' might be achieved. Nevertheless, within these constraints, access historically meant requesting an appointment. A recent study of skill mix change in primary care highlights how much these processes have changed (McDermott et al, 2022). In a large-scale mixed-methods study, the team observed all areas of GP practices which had implemented skill mix change, including in reception areas, back office phone banks and in consultations. They found that obtaining access has become a complicated dance around the need for *categorisation* of patients' problems – what is the problem? – *matching* patients to appropriate practitioners and appointments – who can deal with this problem? – with an underlying need for *flexibility* – being able to move quickly to adjust to resolve any delays or difficulties arising if categorisation and matching went wrong (Spooner et al, 2022).

Thus, in the context of skill mix change in general practice, obtaining access becomes a much more complex task, both for patients and for practices. Moreover, as with remote access, it requires potential patients to both have a 'problem' that can be articulated in a way that can be categorised, and be able to articulate that problem in a way which will trigger the right response. Both of these are potentially problematic. As noted before, general practice has a long history of aspiring to provide holistic and patient-centred care which focuses upon individuals within their family and wider context, rather than as bearers of specific and divisible 'problems' (Toop, 1998). While this ideal is often not achieved, and successive policies over many years have rendered achieving it difficult (Checkland et al, 2008), nevertheless it is undeniable that the undifferentiated issues and complaints which present in primary care are often difficult to reduce to a clearly stated and defined 'problem' which can be straight-forwardly 'matched' to a given practitioners skills. Moreover, Spooner et al (2022) found that patients' articulations of their problems (even those with high health literacy) may be poorly formulated. Perhaps more worryingly, the problem-orientated approach inherent in skill mix change limits the possibility for serendipity, the uncovering of unarticulated or unnoticed problems and the development of therapeutic relationships over time (Balint, 1957). Similarly, undifferentiated and complex health problems that are effectively and comprehensively dealt with, utilising the high level of generalist expertise of GPs, can, when distributed to differently trained practitioners, lead to fragmentation and a reduction in the beneficial aspects of continuity of care (Sibbald, Shen and McBride, 2004).

Like remote triage, current policy around skill mix change in part represents a pragmatic approach to a situation in which it is acknowledged that there is a shortage of GPs. However it also reflects a more positive argument that the provision of care from a team with wider skills will benefit patients (NHS England & BMA, 2019). Two decades ago Sibbald, Shen and McBride (2004) explored these more positive motivations, and argued that broadening a general practice team to include physiotherapists or nurses with advanced skills in diabetes care could improve the quality of care (Renders et al, 2001). However, there was limited evidence that direct *substitution* was possible, or that overall costs would be reduced (Sibbald, Shen and McBride, 2004). Our argument is not that this is wrong, nor that it should not be happening. Indeed, it is not possible within the current context of the NHS to wind back the clock to a simpler time where individual and often single-handed doctors cared lifelong for a stable list of patients. However, our lens of access as 'human fit' highlights the risks and dangers inherent in these ongoing changes. Awareness of these risks and the design of flexible systems that do not irrevocably direct patients in one particular direction may be helpful, alongside appropriate training for all staff which emphasises the importance of generalist expertise and a holistic approach.

Extended access to primary care services

Both skill mix policy and remote-first access represent policy solutions which, while speaking to the issue of access, are not primarily designed around it. The policy most directly relevant to access over the past decade in England has been a requirement for GP practices to open outside of normal hours, in the evenings and at weekends. In return for an additional payment, practices are expected to offer bookable appointments after 6.30 pm and during the day at weekends. The rationale for this policy is that adults of working age struggle to obtain convenient appointments, and that extending surgeries into the evening would improve care and reduce attendance at emergency departments (Department of Health and Social Care, 2011). Initiated in 2011, this policy has continued over time and has recently been incorporated into an ongoing additional contract supporting practices to work together to deliver additional services (NHS England, 2021).

While superficially it might seem that such a policy is compatible with our conceptualisation of access as 'human fit' – those who work long hours need services which 'fit' their timetable – in operation the policy tends to assume that 'one size' will fit all. A diagnosis has been made – that access outside of normal hours is desirable and required – and a policy enacted to address the problem. However, implementing the policy is not necessarily straightforward. Small practices may struggle to open in the evening as their workforce is small; such opening requires administrative staff as well as clinical staff, and enhanced pay may be required. Heating bills will increase, as will electricity costs. In meeting these challenges, many practices have pooled resources to provide extended services. This might, for example, involve one practice providing extended hours services for the patients registered with neighbouring practices. This in turn brings additional complexities, including access to electronic records, information governance, variations in clinical staff scope of practice and logistical challenges with access to linked services such as laboratories (Elvey et al, 2018; Goff et al, 2021). Patients seen in an extended hours centre may need follow-up in their own practice, requiring communication protocols and new pathways to ensure that required care is offered. Duplication is also possible, with problems which cannot be dealt with in a remote location requiring an additional appointment. Evaluation has highlighted all of these issues, with one study finding that the provision of extended access was not associated with increased patient satisfaction, access or a better experience of care (Burch and Whittaker, 2022). The policy costs £250 million per year, and recent extension of the extended access requirement suggests that national policy makers continue to see it as important.

In common with remote-first access and skill mix change, arguing against extended opening hours can be difficult. Those who work during the day do need to be able to see a doctor, and better access can only be a good thing. However, further consideration of the policy raises some deeper concerns relating to the nature of generalist care. The provision of special or separate additional services is often justified on the basis that it is possible – and potentially desirable – to distinguish between acute or time-limited problems and more ongoing chronic care needs. Indeed, a recent report on the future of general practice services in England explicitly suggests establishing separate 'acute' care centres, which would deal with the current excessive demand for appointments, freeing up time to deal with patients with chronic longer term problems who may benefit from more personalised, continuous care (NHS England, 2022). It is suggested that

> Determining which patients benefit most from more personalised continuity of care can depend on a range of medical, psychological or social reasons and should be determined through conversations with patients and using clinical judgement, as well as supported by risk stratification using the wealth of data increasingly available to primary care teams. (NHS England, 2022: 12)

In this vision of primary care, embodied in the current blanket requirement for extended hours services, personalised or holistic generalised care is something which is offered only to those identified, with others offered more transactional problem-focused care. While superficially attractive, we would argue that this approach is an impoverished vision of generalist care. Those requiring same-day or urgent access are often the same people who have ongoing and longer-term health problems, and if access is about 'human fit' between the person and the service then their acute problem must be seen in the wider context of their ongoing health and social circumstances. While it is possible within extended access services to build systems which allow clinicians to view records and transmit information, this is a poor second to being seen in a setting where personal history and context are well known, and where care can be ongoing. While additional funding for improving access to services must be welcome, we would argue that a blanket requirement to open in the evenings and at weekends, regardless of local need and demand, is an inappropriate policy response and may not represent a good use of resources.

Conclusion

In this chapter we have explored three current topical issues in primary care through the lens of 'better access', arguing that conceptualising good access to care as enabling a 'human fit' between the needs of those seeking care and the services provided offers a lens through which to consider the next 75 years of primary care service provision in the NHS. General practice in the UK is sometimes disparagingly referred to as a 'cottage industry' (Mathers and Lester, 2011), unfit for purpose in the modern world. This discourse is not new; more than 10 years ago, UK politician David Miliband referred to the need for public services to develop a more consumer-focused approach, taking inspiration from Amazon or other online retailers (Miliband, 2004). The 'solutions' being offered to current challenges are in keeping with this narrative. Digital and remote access, skill mix changes and extended hours provision, often at a site removed from the patients' registered practice, all represent a conceptualisation of primary care provision which is consumer-focused and reductionist, with assumed unitary 'problems' dealt with in isolation via a one-off consultation. Care is assumed to be substitutable, with emphasis upon the rapid and efficient matching of problems to an available clinician who will deal with a single episode of care. Importantly, care delivered in this way is open to marketisation, with, for example, elements of care available to be contracted out, and emphasis upon choice of time, venue and clinician. Most recently, the opposition Labour Party's health spokesman has upset GPs by suggesting the replacement of the current predominant model of care provided by group partnerships of GPs by a salaried service, with GPs employed by large NHS employers.[6] The not-so-subtle subtext of the argument is that the 'small business' model of care which currently dominates allows GPs to in some way exploit the NHS, and this must be stopped if we are to have a modern service fit for the next 75 years.

At its heart, these debates are not technocratic arguments about the intricacies of the best way in to deliver a service, but rather a more fundamental lack of agreement about what primary care should be, alongside a failure to consider the wider issues facing the NHS as a whole. Bringing these issues into the open and considering them explicitly may offer some pointers towards a meaningful policy for the future.

First, as we have discussed, access as 'human fit' highlights the fact that those commissioning primary care for the future must consider whether its fundamental task is categorising and providing care for discrete problems, or providing holistic care for individuals across the life course. The concept of generalist care relies upon the notion that at its best, primary care is a human endeavour, always seeking to contextualise care within individuals' lives (Rudebeck, 2019). Within this paradigm, more medicine is not always better, and deciding not to seek a diagnosis on occasion can be as rational as the pursuit of technical quality (Heath, 1995, 2016; Heath et al, 2007). Remote-first access, skill mix change and extended hours access can all be inimical to this endeavour, and may embed a biomedical approach which ultimately increases costs and does not reduce suffering.

Second, designing a service to deliver a managerialist approach to care may have unintended consequences. The policy solutions that we have discussed are often justified in terms of their efficiency. A service which is buckling under the strain of excessive demand is ripe for such an approach, and in the context of inadequate supply of staff may be inevitable. However, our analysis would suggest that such an approach should at least be tempered by a considered look at other solutions, including staffing and investment. There is growing evidence that continuity of care by a clinician who knows the patient is both more efficient and effective (Baker et al, 2020). A service designed around continuity of care would look very different than one designed around episodic care, and continuity is a vital component of 'human fit'. The assumption that a subset of the population who 'need' continuity can be identified is as yet untested, and we would caution against an approach that assumes this to be the case. Throughout our lives our medical needs change, and everyone is likely to have the potential to benefit from continuity at some point in their medical journey. Primary care for the next 75 years must engage with this and consider what workforce will be needed to deliver it.

Finally, access as human fit highlights the need for local adaptation and community-focused services. If providers are to truly design their services to maximise the 'fit' with their population needs, they require a deep knowledge of that population and the ability to design services to meet their needs. This in turn suggests less top-down oversight and direction, and more opportunities for local adaptation, with contracts and incentives adjusted to allow and encourage this. As other chapters in this volume have illuminated, there has been a restless policy swing since the inception of the NHS between centralisation and decentralisation of services, autonomy and power. We would argue that for primary care at least this needs to be resolved in favour of local control of services, with a strong focus upon supporting providers to maximise the human fit between what they offer and what their population needs, built upon a strong foundation of generalism and holistic care.

Notes

[1] https://digital.nhs.uk/data-and-information/publications/statistical/nhs-payments-to-general-practice/england-2018-19

[2] https://www.bma.org.uk/advice-and-support/nhs-delivery-and-workforce/pressures/nhs-backlog-data-analysis#:~:text=The%20latest%20figures%20for%20October,slight%20increase%20from%20last%20month

[3] https://www.pressreader.com/uk/daily-mail/20210920/281479279552293

[4] https://www.theguardian.com/society/2021/nov/02/no-10-set-to-break-promise-of-6000-more-gps-in-england-sajid-javid-says

[5] https://www.ipsos.com/en-uk/2022-gp-patient-survey-results-released

[6] https://www.theguardian.com/politics/2023/jan/20/labour-wes-streeting-reform-is-not-a-conservative-word-nhs-health

References

Aday, L.A. and Andersen, R. (1974) 'A framework for the study of access to medical care'. *Health Services Research*, 9, 208–220.

Anonymous. (1965) 'Charter for general practice'. *British Medical Journal*, 1, 669.

Baker, R., Freeman, G.K., Haggerty, J.L., Bankart, M.J. and Nockels, K.H. (2020) 'Primary medical care continuity and patient mortality: A systematic review'. *British Journal of General Practice*, 70, e600–e611.

Balint, M. (1957) *The Doctor, His Patient and the Illness*. London: Pitman Medical Publishing Co.

Bramwell, D., Checkland, K., Allen, P. and Peckham, S. (2014) *Moving Services Out of Hospital: Joining up General Practice and Community Services?* University of Manchester: Policy Research Unit in Commissioning and the Healthcare System (PRUComm).

Bramwell, D., Checkland, K., Shields, J. and Allen, P. (2022) *Understanding Community Nursing Services: An Historical Policy Analysis*. London: Policy Research Unit in Health and Care Systems and Commissioning.

Burch, P. and Whittaker, W. (2022) 'Exploring the impact of the national extended access scheme on patient experience of and satisfaction with general practice: An observational study using the English GP Patient Survey'. *BJGP Open*, 6, 2 (June).

Campbell, J.L., Fletcher, E., Britten, N., Green, C., Holt, T.A., Lattimer, V. et al (2014) 'Telephone triage for management of same-day consultation requests in general practice (the ESTEEM trial): A cluster-randomised controlled trial and cost-consequence analysis'. *Lancet*, 384, 1859–1868.

Campbell, S.M., Kontopantelis, E., Reeves, D., Valderas, J.M., Gaehl, E., Small, N. et al (2010) 'Changes in patient experiences of primary care during health service reforms in England BETWEEN 2003 and 2007'. *The Annals of Family Medicine*, 8, 499.

Chapman, R. and Groom, H. (1999) 'Should we fight to preserve the independent status of general practitioners? For and against'. *BMJ*, 318, 797.

Checkland, K., Harrison, S., McDonald, R., Grant, S., Campbell, S. and Guthrie, B. (2008) 'Biomedicine, holism and general medical practice: Responses to the 2004 General Practitioner contract'. *Sociology of Health & Illness*, 30, 788–803.

Coleman, A., Checkland, K., McDermott, I. and Harrison, S. (2013) 'The limits of market-based reforms in the NHS: The case of alternative providers in primary care'. *BMC Health Services Research*, 13 (Suppl 1).

Cook, J. (2018) 'Technology like Babylon's GP at Hand should be available to all, says health secretary'. GP online. https://www.gponline.com/technol ogy-babylons-gp-hand-available-all-says-health-secretary/article/1488456.

Department of Health and Social Care. (2011) *Guidance: GP Extended Hours Access Scheme Directed Enhanced Service – 1 April 2011 to 31 March 2012*. London: DHSC.

Department of Health and Social Care. (2021) *Health and Care Act*. London: The Stationary Office.

Dixon-Woods, M., Cavers, D., Agarwal, S., Annandale, E., Arthur, A., Harvey, J. et al (2006a) 'Conducting a critical interpretive synthesis of the literature on access to healthcare by vulnerable groups'. *BMC Medical Research Methodology*, 6, 1–13.

Dixon-Woods, M., Cavers, D., Agarwal, S., Annandale, E., Arthur, A., Harvey, J. et al (2006b) 'Conducting a critical interpretive synthesis of the literature on access to healthcare by vulnerable groups'. *BMC Medical Research Methodology*, 6, 35.

Donabedian, A. (1973) *Aspects of Medical Care Administration: Specifying Requirements for Health Care*. Cambridge, MA; Harvard University Press.

Elvey, R., Bailey, S., Checkland, K., McBride, A., Parkin, S., Rothwell, K. et al (2018) 'Implementing new care models: Learning from the Greater Manchester demonstrator pilot experience'. *BMC Family Practice*, 19, 89.

Gillam, S. (2017) 'The Family Doctor Charter: 50 years on'. *British Journal of General Practice*, 67, 227.

Goff, M., Bailey, S., Hodgson, D., Bresnen, M., Elvey, R. and Checkland, K. (2021) 'Ambiguous workarounds in NHS policy piloting: Tensions, trade-offs and legacies of organisational change projects'. *New Technology, Work and Employment*, 36, 17.

Goldzahl, L., Stokes, J. and Sutton, M. (2022) 'The effects of multi-disciplinary integrated care on healthcare utilization: Evidence from a natural experiment in the UK'. *Health Economics*, 31, 2142–2169.

Greer, S.L. (2016) 'Devolution and health in the UK: Policy and its lessons since 1998'. *British Medical Bulletin*, 118, 16–24.

Griffiths, P., Murrells, T., Maben, J., Jones, S. and Ashworth, M. (2010) 'Nurse staffing and quality of care in UK general practice: Cross-sectional study using routinely collected data'. *British Journal of General Practice*, 60, e36.

Hasegawa, H., Reilly, D., Mercer, S.W. and Bikker, A.P. (2005) 'Holism in primary care: The views of Scotland's general practitioners'. *Primary Health Care Research and Development*, 6, 320–329.

Haynes, L. (2022) 'Third of GP appointments consumed by patients asking about delayed hospital care'. GP online. https://www.gponline.com/third-gp-appointments-consumed-patients-asking-delayed-hospital-care/article/1754834.

Heath, I. (1995) *The Mystery of General Practice*. London: The Nuffield Provincial Hospitals Trust.

Heath, I. (2016) 'How medicine has exploited rationality at the expense of humanity: an essay by Iona Heath'. *BMJ*, 355, i5705.

Heath, I., Hippisley-Cox, J. and Smeeth, L. (2007) 'Measuring performance and missing the point?'. *BMJ*, 335, 1075–1076.

Jones, R., Majeed, A., Bhatti, N., Murchie, P., Vautrey, R. and Rosen, R. (2015) 'Should general practice give up the independent contractor status?'. *British Journal of General Practice*, 65, 314.

Joseph, A.E. and Bantock, P.R. (1982) 'Measuring potential physical accessibility to general practitioners in rural areas: A method and case study'. *Social Science & Medicine*, 16, 85–90.

Levesque, J.F., Harris, M.F. and Russell, G. (2013) 'Patient-centred access to health care: Conceptualising access at the interface of health systems and populations'. *International Journal for Equity in Health*, 12, 18.

Lewis, J. (1998) 'The medical profession and the state: GPs and the GP contract in the 1960s and the 1990s'. *Social Policy & Administration*, 32, 132–150.

MacKichan, F., Brangan, E., Wye, L., Checkland, K., Lasserson, D., Huntley, A. et al (2017) 'Why do patients seek primary medical care in emergency departments? An ethnographic exploration of access to general practice'. *BMJ Open*, 7.

Mathers, N. and Lester, H. (2011) 'From cottage industry to post-industrial care? The King's Fund report on quality in general practice'. *British Journal of General Practice*, 61, 602.

McDermott, I., Spooner, S., Goff, M., Gibson, J., Dalgarno, E., Francetic, I. et al (2022) *Scale, Scope and Impact of Skill Mix Change in Primary Care in England: A Mixed-Methods Study*. Southampton: National Institute for Health and Care Research.

Miliband, D. (2004) 'Choice and Voice in Personalised Learning'. Speech by David Miliband DfES Innovation unit / DEMOS. OECD conference on Personalising Education. Paris: OECD Publishing.

Mold, F., Hendy, J., Lai, Y.L. and de Lusignan, S. (2019) 'Electronic consultation in primary care between providers and patients: Systematic review'. *JMIR Medical Informatics*, 7, e13042.

Mroz, G., Papoutsi, C. and Greenhalgh, T. (2022) 'UK newspapers "on the warpath": Media analysis of general practice remote consulting in 2021'. *British Journal of General Practice*, 72 (725), e907–e915.

Murphy, M., Scott, L.J., Salisbury, C., Turner, A., Scott, A., Denholm, R. et al (2021) 'The implementation of remote consulting in UK primary care following the COVID-19 pandemic: A mixed-methods longitudinal study'. *British Journal of General Practice*, 71 (704), e166–e177.

Newman, J. and Vidler, E. (2006) 'Discriminating customers, responsible patients, empowered users: Consumerism and the modernisation of health care'. *Journal of Social Policy*, 35, 193–209.

NHS England. (2019) *Investment and Evolution: A Five-year Framework for GP Contract Reform to Implement the NHS Long Term Plan*. Leeds: NHS England.

NHS England. (2020) *Network Contract Directed Enhanced Service: Contract specification 2020/21 – PCN Requirements and Entitlements*. Leeds: NHS England.

NHS England. (2021) *Network Contract Directed Enhanced Service: Contract Specification 2022/23 – PCN Requirements and Entitlements*. Leeds: NHS England.

NHS England. (2022) *Next Steps for Integrating Primary Care: Fuller Stocktake Report*. Leeds: NHS England.

NHS England and BMA. (2019) *Investment and Evolution: A Five-year Framework for GP Contract Reform to Implement The NHS Long Term Plan*. Leeds: NHS England.

Norman, A.H., Russell, A.J. and Merli, C. (2016) 'The quality and outcomes framework: Body commodification in UK general practice'. *Social Science & Medicine*, 170, 77–86.

Oliver, D. (2021) 'David Oliver: Daily Mail's campaign on general practice won't help GPs or their patients'. *BMJ*, 375, n2532.

Peckham, S. and Exworthy, M. (2003) *Primary Care in the UK*. Basingstoke: Palgrave MacMillan.

Penchansky, R. and Thomas, J.W. (1981) 'The concept of access: Definition and relationship to consumer satisfaction'. *Medical Care*, 19, 2, 127–140.

Potter, C. (2022) 'Face-to-face GP appointments reach highest level since February 2020'. Pulse. https://www.pulsetoday.co.uk/news/break ing-news/fewer-than-a-third-of-gp-appointments-remote-last-month/#:~:text=New%20data%20published%20today%20by,appointments%20w ere%20delivered%20in%20person

Powell, M. and Exworthy, M. (2003) 'Equal access to health care and the British National Health Service'. *Policy Studies*, 24, 51–64.

Renders, C.M., Valk, G.D., Griffin, S. J., Wagner, E.H., Eijk van, J.T. and Assendelft, W.J.J. (2001) 'Interventions to improve the management of diabetes in primary care, outpatient, and community settings: A systematic review'. *Diabetes Care*, 24, 1821–1833.

Roberts, C. (2004) '"Only connect": The centrality of doctor–patient relationships in primary care'. *Family Practice*, 21, 232–233.

Roland, M. and Abel, G. (2012) 'Reducing emergency admissions: Are we on the right track?'. *BMJ: British Medical Journal*, 345.

Roland, M., Barber, N., Howe, A., Imison, C., Rubin, G. and Storey, K. (2015) *The Future of Primary Health Care: Creating Teams for Tomorrow: Report by the Primary Care Workforce Commission*. Leeds: Health Education England.

Royal College of General Practitioners. (2022) *Fit for the Future: Relationship-based Care*. London: RCGP.

Rudebeck, C.E. (2019) 'Relationship based care – how general practice developed and why it is undermined within contemporary healthcare systems'. *Scandinavian Journal of Primary Health Care*, 37, 335–344.

Saint-Pierre, C., Herskovic, V. and Sepúlveda, M. (2018) 'Multidisciplinary collaboration in primary care: A systematic review'. *Family Practice*, 35, 132–141.

Salisbury, C., Goodall, S., Montgomery, A.A., Pickin, D.M., Edwards, S., Sampson, F. et al (2007) 'Does Advanced Access improve access to primary health care? Questionnaire survey of patients'. *British Journal of General Practice*, 57, 615–621.

Shum, C., Humphreys, A., Wheeler, D., Cochrane, M.A., Skoda, S. and Clement, S. (2000) 'Nurse management of patients with minor illnesses in general practice: Multicentre, randomised controlled trial'. *BMJ (Clinical research ed.)*, 320, 1038–1043.

Sibbald, B., Shen, J. and McBride, A. (2004) 'Changing the skill-mix of the health care workforce'. *Journal of Health Services Research & Policy*, 9, 28–38.

Simpson, J.M., Checkland, K., Snow, S., Voorhees, J., Rothwell, K. and Esmail, A. (2015) 'Access to general practice in England: Time for a policy rethink'. *British Journal of General Practice*, 65, 606–607.

Smith, J.W. and Donovan, J.B. (1970) 'The practice nurse – A new look'. *British Medical Journal*, 4, 673.

Spooner, S., McDermott, I., Goff, M., Hodgson, D., McBride, A. and Checkland, K. (2022) 'Processes supporting effective skill-mix implementation in general practice: A qualitative study'. *Journal of Health Services Research & Policy*, 27, 4, 269–277.

Stewart, E., Donaghy, E., Guthrie, B., Henderson, D., Huang, H., Pickersgill, M. et al (2022) 'Transforming primary care in Scotland: A critical policy analysis'. *British Journal of General Practice,* 72, 292.

Stokes, J., Kristensen, S.R., Checkland, K. and Bower, P. (2016) 'Effectiveness of multidisciplinary team case management: Difference-in-differences analysis'. *BMJ Open*, 6.

Toop, L. (1998) 'Patient-centred primary care', in Pringle M. (ed) *Primary Care Core Values*. London: BMJ Books, p 8.

Tudor Hart, J. (1971) 'The inverse care law'. *The Lancet*, 297, 405–412.

Voorhees, J., Bailey, S., Waterman, H. and Checkland, K. (2022) 'Accessing primary care and the importance of "human fit": A qualitative participatory case study'. *British Journal of General Practice*, 72, e342. https://bjgp.org/content/72/718/e342.

Walker, P. (2020) 'All GP consultations should be remote by default, says Matt Hancock'. *The Guardian*, 30 July.

6

NHS hospitals and the bedpan doctrine: the first 75 years

Rod Sheaff and Pauline Allen

Introduction

Since its inception NHS hospital management has been subject to the 'bedpan doctrine'. Although no-one seems certain exactly when, Aneurin Bevan, the founder of the NHS, is often credited with saying that 'If a bedpan is dropped on a hospital floor in Tredegar, I want the noise to reverberate in the corridors of the Palace of Westminster'. Essentially, the government is ultimately responsible for how NHS hospitals are managed or mismanaged. However, there are practical limits upon how far central government can actually anticipate or prevent politically awkward developments and events in NHS hospitals. The tension has existed for 75 years since but as we shall see some health policies exacerbate it. This chapter uses the bedpan doctrine as a framework for examining how the governmental balance between central control and local managerial discretion (see Chapter 1) has played out in NHS hospitals, especially since the 2008 financial crash, a watershed in UK economic development (Cribb and Johnson, 2018), including that of NHS hospitals.

What doctrine implies

Central control

A doctrine which attributes to government the ultimate responsibility for the state of NHS services appears to legitimate extensive government involvement in controlling NHS hospitals, an implication which ambitious or reforming policy-makers might welcome. However, the doctrine also implies that governments are also responsible for how NHS hospitals respond to adverse circumstances or events. In the last 75 years that has happened on a grand scale in three ways. One was, and is, the demographic shift. The proportion of UK population aged over 65 has slowly risen, from 16.0 per cent in 2001–02 to 18.6 per cent in 2019–20 (Office for National Statistics, 2022) with the well-known consequences of increasing demand on NHS hospitals, in particular 'winter pressures'. Rising socio-economic inequality has similar consequences (Kivimäki et al, 2020). Another was the 2008–10 financial crash which was followed by a fiscal policy reversal from expansion to austerity. COVID was the third. Additionally, more transient problems have also recurred, including safety scandals, waiting times and strikes. Even when a government is guiltless in creating such problems, the bedpan doctrine still holds it responsible for making NHS hospitals implement a remedy, and culpable should they appear to fail. The bedpan doctrine may also motivate governments to conceal or massage information that might make them seem culpable.

Responsibilisation

Responsibilisation can be defined as shifting the responsibility for certain policy decisions, implementing a policy or failing to from government onto the policy subjects themselves. In its positive form, it assumes that responsibilisation will enable and stimulate the latter to take corrective action; or, if the policy subjects do not sufficiently respond, representing, or indeed treating, them as the authors of their own misfortune (Pyysiäinen, Halpin and Guilfoyle, 2017). Although the bedpan doctrine may hold governments responsible for the management or mismanagement of NHS hospitals, in practice governments depend heavily on the hospitals and their managers to implement any remedy. Should that fail, governments then have a motive to shift the responsibility, in the sense of blame, for the dropped bedpan (unpopular decisions, service failures) onto the hospitals or their managers: a negative form of responsibilisation in which a government tries to escape the adverse electoral or political consequences which bedpan doctrine may then hold for it. Although 'bedpan *doctrine*' has become the standard term for these assumptions the more modest term 'framing' might be more accurate.

Either way, the bedpan doctrine then motivates governments to be seen to respond to salient NHS hospital problems in ways that at least minimise adverse media attention and electoral consequences. That involves framing or re-framing the problem in a way that justifies the government's preferred intervention. When the government acts not just responsively but on its own initiative, an existing practical 'problem' may be selected, or a new one discovered or even invented, to justify policies pursued for other reasons (for example, marketisation). The electoral imperative gives a reason for governments to act upon the bedpan doctrine in ways that can be implemented within the current election cycle: five years at most, usually fewer. As Greer remarks (Chapter 2) the bedpan doctrine 'creates a market for quick governance and policy fixes among politicians, making it hard to find health policy ideas, whether copied from other health systems or the product of indigenous creativity, that have not at some point been adopted in England'. It also tempts governments, when dealing with the media, to inflate their achievements, down-play (for instance discreetly re-name) any policy reversals, and control what NHS hospitals themselves say to the media.

Policies and events that have triggered the bedpan doctrine

Continuing the metaphor, what has counted as a dropped bedpan in regard to NHS hospital services? This issues which have become politically salient have resulted from what electors, the media, and policy communities think the government is responsible for, and from governments' own policy preferences. Certain issues have been perennial through all 75 years of the NHS. Arguably the most persistent and conspicuous have been waiting times for hospital admission, and concomitantly the effect of private hospitals on them, including the proper role, if any, of pay beds and private practice within NHS hospitals, and the alleged conflicts of interests between consultants' private practice and the reduction of NHS waiting lists (Yates, 1995). As explained below NHS hospital waiting times began to increase after 2013, but dramatically so during and after the COVID-19 pandemics. Another perennial issue, especially at election time, has been the sufficiency of public spending on the NHS, and therefore the necessity for 'rationing'. Medical and nursing care scandals have intermittently moved into and out of the political limelight, triggering applications of the bedpan doctrine. Before the 1990s these scandals seemed particularly to affect long-stay mental and geriatrics hospitals (Martin and Evans, 1984) but then increasingly the acute hospitals too, where the main incidents concerned child surgery (the inquiry into the management of care of children receiving complex heart surgery at the Bristol Royal Infirmary 1984–1995, 2001), nursing care (Healthcare Commission, 2009), gynaecology (Ritchie, 2000) and maternity services (Ockenden, 2022). After strikes and other disputes during the 1970s and early 1980s, some years of relatively calm industrial relations followed but NHS hospital wage levels and industrial relations regained political prominence in 2022–2023.

Since 1989 the most consistent policy package, and one which has provided considerable application for the bedpan doctrine, is what might be called neo-liberal or Washington consensus reforms: the corporatisation of NHS-owned services (explained later), the marketisation of NHS structures, and privatisation. Here, 'corporatisation' means making the organisational structures and managerial practices of (in this case) NHS hospitals mimic what policy-makers think corporate commercial practice is (Nelson and Nikolakis, 2012). Until the 2008 financial crash the shift towards corporatisation continued across a range of NHS hospital activities. Governments increasingly responsibilised NHS hospital managers by increasing both their managerial autonomy and formal accountability; shifted the payment for hospitals services from large combined payments towards more commodified, per-patient payments (by 'Health Resource Groups', modelled on the US Diagnosis Related Group payment system); introduced private financing of hospital infrastructure development (the Private Finance Initiative (PFI)), and encouraged NHS hospitals to seek income from private sources. After 2010, however, some but not all of these corporatising trends halted. The proportion of commodified (HRG) payments stabilised. The Private Finance Initiative stopped.

These were bi-partisan policies. Where the main parties in government differed, at least until 2010, was in fiscal policy towards NHS hospitals. Between 1990 and 1997 the Thatcher and Major governments combined fiscal stringency with neo-liberal reform. Their fiscal strategy was of trying to minimise the growth of spending by means of quasi-market reforms and strengthening hospitals' internal managerial capacity (Flynn, 1992), although in real terms the spending grew nevertheless. Until the financial crash, New Labour governments combined further neo-liberal reforms with fiscal generosity. Public spending on the NHS began to converge upon the European average. The neo-liberal reforms were presented as 'Modernising' the NHS and (so to speak) the price that NHS hospitals had to pay for fiscal growth (Department of Health, 1997). After the 2008–2010 financial crash came another period of austerity with further neo-liberal reforms, a combination to which New Labour switched and the post-2012 Coalition and then Conservative governments intensified.

Consequences for NHS hospitals

A caveat must accompany general statements about the consequences for NHS hospitals of the outlined policy climate. Official data-sets often combine non-hospital community health and mental health services with hospital figures without distinction. Then we have to assume that the general patterns for all trusts also apply to hospitals, but that is not entirely unwarranted. Of the 224 NHS trusts in 2020, 148 were hospitals (93 general acute, 17 specialist, 38 teaching) (NHS Digital, 2020). These trusts took 80 per cent (75 per cent to acute and 5 per cent to specialist hospitals) of the total revenue paid to NHS trusts (Kraindler, Gershlick and Charlesworth, 2019), and employed the majority of general managers (The King's Fund, 2011). In these respects hospitals dominate the population of NHS trusts. To avoid further complicating an already complex picture, only the consequences of the bedpan doctrine for English NHS hospitals is described next. The story differs, in parts, for Northern Ireland, Scotland and Wales.

Central control

Since 2008, indeed 1990, a constant churn of structural 'reform' of the NHS has continued, adding regulatory and performance management systems (Klein, 2019) for the central control of NHS hospitals, a predictable consequence of the bedpan doctrine. An American expert examining UK systems for maintaining patient safety concluded that 'The current NHS regulatory system is bewildering in its complexity and prone to both overlaps of remit and gaps between different agencies' (Berwick, 2013). Monitor and the NHS Trust Development Authority were the agencies supervising hospital (and indeed all) trusts until 2016, when NHS Improvement took on the task, and was then absorbed into NHS England in 2021. From 2010 the Department of Health 'segmented' trusts according to their performance regarding quality of care, finance, operational activity, strategic change, leadership and improvement capability (NHS Improvement, 2018) and 'If the agreed trajectory is missed, then the [NHS England] regional team will intervene' (NHS England and NHS Improvement 2019: 12). By 2018 only 16 per cent of trusts had completely avoided such interventions.

Yet it is not practicable for one national body, whether the Department of Health or an NHS body, to commission and monitor 148 hospital trusts individually, some containing multiple hospitals. For the last 75 years NHS hospitals' relationship to government, and therefore implementation of the bedpan doctrine, has been mediated through regional organisations. In 2022, the Sustainability and Transformation Partnerships were reformed as Integrated Care Systems (ICS). Certain structures complicate central control of NHS hospitals. At national and regional levels of the NHS the main networks representing NHS hospital interests are respectively NHS providers (and the Shelford Group for the ten largest university hospitals) and, within the ICSs, provider collaboratives in which hospitals have a large if not dominant role. At local commissioner level, the contractual relationships between NHS hospitals and their commissioners involve in practice a bilateral dependence of commissioners and NHS hospitals upon each other. Nevertheless the overall result has been a quasi-hierarchy (Exworthy, Powell and Mohan, 1999): a centred (and centralised) network of formally independent organisations, each controlling, monitoring, paying and sanctioning the level below (Sheaff and Schofield, 2016), and ultimately NHS hospitals.

The corresponding, very hierarchical, style of government over NHS hospitals has been called 'targets and terror' (Bevan and Hood, 2006). The targets were expressed in a succession of performance management indicators, balanced scorecards, dashboards and 'metrics', and summarised in annual guidance for the formulation of contracts and operational management (see for example NHS England, 2023a). In addition, the CQC rated hospitals as 'outstanding', 'good', 'Improvement needed' or 'Inadequate'. NHS Improvement (2019b) grouped hospitals into four 'segments', segment 1 having 'no potential support needs identified and therefore receiving the lowest level of central oversight' while segment 4 are 'Providers in special

Table 6.1: NHS trust segmentation, February 2023

Segmentation level	Number of trusts
1: 'No specific support needs'	34
2: 'Flexible support'	94
3: 'Bespoke mandated support'	66
4: 'Mandated intensive support'	18

Source: NHS England (2023)

measures: there is actual or suspected breach of licence with very serious and/or complex issues.'

Table 6.1 shows the distribution of (all) trusts in February 2023 and, in general terms, the corresponding NHSE response.

In especially adverse circumstances, hospital chief executives may receive a ministerial phone call. Most imperative were the so-called 'P45 targets' (named after the P45 tax certificate one receives upon leaving one's job) of which the most important in practice before the COVID-19 pandemic was the requirement for NHS providers to make 2 per cent overall cost savings annually besides more specific savings stated in the Quality Innovation and Productivity Programme (QIPP).

Both the control and responsibilisation implications of the bedpan doctrine require that NHS hospital activity be transparent to external, or at least government, scrutiny. Repeated national-level attempts to buy turnkey NHS hospital IT systems systems (for example, for electronic patient records) through consultancies and outsourcing to corporate suppliers have included some expensive failures, the ones where the bedpan doctrine came most obviously into play being the National Programme for IT, abandoned in 2011 (House of Commons Committee of Public Accounts, 2013; House of Commons Public Accounts Committee, 2020), and the COVID-19 Test-and-Trace system (Jones and Hameiri, 2022). This centralised approach contrasted to the one initially adopted for general practice (see Chapter 5), where certain data standards had to be met but otherwise IT implementation was left to the general practices. (Later however the hospital IT approach was extended to general practices, with similar consequences (National Audit Office, 2018).) Nevertheless, the development of IT since 2000 has greatly facilitated and extended the central collection and analysis of hospital data, indeed to the point where that aspect of NHS IT is arguably more developed than IT within many hospitals. The national-level information resources of NHS Data (formerly HSCIC) now include the Hospital Episode Statistics, National Workforce Data Set, Hospital Estates Statistics, the NHS Outcomes Framework, Patient Reported Outcomes Measures and others. NHSE's Reference Costs database compares hospitals' waiting times and service costs. Referral-to-treatment (that is, hospital waiting times for non-urgent care) data have been reported monthly since 2007. With hospitals' published accounts, these are the main sources informing NHSE/I scrutiny and parliamentary oversight over NHS hospitals, and to that extent the operation of the bedpan doctrine.

Responsibilised management

The responsibilisation of NHS hospital management gathered pace when between 1991 and 1995 all line-managed NHS hospitals (and all other NHS service providers) were converted to NHS trusts (NHST) with greater freedoms to make decisions about managing their services. From 2004 many hospitals became Foundation Trusts (FTs) which had greater managerial autonomy again from the Department of Health – which they 'earned' by achieving above-average performance on a range of the centrally-stipulated performance indicators (Wright et al, 2012). However similar governance, accountability and audit rules, and the same policy priorities, applied to both kinds of trust so that the distinction between them became increasingly nominal. From 2018 it started to disappear from NHSE management practice and many of the current official data-sets.

A landmark event in responsibilising the internal management of NHS hospitals was the Griffiths report (Department of Health and Social Security, 1983), following which hierarchical 'general' management replaced multi-professional consensus as NHS hospitals' internal managerial regime. Since then a gradual corporatisation of NHS hospital management has continued, drawing heavily on New Public Management ideas and practices which, among other things, emphasise the managerial control and oversight of services, and the professionalisation of management (Diefenbach, 2009), with an ongoing 'identity work' which has included re-framing the NHS hospital managers' role in such terms as 'public sector entrepreneurialism' (Exworthy and Lafond, 2021; Hodgson et al, 2021). As an instance of 'responsibilization through threat to personal control' (Pyysiäinen, Halpin and Guilfoyle, 2017: 217) performance related pay (PRP) for hospital managers was introduced in 1989 and extended down to lower middle managers (Dowling and Richardson, 1997). Each manager's pay was linked to achieving targets set by her own line manager or, for top managers, a remuneration committee. The system worked by making local adjustments to national pay-scales which reflected the type of service (acute hospital, mental health and so on), job-grade, time in post and (later) the provider's financial turnover. By 2013 the system had been revised so that up to 25 per cent of very senior managers could receive up to 5 per cent of their base salary as a PRP supplement but remuneration panels could also reduce their pay through 'a requirement to meet agreed performance objectives to earn back an element of base pay (normally at least 10%) placed at risk' (Department of Health, 2013: 16). Chief executives whose trust failed to meet financial targets received no annual pay uplift for inflation: the only publicly-documented performance criterion for which specific personal financial penalties were mandated. In 1998–2003, when the reward systems for NHS hospital managers were already much the same as nowadays, Ballantine, Forker and Greenwood (2008) found that the annual rate of CEO turnover was just over 20 per cent (compared with a turnover for all managers estimated at 10 per cent in 2012 (Veronesi, Kirkpatrick and Altanlar, 2019)). The reasons were undisclosed in 89 out of 161 cases, but where they were reported resignations and golden handshakes together accounted for 12.5 per cent of CEO departures, although the greatest turnover (65 per cent) arose from the replacement of acting CEOs, secondments or moves within the NHS. At whole-hospital level, egregious failures could lead to the trust being dissolved and the hospital merging into another trust (which is what happened to Mid Staffordshire NHS Foundation Trust), in which case the hospital services themselves usually continued but under new management.

Concurrently there appears, at least in Foundation Trusts, to have been a shift of managerial roles towards strategic roles, although no overall expansion of managerial roles (Kirkpatrick, Altanlar and Veronesi, 2017). There is some evidence that the managers had a positive impact on hospital performance in terms of infection rates and patient experience (but not necessarily microeconomic efficiency) (Veronesi, Kirkpatrick and Altanlar, 2019). It would certainly be consistent with the bedpan doctrine to argue that media scrutiny and criticism mediate the development of more corporatised management practices in NHS hospitals. Exworthy, Frosini and Jones (2011) and Kirkpatrick, Altanlar and Veronesi (2017) have suggested that sensitivity to potentially adverse media exposure and regulatory scrutiny is one reason why FT chief executives might have been reluctant to increase the number of FT managers, or to exercise their autonomy too radically (Kirkpatrick, Altanlar and Veronesi, 2017).

The continued and growing responsibilisation of senior doctors in NHS hospitals continues trends that began in the 1980s (Flynn, 1992): those of giving senior doctors control over and responsibility for clinical budgets; introducing clinical information systems (with the varied success noted before); and, at department or speciality level, establishing clinical directorates (a controlling triumvirate of, usually, a doctor, a nurse and a generalist manager). By 2012, 31 per cent of all managers were 'hybrids': clinicians who also held a managerial role (Kirkpatrick, Altanlar and Veronesi, 2022), concentrated at middle management and operational (for example, ward or department managers) levels. There was, and is, the strongest clinical justification for promulgating evidence-based medicine but a side-effect was gradually to expose the mysteries of clinical practice to critical scrutiny by general managers, government and public. Thus the Ockenden enquiry into maternity care at Shrewsbury and Telford Hospital Trust was able to see that 'none of the mothers [who had been injured] had received care in line with best practice at the time and in three-quarters of cases the care could have been significantly improved' (Ockenden, 2022: ix). (The enquiry also found that the rate of caesarian sections was a counter-productive service metric.) Despite that, rising workloads and staff overload made some hospital services more fragile and accident-prone, the Mid-Staffordshire case being a prominent example (Healthcare Commission, 2009). Another centrally initiated attempt to manage patient safety in NHS hospitals was the introduction of Patient Safety Collaboratives, networks designed to share of information and good practice between hospitals (and indeed other providers). But at department or speciality level, sustaining the collaboratives sometimes fell victim to staff and departmental overload (Sheaff et al, 2018). Notwithstanding rearguard defences of professional power and discretion (Currie et al, 2012), the long-term picture was of a gradual exposure of the medical establishment, besides general managers, to the bedpan doctrine.

One thing which did not occur was the privatisation of NHS hospitals (see Chapter 1). Instead, service privatisation occurred through increasing the proportion of NHS spending on private providers, from 3.66 per cent in 2001–2002 (House of Commons Health Committee, 2010) to 10.9 per cent in 2019–2020 (Department of Health and Social Care, 2020). From 1985 the main support services in NHS hospitals (laundry, catering, cleaning and in some hospitals some laboratory work) were outsourced, and in response to the workload crises described later, many hospitals relied increasingly on agency staff, until in 2015 the Department of Health explicitly discouraged this expensive practice. Another managerial way of imitating corporate practice ('business envy') was to engage management consultancies, whose overall contribution to hospital efficiency and cost control was nevertheless negative (Kirkpatrick et al, 2019).

After the 2008 financial crash, fiscal 2008 austerity became, in practice, the dominant policy imperative for NHS hospitals. This imperative and the responsibilisation of NHS hospital managers for dealing with *force majeure* events tended to produce the following patterns of hospital response.

Workload

Ever-increasing demand pressures have in recent years become one of the clearest instances of the bedpan doctrine requiring NHS hospitals to respond to *force majeure* events, whether or not of their own or the government's making.

For inpatient services, NHS hospitals admitted 28 per cent more patients (16.252 million) in 2015–2016 than a decade earlier (Liverpool Heart and

Chest Hospital NHS Foundation Trust, 2018). Due perhaps to the bedpan doctrine, their political salience and continued (although declining: see next) public support (Frankenburg et al, 2021), NHS hospitals were more sheltered from austerity policies than other parts of public sector, especially local government. Social care faced severe overload and fiscal pressures, rising admission thresholds to care, provider bankruptcy and staff turnover, to which from early 2020 the effects of the COVID-19 pandemic were added. The well-known consequences for NHS hospitals have been, above all, a chain reaction of service blockages. Reduced social care makes patient discharges home from hospital slower, so beds and ward remain occupied longer, slowing down the reception of new patients from A&E. That slows down patient acceptance into A&E, including the acceptance of patients in ambulances, leading to slower ambulance response times. For non-urgent care mean referral-to-treatment waiting time in October 2022 was 12.5 weeks compared with a norm of 18 weeks wait or less, but even so 27,460 patients (9.7 per cent of the total) had waited 52 weeks or longer (NHS England, 2022a). During December 2021–March 2022 at least 16,700 and occasionally over 17,500 beds were occupied by patients who had been there more than three weeks (NHS England, 2022b). Some of these long stays will have been clinically necessary but it appears likely that most were not. Individual hospitals have responded *ad hoc* by declaring 'black alert' days. Although over 500, and exceptionally more than 1000, A&E admissions per day from ambulances have been delayed by more than an hour, only a handful of hospitals at once have ever diverted A&E admissions (and ambulances) to other hospitals (NHS England, 2022b). Many hospitals created discharge support teams to expedite patient transfers out of hospital, often involving social workers (employed by local government not the NHS in England). NHS England advised NHS hospitals on how to use hotel spaces as step-down accommodation for recovering patients, where insufficient social care is available (NHS England, 2021). During periods of severe winter pressures the government has, as the bedpan doctrine might lead one to expect, demanded weekly situation reports (see https://www.england.nhs.uk/statistics/statisti cal-work-areas/uec-sitrep/urgent-and-emergency-care-daily-situation-repo rts-2020-21/) from hospitals, to enable it both to manage their responses and anticipate media attention. The COVID-19 pandemics exacerbated these pressures, although in bedpan doctrine terms the political salience of hospitals was at times eclipsed by PPE supply, vaccination, test-and-trace and other non-hospital issues.

Similarly, annual accident and emergency (A&E) department attendances rose by 23.5 per cent over the decade to 2016–2017 to 23.372 million (Liverpool Heart and Chest Hospital NHS Foundation Trust, 2018). In 2021–2022 there were 24.4 million A&E attendances (NHS Digital, 2022a), producing 6.21 million emergency admissions (NHS Digital, 2022b). Because of COVID-19 the patient numbers for the two periods reflect quite different case-mixes, but are sufficient to show the continually increased number of patients needing urgent hospital care. Partly these changes reflected the demographic shift to an older population, but they may also reflect the increasing pressures on general practice and other NHS primary care services (see Chapter 5).

Workforce

It is hardly surprising that continually increasing workloads, fiscal austerity, the COVID-19 pandemics and their high exposure to COVID-19 itself had adverse consequences for NHS hospital workers.

Because wages were 46.6 per cent of spending in 2019–2020 across all NHS trusts, and a gradually increasing proportion at that (Department of Health and Social Care, 2021), they were bound to be a prime target for fiscal control. Due mainly to the cap on public sector pay increases between 2010 and 2018 nurses' remuneration fell by over 5 per cent in real terms. By 2021 UK nurses were paid almost exactly the national average wage (compared with a mean of 1.2 times the average across the 32 OECD countries) (OECD, 2021). Nurse turnover especially increased where house prices were high (Propper, Stockton and Stoye, 2021), reaching 14.6 per cent in London in 2018 (National Audit Office, 2019). Given fiscal austerity, one common response at hospital level was to delay (sometimes indefinitely) the filling of vacancies. Another was that NHS trusts increasingly used temporary contracts, 'bank' staff (NHS Improvement, 2019b) (effectively zero-hours contracts but at NHS pay rates) and agency staff, until the Department of Health restricted the latter practice from 2015. The same wage policies and workload pressures applied to most other categories of NHS hospital staff. In the form of nurses' strikes the industrial relations consequences of these long-term pressures became evident by the winter of 2022–2023.

Workforce planning and supply is a national-level NHS activity, or at times inactivity, but it remains the hospitals who have had to deal with its consequences. Twelve new medical schools opened between 2000 and 2018, when the opening of five more was announced. As a result the number of full-time equivalent consultants (most but not all in NHS hospitals) rose by 22 per cent between 2010 and 2016 (Lafond, Charlesworth and Roberts, 2017). Student nurses continue to receive a means-tested NHS bursary (a grant) but their repayment charges for any supplementary student loan are to increase from 2023. NHS hospitals continued to rely heavily on recruiting nurses from developing countries, although with a post-Brexit shift away from EU to non-EU nurses (Gillin and Smith, 2020).

As an instance of the negative responsibilisation of staff groups for policy failures, government and mass media representation of NHS hospital managers since the Griffiths report have sometimes represented – even scapegoated – them as incapable or a bureaucratic dead-weight (Veronesi, Kirkpatrick and Altanlar, 2019). Across all NHS trusts managers were however just over 2 per cent of the workforce early in 2022 (NHS Digital, 2022c), a low proportion compared with the UK workforce generally.

Hospital infrastructure

NHS hospitals include much infrastructure which despite its historical or architectural interest is outdated in practical terms. By gross internal area 46 per cent of the NHS estate, predominantly hospitals, was over 33 years old in 2019. Another consequence of fiscal austerity, exacerbated in some hospitals by transferring money from capital to revenue budgets, was delayed and reduced building maintenance which grew by 139 per cent between 2014–15 and 2018–19, when its total value was estimated at £6.5 billion (National Audit Office, 2020). Acute and specialist hospitals contributed 93 per cent of the backlog in 2017–18 (Kraindler, Gershlick and Charlesworth, 2019). Of that sum, £1.1 billion represented high-risk maintenance 'where repairs/ replacement must be addressed with urgent priority in order to prevent catastrophic failure, major disruption to clinical services or deficiencies in safety liable to cause serious injury and/or prosecution' (National Audit Office, 2020).

After reaching 98 per cent in 2008–09, the proportion of profitable trusts had by 2020 reverted to the 1995 level of 77 per cent, but even at their highest, trusts' collective gross operating profits were approximately 1.6 per cent of operating income, insufficient to fund much infrastructure development. In response to the perennial bedpan doctrine concerns about hospital waiting times, Independent Sector Treatment Centres were opened from 2003. Initially these were privately owned (NHS hospitals were not allowed to set them up), but when the non-NHS providers' contracts began to expire from 2008, NHS hospitals took over at least 14 of the 48 centres (Naylor and Gregory, 2009). Otherwise, new hospital infrastructure was from 1998 mostly funded through Private Finance Initiatives (PFI), corporate consortia which lent trusts capital and held the support service (maintenance, cleaning and so on) contracts for those projects for between 15 and 52 years afterwards (Shaoul Stafford and Stapleton, 2008). High interest charges (Hellowell and Pollock, 2007; Pollock, Price and Liebe, 2011) compromised this way of introducing capitalised infrastructure and it ceased in 2018 (Department of Health and Social Care, 2019), by which time above 19 per cent of NHS capital stock had been PFI-funded (Kraindler, Gershlick and Charlesworth, 2019). From 2009–10 these liabilities were added to NHS hospital balance sheets, which exposed the scale of hospitals' financial liability (Ellwood and Garcia-Lacalle, 2012). Of the 156 PFI and

Local Improvement and Finance Trust schemes, 26 each had a total future commitment exceeding £500 million (National Audit Office, 2020).

The Department of Health and Social Care (DHSC) capital budget replaced PFI, but on a smaller scale. Acute hospitals accounted for 78 per cent of all capital spending 2017–2018 (Kraindler, Gershlick and Charlesworth, 2019). This spending fluctuated, changing by between +12.7 per cent and -8.7 per cent year-on-year during 2010–2020, but declined overall by 7 per cent in real terms to £5.8 billion (4.2 per cent of total NHS spending) from 2010–2011 to 2017–2018. Of this money, NHS trusts spent about 60 per cent (Kraindler, Gershlick and Charlesworth, 2019). Twenty new capital projects were announced in 2019 (National Audit Office, 2020) and a Health Infrastructure Plan (HIP1) for 2020–2025 anticipated five more. As the bedpan doctrine might lead one to expect, Boris Johnson, then prime minister, announced a commitment to 40, or perhaps 48 (Hansard, 2022), new hospitals but eight of these projects were already in progress, 25 were rebuilding and 12 extensions of existing hospitals, and three were new hospitals, two of which had initially been funded through PFI but delayed when the corporation building them failed (Barrett and Palumbo, 2021). More definitely, from 2021, 40 local diagnostic centres would be established to replace hospital-based with ambulatory testing.

Private income

Another sphere of hospital management responsibilisation since 1990 was that policy-makers encouraged NHS hospitals to mitigate the pressures of fiscal austerity by seeking supplementary income from private sources. In 2015–2016 these sources contributed 7.7 per cent of NHS hospital income (Exworthy and Lafond, 2021) coming, in descending order of size, from hosting research, education and training (5.5 per cent of hospital income), services for local government agencies (1.0 per cent), and commercial income from on-site shops and car-parking (below 1 per cent). The Health and Social Care Act 2012 permitted NHS hospitals to earn up to 49 per cent of their income from private patients, which allowed some London teaching hospitals to increase such income substantially (more than 20 per cent) (Bayliss, n.d.), but across NHS hospitals that relaxation made little difference. For all NHS trusts combined, private patient income fluctuated around 1 per cent of income between 1995 and 2019. (The figure for hospitals taken alone may be a little higher since non-hospital services have fewer private patients.) Nine NHS hospitals made a loss on treating private patients during at least one financial year between 2010–2016 but FOI requests in 2015–2016 found that 73 more could not report the cost of treating private patients nor, therefore, whether that made a profit or loss (Walpole, 2018). Just over half the private patient income came from hospitals in London (Bayliss,

2016) where it accounted for 9.0 per cent of non–NHS income (Exworthy and Lafond, 2021). There was a similar geographical concentration in the partnerships between NHS hospitals and corporate hospitals. Consultants at three cancer hospitals became shareholders who received a share in profits (*Guardian*, 1 July 2019). The other main source of supplementary income was the sale of land and other assets, which increased by 99 per cent between 2016–2017 and 2018–2019 (when they raised £441 million) (National Audit Office, 2020).

Efficiency and performance

This brings us to the question of how NHS hospitals have performed, especially since 2008, in the terms that the bedpan doctrine made salient: the inherent goals of healthcare, that is patients' access to, outcomes and experiences of hospital care; and the extrinsic goals set by government, since 2010 fiscal austerity above all.

To begin with technical (not microeconomic) efficiency, the number of NHS hospital beds has declined steadily since at least 1985, and those remaining have been concentrated in district general hospitals which in April 2010 had 110,568 general and acute beds (86 per cent of them occupied) and 7,906 maternity beds (60 per cent occupied) (NHS England, 2022c). By March 2022 the respective figures were 91,862 acute beds (94 per cent occupied) (NHS England, 2022b) and 7,562 maternity beds (59 per cent occupied) (NHS England, 2022d). Indeed the 2020–2021 planning guidance recommended *reducing* bed occupancy rates to 92 per cent. (The 8 per cent margin accommodates fluctuations in urgent care and temporary closures for maintenance.) The number of admissions increased by 15 per cent over that decade while mean length of stay fell from 6 days to 4.4 (NHS Digital, 2022b). The increased technical efficiency also appears to be partly explained by the growth of planned day case admissions which continually increased both numerically and as a proportion of all planned elective hospital admissions (93 per cent by January 2019) (NHS England, 2022e), until the onset of COVID-19 in 2020 almost halved the proportion of day cases but caused hospitals to increase the number of critical care beds by almost a half. During 2009–2016 there was also a decrease (of 0.8 per cent) from emergency long-stay admissions alongside an increase (of 4 per cent) in emergency short-stay care, with the side-effect of slightly relieving the cost pressures on A&E services too (Lafond, Charlesworth and Roberts, 2017). More recently NHS hospitals began shifting some urgent care out of A&E departments into community settings (NHS England, 2022f). The rising workloads described earlier also increased the pressure on NHS hospitals to assist service 'integration' in the sense of substituting primary for secondary care: that is, to encourage general practice, community health and other primary care services to take on some kinds of clinical work hitherto done in hospital (see Chapter 5).

Over the last 75 years hospital waiting times have perhaps been the topic which exercised the bedpan doctrine most consistently. There is some evidence that the implementation of waiting times targets through 'targets and terror' helped reduce waiting times for English NHS hospital patients, compared with Scotland where no such system existed (Bevan and Hood, 2006; Propper et al, 2008). The NHS Constitution (2016) stated that at least 95 per cent of patients should start treatment within 18 weeks of referral to a hospital consultant. In 2007, 57.2 per cent of patients were treated that soon, above 90 per cent between 2009 and 2017, and peaking at 94.8 per cent in May 2013. During the later 2000s NHS hospitals were beginning to challenge the private hospitals' main selling point of faster treatment than the NHS offered. Compliance with the 18-week target fell to a COVID-19-induced 46 per cent in July 2020, recovering to around 60 per cent at present (NHS England, 2022a), but hospitals' performance against that target had been decreasing, though more slowly, before the COVID-19 pandemics, partly for fiscal and partly for demographic reasons (discussed earlier). Yet throughout 1994–2019 (start of the COVID-19 pandemics), and again after October 2021, the proportion of cancelled operations remained between 0.7 per cent and (early in 2001) 1.8 per cent of planned elective operations (NHS England, 2022g).

When a maximum A&E waiting time target of four hours was introduced in 2011, 97.1 per cent of patients were seen that quickly (NHS England, 2022h). In the year (2017–2018) immediately before the COVID-19 pandemics the figure had slipped to 88.4 per cent (NHS England, 2018). Even during the pandemic (2019–2020) it remained at 84 per cent, but as the pandemic abated declined to 73 per cent (March 2022) (NHS England, 2022h). One apparent explanation is the multiple backlogs as already described.

Following, and partly because of, the COVID-19 pandemic, public satisfaction with NHS hospital services declined markedly. The British Social Attitudes Survey net satisfaction scores (percentage of satisfied minus percentage of unsatisfied respondents) for NHS inpatient services fell from 55 per cent to 30 per cent from 2019 to 2021, from 60 per cent to 35 per cent for outpatient services, and from 31 per cent to 9 per cent for A&E, although these declines were less than for other NHS services. The most frequent cause of dissatisfaction was waiting time for treatment, followed by the insufficiency of NHS staffing and funding (although the belief that money was being wasted in the NHS scored almost as high). Satisfaction rates were higher among respondents who actually had recent contact with NHS hospitals (especially as outpatients) than those who had not (Frankenburg et al, 2021).

By way of fiscal responsibilisation, and thus economy, NHS trusts had a statutory duty to break even taking one year with another: their only quantified statutory obligation. Trust profitability was defined as a surplus of operating income over operating expenses (Harris and Neely, 2021), which just 34 per cent of acute trusts achieved in 2018–2019 (National Audit Office, 2020). In bedpan doctrine terms discreet subsidies to unprofitable hospitals were a lesser evil for governments than hospital closures or part-closures (cf. Sheaff et al, 2015), and so from 2008 the Department of Health began to provide loans as 'interim' financial support 'for NHS providers in financial distress to support the continued delivery of services' (National Audit Office, 2020). 'Control total incentive payments' were made to trusts that were judged to be trying to reduce their deficits (National Audit Office, 2016). A Sustainability and Transformation Fund followed, and then (2018–2019) a Provider Sustainability Fund, without which the 88 non-specialist trusts' collective deficit of £1277 million would have been £3258 million (Comptroller and Auditor General 2020). These deficits were concentrated in hospital trusts. However extra funding allocated in response to COVID-19 brought NHS trusts collectively into surplus by £0.65 billion in 2020–2021, the first such in eight years (Kings Fund, 2022).

Evaluating the bedpan doctrine and its consequences

For NHS hospitals, the centralising and responsibilising components of the bedpan doctrine have been complementary. Policy rhetoric about decentralisation referred in practice to responsibilisation, not the relaxation of central control. By 1990 the structures for managing NHS hospitals were already more centralised than those of the USSR. Subsequent major NHS reform policy statements have stated that NHS hospitals shouldn't be controlled from Whitehall, while proposing further structures to ensure that they were.

Klein (2019) argues that NHS accountability to parliament, and by implication the bedpan doctrine, results from the NHS being funded from taxation. This is true insofar as electors or the media hold governments accountable for fiscal events. Furthermore, governing parties have themselves made tight fiscal policy either an article of ideological faith (parts of the Conservative Party) or a badge of fiscal responsibility and prudence (New Labour) in response to hostile media coverage which often equated fiscal responsibility not just with judicious, but with low taxation and spending. To varying extents these conditions apply all across the public sector but additional non-fiscal reasons make the bedpan doctrine especially applicable to NHS hospitals: their status as an emergency service, the level of public support for them (Frankenburg et al, 2021), and their fairly uniform nationwide coverage (see Chapter 4).

Intrinsic practical characteristics of hospital management make the bedpan doctrine a permanent source of political (electoral, media) risk for governments. Where access to hospital care is based on need, hospitals have to respond not only to changes which they can foresee (for example, demographic shift, winter pressures, workforce change) but also changes they can neither predict nor control (for example, pandemics). Governments themselves have created some of these problems through policy messes (conflicting policies such as cost control *versus* PFI), implementation failures (for example, the attempts to increase nurse training and recruitment); and governments' technical and procurement incapacity (for example, for NHS hospital information systems). Neither have all government responses motivated by the bedpan doctrine been counter-productive. Depending on circumstances, the bedpan doctrine can and has motivated initiatives to make NHS hospital management more effective and care safer (for example, Patient Safety Collaboratives (Sheaff et al, 2018)) and, under favourable conditions, reduced hospital waiting times. In some cases (Healthcare Commission, 2009; Ockenden, 2022) the facts also justified the responsibilisation of NHS hospital management for defects in patient care. The Francis report described the bullying of whistle-blowers, falsification of evidence of harm to patients, and an 'insidious' tolerance of poor quality and safety standards (Healthcare Commission, 2009).

So it is open to debate whether the bedpan doctrine is a structural defect of NHS hospital management or the opposite. Underpinning the bedpan doctrine is governments' fear of accountability to parliament and ultimately the electorate. Whether the bedpan doctrine is a defect or strength therefore partly depends on how well informed the electorate is, hence upon whether government and media manage to inform or to mislead the electorate in matters of health policy and management. As noted, the bedpan doctrine also gives governments a reason not to publicise, even to conceal, information which seems to suggest government culpability. Certain of the debates that have triggered or resulted from application of the bedpan doctrine have been simplistic, for instance to demand more spending on the NHS as though that *alone* would solve many of the problems mentioned before. As Klein noted, 'Changing the distribution of resources, it turns out, is relatively easy; changing the way those resources are used and the way doctors practice is a very different matter' (Klein 2019: 3). The bedpan doctrine operates perforce within the electoral cycle, a short timescale for addressing such matters as hospital infrastructure development and the scale of medical training. As a major part of the public sector, NHS hospitals have also been a venue in which governments have normalised and implemented policies whose rationale lies not in healthcare so much as wider ideologies: those of marketisation, corporatisation, privatisation and austerity.

Nevertheless the last 75 years also offer evidence of how some of the adverse consequences noted earlier can be mitigated. A first step in remedying clinical safety mistakes or risks is to acknowledge them, which requires that staff not be blamed or penalised for doing so provided that the risk or mistake arose by chance or unforeseen causes (not malice or gross incompetence) and that practical lessons be drawn (Carmeli and Gittell, 2009; Wachter and Pronovost, 2009; Dekker et al, 2010). That involves the information which exposes such events and their causes being more widely and openly available than to government and managers alone. Optimistic, even naïve, though it may be to expect them to approach policy and managerial failures that way, the same would appear to apply to them and to media reporting. Over its 75 years there have been periods when NHS hospital infrastructure, foreseeable developments such as demographic shift and (though less successfully) workforce provision were consistently planned for on a long-term basis (five years or longer). Since this was already done before 1990, it is known to be feasible. Finally, some policy messes remain to be cleared up: the tensions between fiscal austerity and (on the other hand) sufficient hospital staffing and social care provision to relieve bed-blocking.

The bedpan doctrine has proved remarkably durable and at times politically hazardous for governments, but that is not necessarily a bad thing, at least for those who use and pay for the NHS. The dropped bedpan is very much a hospital metaphor but (perhaps using different metaphors) a similar doctrine would apply wherever government is held publicly accountable for the performance of the services it funds. If so, the bedpan doctrine may hold lessons for other public services too.

References

Ballantine, J., Forker, J. and Greenwood, M. (2008) 'The governance of CEO incentives in English NHS hospital trusts'. *Financial Accountability & Management*, 24, 4, 385–410. DOI: 10.1111/j.1468-0408.2008.00459.x

Barrett, N. and Palumbo, D. (2021) 'What's happened to the 40 new hospitals pledge?', *BBC News*, 1 December. https://www.bbc.com/news/59372 348 .

Bayliss, K. (2016) *The Financialisation of Health in England: Lessons from the Water Sector*. Leeds: Leeds Business School.

Berwick, D. (2013) *A Promise to Learn – a Commitment to Act: Improving the Safety of Patients in England*. London: National Advisory Group on the Safety of Patients in England.

Bevan, G. and Hood, C. (2006) 'Have targets improved performance in the English NHS?' *BMJ*, British Medical Journal Publishing Group, 332, 7538, 419–422.

Carmeli, A. and Gittell, J.H. (2009) 'High-quality relationships, psychological safety, and learning from failures in work organizations'. *Journal of Organizational Behavior*, 30, 6, 709–729. DOI: 10.1002/job.565

Comptroller and Auditor General. (2020) *Review of Capital Expenditure in the NHS*. London: National Audit Office.

Cribb, J. and Johnson, P. (2018) *10 Years On – Have We Recovered from the Financial Crisis?* London: Comment, Institute for Fiscal Studies.

Currie, G., Lockett, A., Finn, R., Martin, G. and Waring, J. (2012) 'Institutional work to maintain professional power: Recreating the model of medical professionalism'. *Organization Studies*, 33, 7, 937–962. DOI: 10.1177/0170840612445116

Dekker, S.W., Hugh, T.B., Wachter, R.M., Pronovost, P.J., Dekker, S., Laursen, T. et al (2010) 'Balancing no blame with accountability in patient safety'. *New England Journal of Medicine*, 362, 3, 275.

Department of Health. (1997) *The New NHS: Modern, Dependable*. London: HMSO.

Department of Health. (2013) 'Pay framework for very senior managers in strategic and special health authorities, primary care trusts and ambulance trusts'. London: Department of Health.

Department of Health and Social Care. (2019) *Annual Report and Accounts 2018–19*, No. HC2344. London: House of Commons.

Department of Health and Social Care. (2020) *Annual Report and Accounts 2018–20*. London: Department of Health and Social Care.

Department of Health and Social Care. (2021) *The Department of Health and Social Care's Written Evidence to the NHS Pay Review Body (NHSPRB) for the 2021/22 Pay Round*. London: Department of Health and Social Care.

Department of Health and Social Security. (1983) *NHS Management Enquiry. Report*. London: Department of Health and Social Security.

Diefenbach, T. (2009) 'New Public Management in public sector organizations: The dark sides of managerialistic "enlightenment"'. *Public Administration*, Wiley Online Library, 87, 4, 892–909.

Dowling, B. and Richardson, R. (1997) 'Evaluating performance-related pay for managers in the National Health Service'. *The International Journal of Human Resource Management*, Routledge, 8, 3, 348–366. DOI: 10.1080/095851997341685

Ellwood, S. and Garcia-Lacalle, J. (2012) 'Old wine in new bottles: IFRS adoption in NHS foundation trusts'. *Public Money & Management*, 32, 5, 335–342.

Exworthy, M., Frosini, F. and Jones, L. (2011) 'Are NHS foundation trusts able and willing to exercise autonomy? "You can take a horse to water …"'. *Journal of Health Services Research & Policy*, 16, 4, 232–237. DOI: 10.1258/jhsrp.2011.010077

Exworthy, M. and Lafond, S. (2021) 'New development: Commercialization of the English National Health Service: a necessity in times of financial austerity?' *Public Money & Management*, Taylor & Francis, 41, 1, 81–84.

Exworthy, M., Powell, M. and Mohan, J. (1999) 'The NHS: Quasi-market, quasi-hierarchy and quasi-network?' *Public Money and Management*, 19, 4, 15–22.

Flynn, R. (1992) *Structures of Control in Health Management*. London: Routledge.

Frankenburg, S., Howe, S., Popa, A. and Woods Rogan, R. (2021) *British Social Attitudes 39*. London: National Centre for Social Research.

Gillin, N. and Smith, D. (2020) 'Overseas recruitment activities of NHS trusts 2015–2018: Findings from FOI requests to 19 Acute NHS trusts in England'. *Nursing Inquiry*, Wiley Online Library, 27, 1, e12320.

Hansard (2022)*Engagements Debated on Wednesday 8th June 2022*, Volume 715, London: Parliament.

Harris, E.E. and Neely, D. (2021) 'Determinants and consequences of nonprofit transparency'. *Journal of Accounting, Auditing & Finance*, Sage Publications Inc., 36, 1, 195–220. DOI: 10.1177/0148558X18814134

Healthcare Commission. (2009) *Investigation into Mid Staffordshire NHS Foundation Trust*. London: Healthcare Commission.

Hellowell, M. and Pollock, A.M. (2007) 'Private finance, public deficits'. *A Report on the Cost of PFI and Its Impact on Health Services in England*. Edinburgh: Centre for International Health Policy, University of Edinburgh.

Hodgson, D., Bailey, S., Exworthy, M., Bresnen, M., Hassard, J. and Hyde, P. (2021) 'On the character of the new entrepreneurial National Health Service in England: Reforming health care from within?'. *Public Administration*, 100, 2: Symposium, pp 1–18. DOI: 10.1111/padm.12797.

House of Commons Committee of Public Accounts. (2013) *The Dismantled National Programme for IT in the NHS*, No. HC294. London: House of Commons.

House of Commons Health Committee. (2010) *Public Expenditure on Health and Personal Social Services 2009*. London: House of Commons.

House of Commons Public Accounts Committee. (2020) *Digital Transformation in the NHS*, No. HC680. London: House of Commons.

Jones, L. and Hameiri, S. (2022) 'COVID-19 and the failure of the neoliberal regulatory state'. *Review of International Political Economy*, Taylor & Francis, 29, 4, 1027–1052.

Kings Fund. (2022) *NHS Trusts in Deficit*. The King's Fund. https://www.kingsfund.org.uk/projects/nhs-in-a-nutshell/trusts-deficit

Kirkpatrick, I., Altanlar, A. and Veronesi, G. (2017) 'Corporatisation and the emergence of (under-managed) managed organisations: The case of English public hospitals'. *Organization Studies*, 38, 12, 1687–1708. DOI: 10.1177/0170840617693273

Kirkpatrick, I., Altanlar, A. and Veronesi, G. (2022) 'Hybrid professional managers in healthcare: An expanding or thwarted occupational interest?'. *Public Management Review*, pp 1–20. DOI: 10.1080/14719037.2021.1996777

Kirkpatrick, I., Sturdy, A.J., Alvarado, N.R., Blanco-Oliver, A. and Veronesi, G. (2019) 'The impact of management consultants on public service efficiency'. *Policy & Politics*, Policy Press, 47, 1, 77–95.

Kivimäki, M., Batty, G.D., Pentti, J., Shipley, M.J., Sipilä, P.N., Nyberg, S.T. et al (2020) 'Association between socioeconomic status and the development of mental and physical health conditions in adulthood: A multi-cohort study'. *The Lancet Public Health*, 5, 3, e140–e149.

Klein, R. (2019) 'The National Health Service (NHS) at 70: Bevan's double-edged legacy'. *Health Economics, Policy and Law*, 14, 1, 1–10.

Kraindler, J., Gershlick, B. and Charlesworth, A. (2019) *Failing to Capitalise*, London: Briefing, Health Foundation.

Lafond, S., Charlesworth, A. and Roberts, A. (2017) *A Year of Plenty? An Analysis of NHS Finances and Consultant Productivity*. London: Health Foundation.

Liverpool Heart and Chest Hospital NHS Foundation Trust. (2018) '70 years of the NHS 1948–2018'. Liverpool: Liverpool Health and Chest Hospital. https://www.lhch.nhs.uk/news-archive/2018/july/celebrating-nhs70-at-liverpool-heart-and-chest-hospital/

Martin, J. and Evans, D. (1984) *Hospitals in Trouble*. Oxford: Blackwell.

National Audit Office. (2016) *Financial Sustainability of the NHS*. Report by the Comptroller and Auditor General No. HC785. London: National Audit Office.

National Audit Office. (2018) *NHS England's Management of the Primary Care Support Services Contract with Capita*, No. HC632. London: National Audit Office.

National Audit Office. (2019) *NHS Financial Sustainability*, Report by the Comptroller and Auditor General, No. HC1867. London: National Audit Office.

National Audit Office. (2020) *Review of Capital Expenditure in the NHS*, No. HC43. London: House of Commons.

Naylor, C. and Gregory, S. (2009) *Independent Sector Treatment Centres*, Briefing. London: Kings Fund.

Nelson, H. and Nikolakis, W. (2012) 'How does corporatization improve the performance of government agencies? Lessons from the restructuring of state-owned forest agencies in Australia'. *International Public Management Journal*, 15, 3, 364–391. DOI: 10.1080/10967494.2012.725323

NHS Digital. (2020) 'Estates Return Information Collection (ERIC) 2019/20'. NHS Digital.

NHS Digital. (2022a) 'Hospital Accident & Emergency Activity 2021–22'. *NDRS*. https://digital.nhs.uk/data-and-information/publications/statistical/hospital-accident--emergency-activity/2021-22

NHS Digital. (2022b) 'Hospital Admitted Patient Care Activity, 2021–2'. *NDRS*. https://digital.nhs.uk/data-and-information/publications/statistical/hospital-admitted-patient-care-activity/2021-22

NHS Digital. (2022c) 'NHS Workforce Statistics – January 2022 (Including selected provisional statistics for February 2022)'. *NDRS*. https://digital.nhs.uk/data-and-information/publications/statistical/nhs-workforce-statistics/january-2022

NHS England. (2018) *Annual Report 2017/18 Performance Report*. London: NHSE.

NHS England. (2021) 'Hotel space: How to guide'. Leeds: NHS England.

NHS England. (2022a) 'Consultant-led referral to treatment waiting times data 2022–23'. Statistics. https://www.england.nhs.uk/statistics/statistical-work-areas/rtt-waiting-times/rtt-data-2022-23/

NHS England. (2022b) 'Urgent and emergency care daily situation reports 2021–22'. Statistics. https://www.england.nhs.uk/statistics/statistical-work-areas/uec-sitrep/urgent-and-emergency-care-daily-situation-reports-2021-22/

NHS England. (2022c) 'Average daily available and occupied beds timeseries'. Leeds: NHS England.

NHS England. (2022d) 'Bed availability and occupancy data – Overnight'. Statistics. https://www.england.nhs.uk/statistics/statistical-work-areas/bed-availability-and-occupancy/bed-data-overnight/

NHS England. (2022e) 'Monthly hospital activity data'. Statistics. https://www.england.nhs.uk/statistics/statistical-work-areas/hospital-activity/monthly-hospital-activity/mar-data/

NHS England. (2022f) 'Hospital activity'. Statistics. https://www.england.nhs.uk/statistics/statistical-work-areas/hospital-activity/ .

NHS England. (2022g) 'Cancelled elective operations data'. Statistics. https://www.england.nhs.uk/statistics/statistical-work-areas/cancelled-elective-operations/cancelled-ops-data/

NHS England. (2022h) 'A&E attendances and emergency admissions'. Statistics. https://www.england.nhs.uk/statistics/statistical-work-areas/ae-waiting-times-and-activity/

NHS England. (2023a) '2023/24 priorities and operational planning guidance'. NHS England.

NHS England. (2023b) 'NHS oversight framework segmentation'. https://www.england.nhs.uk/publication/nhs-oversight-framework-segmentation/

NHS England and NHS Improvement. (2019) 'NHS Operational Planning and Contracting Guidance 2019/20'. Leeds: NHS England.

NHS Improvement. (2018) 'Single Oversight Framework'. NHS Improvement.

NHS Improvement. (2019a) 'NHS Oversight Framework for 2019/20: Provider trust segmentation'. NHS Improvement.

NHS Improvement. (2019b) Consolidated NHS Provider Accounts 2018/19, No. HC2376. London: NHS Trust Development Authority.

Ockenden, D. (2022) *Findings, Conclusions and Essential Actions from the Independent Review of Maternity Services at The Shrewsbury and Telford Hospital NHS Trust*. London: House of Commons.

OECD. (2021) *Health at a Glance 2021: OECD Indicators*. Paris: OECD Publishing.

Office for National Statistics. (2022) 'Estimates of the population for the UK, England, Wales, Scotland and Northern Ireland – Office for National Statistics'. https://www.ons.gov.uk/peoplepopulationandcommunity/populationandmigration/populationestimates/datasets/populationestimatesforukenglandandwalesscotlandandnorthernireland

Pollock, A.M., Price, D. and Liebe, M. (2011) 'Private finance initiatives during NHS austerity'. *BMJ*, 342, d324.

Propper, C., Stockton, I. and Stoye, G. (2021) *Cost of Living and the Impact on Nursing Labour Outcomes in NHS Acute Trusts*. London: Institute for Fiscal Studies.

Propper, C., Sutton, M., Whitnall, C. and Windmeijer, F. (2008) 'Did "targets and terror" reduce waiting times in England for hospital care?'. *The BE Journal of Economic Analysis & Policy*, De Gruyter, 8, 2.

Pyysiäinen, J., Halpin, D. and Guilfoyle, A. (2017) 'Neoliberal governance and "responsibilization" of agents: Reassessing the mechanisms of responsibility-shift in neoliberal discursive environments'. *Distinktion: Journal of Social Theory*, 18, 2, 215–235.

Ritchie, J. (2000) *An Inquiry into Quality and Practice within the National Health Service Arising from the Actions of Rodney Ledward*, Ashford: Department of Health.

Shaoul, J., Stafford, A. and Stapleton, P. (2008) 'The cost of using private finance to build, finance and operate hospitals'. *Public Money and Management*, 28, 2, 101–108.

Sheaff, R., Bethune, R., Doran, N., Ball, S., Medina-Lara, A., Lang et al (2018) *The Patient Safety Collaborative Evaluation Study (The PiSCES Study)*, No. PR-R11-0914-12002. London: NIHR.

Sheaff, R., Charles, N., Mahon, A., Chambers, N., Morando, V., Exworthy, M. et al (2015) 'NHS commissioning practice and health system governance: A mixed-methods realistic evaluation'. *Health Services and Delivery Research*, 3, 10, 1–184. DOI: 10.3310/hsdr03100

Sheaff, R. and Schofield, J. (2016) 'Inter-organizational networks in health-care: Program networks, care networks and integrated care', in E., Ferlie, A. Pedersen and K. Montgomery (eds) *Oxford Handbook of Health Care Management*. Oxford: Oxford University Press.

The Inquiry into the management of care of children receiving complex heart surgery at the Bristol Royal Infirmary 1984–1995. (2001) *Learning from Bristol: The Report of the Public Inquiry into Children's Heart Surgery at the Bristol Royal Infirmary 1984–1995*, No. Cm5207. London: HMSO.

The King's Fund. (2011) *The Future of Leadership and Management in the NHS: No More Heroes*. London: Kings Fund.

Veronesi, G., Kirkpatrick, I. and Altanlar, A. (2019) 'Are public sector managers a "Bureaucratic Burden"? The case of English public hospitals'. *Journal of Public Administration Research and Theory*, 29, 2, 193–209. DOI: 10.1093/jopart/muy072

Wachter, R.M. and Pronovost, P.J. (2009) 'Balancing "no blame" with accountability in patient safety'. *New England Journal of Medicine*, 361, 14, 1401–1406.

Walpole, S. (2018) *NHS Treatment of Private Patients: The Impact on NHS Finances and NHS Patient Care*. London: Centre for Health and the Public Interest.

Wright, J.S.F., Dempster, P.G., Keen, J., Allen, P. and Hutchings, A. (2012) 'The new governance arrangements for NHS Foundation Trust Hospitals: Reframing governors as meta-regulators'. *Public Administration*, 90, 2, 351–369. DOI: 10.1111/j.1467-9299.2011.01975.x

Yates, J. (1995) *Private Eye, Heart and Hip: Surgical Consultants, the National Health Service and Private Medicine*. Edinburgh: Churchill.

7

Quality and the NHS: fair-weather friends or a longstanding relationship?

Ross Millar, Justin Waring and Mirza Lalani

Introduction

The quality and safety of healthcare remains a global health policy priority with the likes of the World Health Organization and major international forums promoting standards and methods for improving care quality (WHO 2022). The English National Health Service (NHS) exemplifies such trends where the significance of quality as an NHS priority has been framed, in a large part, by the many high-profile failings and scandals in care quality dating back to the late 1960s. Scandals around long-term care at Ely, unsafe paediatric heart surgery at Bristol Royal Infirmary, the systematic neglect of patients at Mid-Staffordshire hospital and very recently, the prominent failings at multiple maternity units provide a disturbing backdrop to the NHS and the quality of care (Mannion et al, 2018; Knight and Stafford, 2022). Such events have often been followed by investigations and Public Inquiries and led to extensive recommendations, many of which look similar from one report to the next, arguing for increased transparency, support for speaking up and whistleblowing, culture change, better governance and reforms of professional regulation (Powell, 2019).

The response to quality failings has instigated a range of regulatory responses and the need for greater quality assurance (Waring et al, 2010). National improvement and performance management programmes from the early 2000s onwards have been implemented by a succession of regulatory bodies from the Centre for Healthcare Improvement (CHI) followed by the Healthcare Commission and then the CQC. In responding to such events, the NHS has also been the testbed for many innovations in quality improvement and management, often drawing from the experiences of other safety-critical or high-quality industries (Waring and Bishop, 2010; Millar, 2013). This is exemplified by the growth of specialist agencies and charities committed to promoting care quality such as the Modernisation Agency, the Institute for Innovation and Improvement, NHS Improvement and The Health Foundation (The Health Foundation, 2021).

And yet despite such an emphasis and policy innovation, the commitment to quality and quality improvement has not been constant. The focus on quality and quality improvement has competed for attention among other policy priorities, especially cost and responding to exogenous events such as the COVID-19 pandemic. Such variable traction and success have led to the quality agenda appearing more like fads and fashions rather than a sustained policy approach (Ham, Berwick and Dixon, 2016; Molloy, Martin and Gardner, 2016).

This chapter introduces the themes of quality and quality improvement in the NHS. It outlines prominent conceptualisation and definitions of quality and places quality in its historical context, thereby showing its changing significance. This historical viewpoint also allows for more critical consideration of the changing ideas and assumptions that have informed the quality agenda, especially the shift towards managerial approaches. The chapter argues that quality remains a significant policy priority and that service leaders are often in search of the 'next big thing' to improve quality, but that the relevance and fit of these innovations often does not achieve the desired goals or outcomes. We argue that how we define or know quality carries with it certain assumptions about the sources and threats to quality and, in turn, how quality (and those threats and sources) should be governed. While quality represents a focal issue for policy and practice, it has lacked a coherent strategy up to this point. Moving forward, the chapter concludes with a prospective analysis for quality within a context for whole-systems working and integrated care. It argues that given what history tells us, any future agenda for quality remains unstable, with the achievement of system-wide process improvement still to be realised.

Quality: its definition and operationalisation in the NHS

Quality is one of those peculiar concepts that most people will have a view about, but which often alludes universal or precise definition. In general, it relates to how 'good' something is at meeting some given expectations, but where quality is inherently relative to the particular activity, given expectations which are themselves relative a given time, people or culture. Take, for example, our contemporary expectations about the quality of something like a car and compare that with ten or twenty years ago. It is for this reason that many approaches to quality still focus on the idea of it being a subjective definition.

In the early 1980s, Donabedian made a significant early contribution to current thinking about healthcare quality by distinguishing between the more technical (clinical) and the interpersonal (non-clinical) aspects of care. Importantly he stressed that any definition of technical effectiveness can only be judged against the current evidence and standards of care, while interpersonal quality needs to meet broader social expectations. His other significant contribution was showing how the assessment of quality can be classified in terms of structures, processes and outcomes (Donabedian, 1988). That is, the resources and infrastructure needed deliver effective care, the processes of providing care, and the outcomes of care.

Based on these ideas, Maxwell (1992) further elaborated the definition of quality along six dimensions. Effectiveness of treatment in terms of providing the best available care; acceptability in terms of whether the care is seen as appropriate by patients and other stakeholders; efficiency in terms of whether the relative costs and benefits of care; access in terms of barriers to timely care; equity in terms of fair treatment for social groups; and relevance or taking account of the needs of wider society.

In contemporary policy discourse, quality is often understood in terms of the degree to which health services increase the likelihood of health outcome. The Institute of Medicine's Crossing the Quality Chasm (Institute of Medicine, 1999), popularised by Don Berwick and the Institute for Health Improvement in the US, described quality along six dimensions:

1. Safety – avoiding harm to people
2. Effectiveness – providing the best available evidence-based care
3. Patient-centredness – care that meets the preferences, needs and values of individuals
4. Timeliness – reduce the need to wait and delay care
5. Efficiency – optimal use of resources
6. Equity – care that does not vary on the basis of gender, ethnicity, location or socio-economic status.

The WHO (2023) characterises this list as comprising the three primary goals of effectiveness, safety and patient-centred which should always be characterised as timely, efficient, equitable and 'integrated' (using services throughout the life course). Yet, some might argue that the issue of efficiency or even equity might not necessarily be central to quality; depending, for example, if a highly individualised or socialised view of quality is taken.

Although there might now be some consensus about what defines healthcare quality, the relative significance of these dimensions is not always consistent, and the methods used to improve or manage quality remains highly changeable. It is also worth considering whether any definition of quality implies often implicitly other deeper assumptions about the sources and threats to quality, and the preferred ways in which quality can be improved or assured. With this in mind, it is important to look closer the history of quality in the NHS, not only to understand how ideas or definitions have change over time, but also to surface the underlying political, economic or social drivers that shape any conceptualisation and, in subtle ways, influence how efforts to improve quality become manifest in day-to-day practice.

A brief history of quality in the NHS

The following section will offer a brief overview of changes witnessed mainly over the last 30 years. A timeline is offered next as less on the basis of demarcated definitions of quality or approaches to quality improvement, but more on seeking to highlight underlying social, economic or political factors that shape the changing understandings of quality. As such, there are clear echoes with broader reform periods and governmental programmes associated with the UK electoral cycle as well as major scandals in healthcare quality.

Throughout the 1990s, the issue of quality gained sustained public, professional and political attention. Research on the internal market reforms showed, for example, the shortcomings of market mechanisms to treat quality with the same significance as cost, especially when it was difficult to measure or compare the quality of care and there was limited information on which to base decision-making. There was also growing national and international evidence about sub-standard clinical performance, not just manifest in long waiting times and variable outcomes, but also mounting evidence of clinical risk and harm. And beyond the UK, a number of significant reports and studies were articulating a new approach to healthcare quality with a focus on evidence-based care, standardisation and more robust systems of improvement (Leape, 1994).

For much of the early history of the NHS, care quality was more assumed than assured. The standards and assessment of care quality were largely embedded within long-established systems of professional regulation and enshrined within notions of professional autonomy that characterised most developed health systems from the mid-twentieth century. This rested on the idea that professionals are best placed to both define and assess the quality of care based on their exclusive expertise and frontline clinical experience. In the main, these systems relied on assuring professional 'entry' through new professionals meeting the agreed standards of qualification and on professional 'exit' where questions of gross misconduct in relation to professional standards led to the removal of license.

The early literature showed how professional autonomy and collegiality allowed many instances of poor practice to go undetected or unaddressed because of the cultural norms and ceremonies of health professions in which making mistakes was often seen as a developmental rite of passage and professional norms were orientated towards protecting professional credibility. These ideas were effectively summarised by Friedson (1970) and later Rosenthal (1995) who talked of the hidden routines and rituals for safeguarding the legitimacy and autonomy of medical professionalism in the face of external scrutiny. The point to emphasise is that for much of the history of the NHS, and continuing to this day, there is an argument that the definition and improvement of professional practice should be led by members of the profession itself because only members of the profession have the relevant expertise and because of associated concerns about inappropriate external scrutiny and management.

It is important to acknowledge that alongside the system of professional self-regulation, service users have and remain able to utilise formal complaints procedures to raise concerns about quality and, in more extreme instances of sub-standard care, to pursue legal action and seek redress through litigation. At the time of writing, the estimated litigation costs for outstanding claims against the NHS totals £2.5 billion (as of 2021–2022) (NHS Resolution, 2022). The early systems for governing care quality were far from complementary and coherent, nor designed to make it easy for people to raise concern, and nor are they especially effective at improving the quality of care (Mannion et al, 2018). NHS complaint systems both in terms of its mechanisms to handle complaints and to use complaints data to driver improvement have continued to remain inadequate (van Dael et al, 2022).

The seeds of change emerged in the early 1980s with a shift in political attitudes towards welfare services and the introduction of what is widely known as New Public Management (NPM). From the mid-1980s onwards, the hilstation and delivery of healthcare became the concern of a new and growing cadre of managers. Part of NPM's mission is to set the performance standards more explicitly for public services, to hilst private sector management techniques to improve and demonstrate performance against these standards and monitor compliance to standards through new forms of monitoring and regulation (McNulty and Ferlie, 2004).

At the same time, established systems of professional regulation became increasingly distrusted on the grounds of being opaque, hilstation professional interests rather than public standards, and not being responsive to service users (Waring and Bishop, 2010). Concerns centred on professional regulation intensified following revelations from the Shipman inquiry (Smith, 2004). The findings resulted in years of discourse about how to improve the regulation of doctors to root out poor performers. The profession argued that their professionalism would ensure care quality whereas politicians were keen for greater external scrutiny and oversight. In 2012, Medical Revalidation was introduced to address longstanding concerns about the accountability of doctors and the quality of medical care. It involved assessing a doctor's performance through collection, reporting and reflection on relevant information produced for annual appraisal (Walshe et al, 2017). Doctors were required to regularly present supporting information of continuing professional development (CPD), quality improvement activities, significant events, feedback from patients and colleagues and a review of compliments and complaints, to demonstrate their competence and that their ongoing performance was meeting regulatory standards. It is thought that revalidation has stimulated improvements in clinical governance and clinical practice for doctors whose practice had raised concerns, but its value has been less clear in further improving the practice of well performing doctors (Walshe et al, 2017).

The succession of high-profile scandals and Public Inquiries further questioned the prevailing system of professional and hilstation regulation throughout the 1990s and 1980s, supporting further calls for a new regulatory settlement. The important point to make is that from the 1980s onwards a broader shift in political ideology and public values provided the backdrop for calls for a new approach to healthcare quality. It is noteworthy that the late 1980s and early 1990s saw a growth in professional and academic interest with the issue of care quality and the introduction of specialist journals, such as *International Journal for Quality in Health Care* (1989) and *Quality in Health Care* (1992).

In the early 1990s, the NHS experienced profound structural reforms in which the top-down model of resource planning and allocation was replaced with an internal market. In this system, acute and specialist services were purchased from a competitive market of healthcare providers. The rationale for markets is that purchasers contract services on the broad parameters of better quality and lower cost, and so quality now took on an entirely different logic and purpose. As discussed in other chapters, these governance changes reshaped the NHS landscape where the principles of better management now evolved to better market management, and with additional capabilities were needed in contracting, business planning and accounting. For some, these reforms were a further attempt to wrest the control over resources away from the bureaucratic machinery dominated by doctors, and instead to give managers and service users greater influence over the allocation of taxpayers' money.

As part of these reforms, explicit attention was given the hilstationa of quality improvement and assurance techniques. These included those more commonly associated with professional education and development and new approaches more commonly associated with private business and industry such as Total Quality Management (TQM) (Pollitt, 1993). TQM, along with others such as Business Process Reengineering (BPR) (McNulty and Ferlie, 2002), sought to import industry thinking from Deming and others regarding how to improve systems and processes of production.

While 'audit and feedback' have long been a feature of professional practice development, in which professionals systematically review aspects of their practice to identify potential areas for learning and improvement, the early 1990s onwards witnessed greater hilstationa with the NHS reforms of the early 1990s, with its explicit approach to quality improvement being defined in the 1989 White Paper as (Department of Health, 1989). Audit represented an explicit attempt to define the standards of medical work, gather systematic information about performance and compare performance among peer groups and identify deficiencies (Walshe, 1999). Although professionals desired a voluntary, confidential, internal and educational in approach (Harrison and Pollitt, 1995), the implemented system was compulsory and involved the systematic collection and analysis of performance data. Audit as a mechanism for quality assurance was in part a response to the Bristol inquiry which identified a lack of transparency of mortality data. Despite the hilstation producing ward level clinical data, the data was rarely assessed, audited or questioned by the Trust board. Moreover, learning may have been hastened if there had been opportunities to compare such data with that of other organisations (Walshe and Offen, 2001).

The alarming nature of the quality of care failures at Bristol – deaths of children following cardiac surgery – caused significant public and media clamour prompting the Health Secretary Frank Dobson to announce that Hospital Mortality Statistics would be published annually and that mortality tables would provide an early warning system for failure (Street, 2002). Soon after, the Hospital Standardised Mortality Ratio (HSMR), introduced as a comparative mortality measure in the *Dr Foster's Hospital Guides* emerged as a prominent methodology for measuring mortality. The central diktat to adopt measures such as audit while also collecting data against performance indicators such as mortality prompted some professionals to argue that it reduced their clinical freedom, yet the actual format remained predominantly based within the established systems of medical work (Dent, 1995). The trend towards collecting performance data on services and individual clinicians has continued to shape the governance of services and the allocation of resources (Exworthy et al, 2019).

If audit was intended to improve the quality of clinical practice, quality management techniques were intended to address broader quality improvement challenges found in the hilstation of care. This saw the early adoption of TQM and associated techniques for Plan–Do–Study–Act within the NHS (Joss and Kogan, 1995). For Pollitt (1993) this represented a broader feature of NPM in which the global 'religious cult' of TQM had spread from global industry into public policy discourse. The specific features of TQM represented a developed methodology for the systematic measurement and improvement of quality drawing upon managerialist ideas and practices drawn from outside of healthcare.

When returned to office in 1997, the Labour government's proposals for a New NHS included more explicit and direct focus on the governance and improvement of care quality (Department of Health, 1997). At the national level this involved by the introduction of the NICE (now National Institute for Health and Care Excellence) which is responsible for approving treatment options and procedures based upon expert review of clinical evidence and systematic reviews. At the hospital level, a new approach to quality improvement was submitted called 'clinical governance' which introduced new obligations for professionals and managers to assure the improve quality. An important feature of clinical governance is the statutory duty on the part of hospital management for service quality, making hospital leaders legally responsible for the quality of care. This discharge of this duty includes promoting more rigorous forms of quality improvement through the hilstation, fostering a new culture of quality (Department of Health, 1998) and establishing new accountability relationships. This replicated the principles of corporate governance for financial management and elevated the hilstation status of quality to that of efficiency.

The implementation policy *A First Class Service* (Department of Health, 1998) set out four components of quality improvement associated with clinical governance; these include:

- 'Clear lines of responsibility and accountability' for quality – ultimately carried by the Chief Executive but dispatched through a range of hilstational mechanisms and agents, such as a clinical lead and a subcommittee of the Trust board;
- 'A comprehensive programme for quality activities' – including full participation in clinical audit and external reviews, the application of evidence-based guidance and the National Service Frameworks, comprehensive workforce planning and continual professional development;
- The management of risks – through proactive risk assessment and self-assessment;
- Procedures for all professional to identify and remedy poor performance – including reactive measures to report incidents and complaints.

At the time, Scally and Donaldson (1998) suggested that as a mechanism for quality improvement clinical governance 'is by far the most ambitious quality initiative that will ever have been implemented in the NHS' (1998: 61). Buetow and Roland (1999) show that the clinical governance framework was based upon tried and tested managerial and professional techniques of quality improvement, such as 'clinical audit' that was an established technique for professional development; while also influenced by methods of 'quality assurance' derived from management theories and 'systems re-engineering'. Clinical governance therefore represents the coming together of both established professional forms of internal regulation, with more recent and emerging forms external managerial techniques for quality assurance.

In 2001, the NHS Modernisation Agency was created to develop and spread new approaches to service improvement. This supported in particular the systematic adoption and application of improvement methodologies more commonly found in other industries, such as process mapping, Plan Do Study Act (PDSA) and statistical process control (SPC) as well as framing itself as a type of social movement for change within the NHS. Its work focused on particular service priorities for improvement, such as waiting times and increasing patient choice, developing new roles and ways of working and addressing structural inequalities in care. The launch of quality improvement collaboratives for priority areas would draw on the IHI Breakthrough Collaborative methodology to facilitate these efforts (Nadeem et al 2013).

In 2005, the Agency was superseded by the NHS Institute for Innovation and Improvement which had the mission of transforming the health service through rapidly spreading new ways of working, technologies, and leadership. This often involved learning from international exemplars of high-quality care provision, and the adoption of quality improvement techniques derived from other industries. The Productive Series, for example, was a suite of improvement methodologies largely informed by the Toyota Production System or what is more often called Lean Thinking. This focused on applying the principles of process mapping, appraisal and continuous improvement to reduce waste and increased value-adding activities across care pathways and processes. Such activities have since been 'homed' in various parts of the NHS England infrastructure (Waring and Bishop, 2010).

Outside of the NHS a range of other foundations and agencies have contributed to the provide critical insight and new ways of thinking about the quality of NHS. Notable groups include the King's Fund, The Health Foundation and the Nuffield Trust, as well as more regionalised improvement networks such as AQUA. In different ways, these organisations function as think tanks, policy advisory groups, research and evaluation services and educational platforms and contribute to the promotion of quality improvement. The Health Foundation has been especially active in development the 'science' of improvement through combining the principles of evidence-based healthcare, with proven methods of quality improvement, and more systematic and theory-based evaluations of improvement initiatives. This parallels similar approaches to quality improvement championed by the likes of the US Institute for Healthcare Improvement.

In an attempt to reconnect policy concerns with quality improvement and continued commitments to market-like mechanisms, the late 2000s saw increasing attentions and emphasis on quality assurance through greater regulation and compliance. The introduction of Commissioning for Quality and Innovation (CQUINs) aimed to make an element of healthcare providers income condition on meeting indicators of quality around targeted service priority issues. They employed a range of approaches to bring quality outliers into line. Alongside inspections, CHI developed star-ratings according to the performance of NHS hospitals against national targets. Organisations that were zero-rated or failing on inspection were publicly named (and shamed).

Better performing organisations were rewarded with 'earned autonomy' which amounted to greater control over financial management, fewer inspections and eligibility to apply for Foundation status (Mannion, 2007; Bevan, 2011). This regime was superseded by the Annual Health Check, which adopted a more comprehensive approach to assessment and inspection, incorporating core and developmental standards in areas such as patient focus and the healthcare environment (Haslam, 2007). The formation of the CQC signalled a more relational approach, gradually shifting the balance of assessment from intermittent inspection to regular contact, illuminating more clearly local organisational context and culture.

These ideas have continued into the 'Lansley' NHS reforms of the 2010s. The main challenge to quality during this time was less the proper functioning of the market mechanisms, but rather the fragmentation of care services, especially health and social care services, and the failure to provide coordinated patient-centred care. This problem was exacerbated by the broader context of austerity measures introduced in the wake of the financial crisis of 2008 and which were unevenly felt by the social care sector. The Berwick Review (2013) in response to the Mid Staffordshire Inquiry provided a reemphasis on quality improvement tools and techniques to improve quality and safety. Greater emphasis on collaboration and partnering also became apparent during this period (Miller and Millar, 2017; Millar et al, 2023) and from around 2014 efforts to address market fragmentation were manifest in a range of initiatives such Integrated Care Pilots (later 'Pioneers') and New Care Models ('Vanguards'), which laid the foundations for the introduction of broader and more inclusive Sustainability and Transformation Partnerships (STPs) and now Integrated Care Systems (ICSs).

The formation of the CQC heralded an opportunity for a regulator to take a direct interventionist approach to identify quality problems and support remedial action through stimulating quality improvement. The Special Measures and Challenged Provider (SMCP) regime was introduced in 2013 to support trusts where serious quality failings had been identified. Drawing strong parallels with the approach of periodic inspections and targeted interventions in education for struggling schools (Vindrola-Padros et al, 2022), the SMCP regime was designed to be supportive and encourage relationship building between the CQC and struggling trusts, extending beyond performance oversight and regulation to include direct intervention to stimulate improvement (Lalani, 2022).

Alongside these developments, quality improvement approaches continued with the launch of the Virginia Mason Institute Partnership in 2017, a five-year partnership between Virginia Mason Institute and five NHS trusts to support the development of lean cultures of continuous improvement. At the same time NHSE were keen to implement a more centralised approach to quality improvement across all trusts but particularly acute providers.

Overseen by the Academic Health Sciences Networks (AHSN), the focus would be on clinical conditions in which risk of quality failures were highest such as deteriorating patients presenting in hospital with signs and symptoms of acute kidney injury and sepsis (Lalani et al, 2022).

More recent developments have been set against the backdrop of the COVID-19 pandemic. The period heralded opportunities to further harness quality improvement (QI) approaches in the NHS (Kings Fund, 2023) and also provided greater emphasis on quality management systems (Shah, 2020). With the advent of Integrated Care Systems, regulation and compliance with quality standards has turned to system-wide approaches with CQC proposing the introduction of a single assessment framework. The framework sets out an intention to base assessment on a wider range of quality outcomes across safety, experience, equity and access while also assessing progress on certain features of integration such as partnership working and patient/public involvement in service planning and design (CQC, 2022).

Making sense of quality in the NHS

Quality and quality improvement has taken many different shapes and forms in the NHS. But as we are all too aware, the implementation of such approaches and methods has been far from straightforward. Ongoing issues and dilemmas remain with regards to whether quality and quality improvement have been able to achieve the goals and outcomes much anticipated. The following section presents a thematic summary of what we consider are the challenges and fault lines facing quality and its relationship with the NHS.

Quality ingredients without a recipe?

Despite the emphasis and attention given to quality in the NHS, problems have long been documented with regards to its adoption and spread. Reflecting on business approaches to quality improvement and 'why they are hard for the NHS to swallow', Pollitt (1996) noted the 'bolted on' nature of QI tools and approaches that were often delivered by management teams into clinical settings. Arguably we have come a long way since then with a range of evidence produced emphasising the importance of context (Fulop and Robert, 2015) and the human dimensions of change (NHS Modernisation Agency 2002) to achieve quality. But deeper questions remain regarding whether or not quality and quality improvement can achieve what its goals and methods set out to do. For example, Dixon-Woods et al (2013) found an almost universal desire to provide the best quality of care across NHS staff, along with 'bright spots' of excellent caring and practice and high-quality innovation. But these authors also identified considerable inconsistency where high-quality care was challenged by unclear goals, overlapping priorities, compliance-oriented bureaucratised management and a regulatory environment populated by multiple external bodies serving different but overlapping functions. In posing the question 'does quality improvement improve quality?', Dixon Woods and Martin (2016) draw attention the misapplication of ideas and methods, the lack of time, expertise, resources to instigate changes, as well as the limited lesson sharing of successes and failures within the NHS.

These, and many other contributions, point to the need for greater coherence and support for achieve an effective quality strategy. System-wide considerations of quality are called for that integrate macro, meso, and micro perspectives (Fulop and Ramsey, 2019). Furthermore, to build cultures of high-quality care in the NHS requires greater attention to cultural readiness, along with greater investment into improvement capabilities and accountabilities (Furnival, Boaden and Walshe, 2018; Burgess et al, 2022). Recent attention paid to 'safety II' approaches promoting strengths-based approaches to improvement represent an additional 'new horizon' for quality in the NHS (Mannion and Braithwaite, 2017). However, until policy provides the NHS with a coherent strategy to build from, the ingredients for success are likely to remain in search of a recipe to work with.

Quality strategies must also consider an increasingly challenging workplace environment for healthcare staff with unprecedented patient demand juxtaposed with workforce shortages of medical, nursing and other health and care professionals. Such issues along with poor workplace culture are contributory factors for staff burnout and stress which have been cited as impacting on quality and safety outcomes (Salyers et al, 2017). As staff experience greater levels of physical and mental exhaustion, they may depersonalise their care with less patient-centredness and suffer cognitive impairment increasing the risk of errors of commission and omission.

Quality as craft or science?

One way of analysing the changing governance of quality is to think about the forms of knowledge and expertise through quality is defined and managed, and in turn how these afford opportunities for new expert jurisdictions in the healthcare division of labour and wider research community (Waring and Bishop, 2019). Here we elaborate a distinction between the craft, science and art of quality.

We use the term 'craft' in the sense of work being based upon embodied skills that are honed through many years of problem-solving and experiential learning. Although training in abstract knowledge may provide some of the foundations to expert work, the craft of work is matured through experience. This contrast with a more rational or 'scientific' approach to work in which relatively standardised and evidence-based rules for practice are prescribed, as a type of cook-book guide to work (McDonald, Waring and Harrison, 2006). In some ways, professional practice is inherently a craft based upon years of experiential learning and the ability to apply abstract teachings to tangible problems in ways that cannot adhere to tightly prescribed rules. And yet, over the last three decades there has been a growing emphasis in evidence-based medicine (EBM) and the formulation of clear guidelines for clinical decision-making and treatment.

The definition and governance of quality interacts with such contexts. While quality improvement methods, such as PDSA cycles and process mapping, promote structured experiential learning that challenges established hierarchies of evidence rooted in positivist thinking (Berwick, 1996), the esoteric and tacit aspects of professional craft have traditionally made it difficult for non-professionals to define and assess the quality of work.

However, the growing 'science of improvement' as manifest in the burdening literature on the role of theory and robust measurement signals a new way of thinking about and governing quality. This echoes the idea that many aspects of healthcare quality can be subject to and improved through the development and adherence to formulaic step-by-step guidance. This is exemplified by the idea of the checklist. We do not want to suggest that such techniques do not improve quality or should not be adopted, rather we want to emphasise that they signal a fundamental change in the basis of understanding the quality of work from one based on craft to one based on science. However, given the inherent complexity of healthcare organisations and the variability of clinical cases questions need to be asked about the scope for cook-book methods to effectively prescribe the quality of care, and the need for localised discretion and adaptation.

The (problematic) borrowing of quality improvement methods

The contemporary rise of quality improvement is located within a wider shift in public policy associated with NPM, in which management ideas and practices drawn from private business have come to redefine the organisation and governance of public services. This broad trend is exemplified by the quality improvement where national and international agencies have promoted approaches to quality improvement more commonly found in production industries or other safety-critical sectors. Techniques such as Statistical Process Control and Plan-Do-Study-Action were initially developed in industries such as electrical engineering, as devised by the likes of Shewhart, and were developed and systematised further by Deming through his work on Japanese and US automotive industries. These are encapsulated in the idea of TQM and have since become mainstays of healthcare quality improvement. In a similar way, Toyota Production System was famously characterised by Womack and Jones as Lean Thinking and went on to transform many US hospital's such as Virginia Mason, which in turn became a global exemplar for process re-engineering. In the area of patient safety, incident reporting and investigations procedures, as well as training processes such as Crew Resource Management, were largely drawn from other safety-critical sectors such as aviation and the nuclear energy sector.

Prominent agencies, such as the Modernisation Agency and IHI, have carefully translated these techniques for application in healthcare and supported their spread and adoption by healthcare providers (Millar, 2013). Notwithstanding the importance of generalised quality improvement methodologies, questions still remain about the relevance and appropriateness of techniques that were developed and applied in largely linear production processes, rather than more complex systems where care processes and outcomes are highly variable and difficult to standardise. Research on the introduction of Lean Thinking that it can often been introduced a relatively superficial or technical way to address rather discrete problems with waste rather than as a more developed philosophy of continuous improvement (Radnor, Holweg and Waring, 2012). The implementation of Lean is also shown to disrupt established ways of working and trigger conflict and disputes in the workplace. The borrowing ideas extends beyond industry to include the adoption of approaches to community transformation and political change associated with social movement (Bate, Robert and Bevan, 2004). This has involved the development of almost prescriptive guides on how to frame arguments for change and mobilise social groups in coordinated quality improvement activities. But as shown by Waring and Crompton (2017) the use of these techniques can be used to enrol clinicians in pre-determined 'top-down' change rather than foster cultural change and willingness for clinicians in bottom-up improvement work.

The adoption of management techniques derived from non-healthcare industries may ostensibly be concerned improving quality, but the use and implementation by managers and quality improvement specialists needs to be located in the particular cultural and political history of healthcare service. By this we need to recognise that novel improvement methods typically operate on the premise of criticising long-established modes of working and governing quality and are shaped by long-established disputes and lines of power in the healthcare division of labour.

Quality and control

The rise of healthcare quality as a distinct and sustained policy issues issue plays into broader debates on the politics and power of healthcare services (Waring, 2005; Waring and Currie, 2009). There is a well-developed literature characterising healthcare organisations as complex political landscapes in which actors compete to influence how services are organised and delivery, and in which entrenched interests and institutionalised lines of power pervade the organisation of care. Much of this literature foregrounds the elevated status and power of healthcare professionals, especially medicine, in the organisation of care, with early commentators talking of medical dominance. However, the managerialisation and marketisation of care has been widely interpreted as challenging the structural interests of medicine, with managers assuming new powers and authority in the organisation of care. More recently, the shift towards collaborative governance and the growing emphasis on co-production has seen additional social actors, such as patients enter more directly into the healthcare political landscape.

The governance of quality plays directly into these wider debates. As noted before, there has been a marked shift in the governance of quality from one based primarily on professional regulation and informal collegial routines, to a system more explicitly based on management control of quality through the introduction of quality improvement techniques derived from other sectors. This shift in the governance of quality represents one of the most significant and fundamental challenges to professional power. As discussed, professional self-regulation has traditionally been premised on the idea that only those with the relevant expertise and knowledge can determine and assess the standards of care work. The introduction of quality improvement methodologies establishes new forms of expertise for defining, assessing and assuring quality based upon techniques of quality control derived from other sectors. For example, the effective introduction of Lean Thinking to healthcare requires developed expertise of the techniques in mapping operational processes, identifying and measuring different wastes, devising processes re-engineering solutions, and then implementing strategic organisational change (Waring and Bishop, 2010). Similarly, the introduction of patient safety reporting and learning systems requires advanced understanding of human factors thinking and the ability to effectively identify and analyse the causal relationships between system factors and frontline safety events. In other words, quality improvement methods introduce new ways of knowing or defining quality based on theories and corresponding procedures for controlling the sources of quality, drawing on management techniques developed outside of healthcare. Given that questions of quality have traditionally been coupled with professional expertise, this new ability to define quality from alternate sources of expertise represents a fundamental challenge to professional status and power because questions of quality fall within the jurisdiction of non-professionals.

In many instances, the borrowing and introduction of these quality improvement techniques have been initiated and lead by clinicians and non-clinicians, but have often been associated with those in specialist agencies, or in other cases they have been taken up by clinicians as a form of delegated empowerment. Both implementation approaches imply new relations of power through changing the definition and control of quality either through established new managerial hierarchies over professional work or by established managerial imperative within professional work. Either way it transforms the governance of quality and represents new expressions of control of professional work.

New abilities to define quality from alternate sources of expertise also draw attention to the ongoing and changing relationship between quality and the role of inner and outer contexts. Much continues to be made of the cultural, structural and political factors that shape quality efforts (Waring, 2022). Recent attention to trends in incident reporting showing how certain population groups, principally ethnic minorities, and those with learning disabilities, are disproportionately harmed within care systems illustrates both the potential for quality improvement to identify key trends and issues (Wade et al, 2022), but also the potential limits to quality approaches in controlling for the multitude of factors shaping care provision.

Conclusion

Quality in the NHS has taken on a range of different features and phases that are reflective of wider trends in both policy and governance. From procedures for defining and assuring quality within professional regulation, to increasingly specialised forms of quality management drawing on techniques found in other business sectors, and a raft of regulatory regimes promoting assurance, compliance, and improvement, quality in the NHS represents a complex and sedimented picture.

This chapter has provided an overview of its history and in doing so has raised important questions with regards to current approaches and the implications these have for policy and practice. As we look beyond 75 years of the NHS, this chapter also provides a platform for considering the future for quality in the NHS.

The 2019 NHS Long Term Plan launch of Integrated Care Systems (ICSs) that aims to bring health and care organisations and services together to work more effectively on a broad whole population health agenda has a remit to improve quality of care outcomes for populations. With growing evidence of variability in health and clinical outcomes across the country, particularly among underserved groups (Wade et al, 2022), clearly there is a pressing need for quality management to address disparities (PHE, 2015). Yet the contributions to quality in the NHS up to this point have been unable to provide whole-systems approaches for managing quality and facilitated quality improvement at the required scale (Braithwaite, 2018). An approach currently being advocated – a Quality Management System (QMS) – aims to support the delivery of good quality care with benefits extending beyond quality improvement to include other key components of quality; planning, control and assurance which together form a comprehensive approach to quality at all levels of an organisation or system (Shah, 2021). But given what history tells us, such an approach to implementation that ambitiously combine various elements, that engages the workforce, and achieves an appropriate balance between assurance and improvement will be far from straightforward.

References

Bate, P., Robert, G. and Bevan, H. (2004) 'The next phase of health care improvement: What can we learn from social movements?'. *Quality and Safety in Health Care*, 13, 62–66.

Bevan, G. (2011) 'Regulation and system management,' in A. Dixon and N. Mays (eds) *Understanding New Labour's Market Reforms of the English NHS*. London: The King's Fund, pp 89–111.

Berwick, D. (1996) 'A primer on leading the improvement of systems'. *BMJ*, 312, 619. DOI:10.1136/bmj.312.7031.619

Berwick, D. (2013) 'A promise to learn – a commitment to act. Improving the safety of patients in England'. https://www.gov.uk/government/publi cations/berwick-review-into-patient-safety

Braithwaite, J. (2018) 'Changing how we think about healthcare improvement'. *BMJ*, 361, k2014. https://doi.org/10.1136/bmj.k2014

Buetow, S.A. and Roland, M. (1999) 'Clinical governance: Bridging the gap between managerial and clinical approaches to quality of care'. *BMJ Quality & Safety*, 8, 184–190.

Burgess, N., Currie, G., Crump, B. and Dawson, A. (2022) *Leading Change Across a Healthcare System: How to Build Improvement Capability and Foster a Culture of Continuous Improvement*. Coventry: Warwick Business School.

Care Quality Commission. (2022) Single Assessment Framework. https://www.cqc.org.uk/about-us/how-we-will-regulate/single-assessment-framework

Dent, M. (1995) 'The new National Health Service: A case of postmodernism'. *Organization Studies*, 16, 875–899.

Department of Health. (1989) *Secretaries of State for Health, Wales, Northern Ireland and Scotland: Working for Patients*. Cm 555. London: HMSO.

Department of Health. (1997) *The New NHS: Modem, Dependable*. London: HMSO. Cm 3807.

Department of Health. (1998) *A First Class Service: Quality in the New NHS*. London: Department of Health. HSC 1998/113.

Donabedian, A. (1988) 'The quality of care. How can it be assessed?'. *JAMA*, 260, 12, 1743–1748.

Dixon-Woods, M., Baker, R., Charles, K., Dawson, J., Jerzembek, G., Martin, G. et al (2013) 'Culture and behaviour in the English National Health Service: overview of lessons from a large multimethod study'. *BMJ Quality & Safety*, 23, 2, 106–115.

Dixon-Woods, M. and Martin, G. (2016) 'Does quality improvement improve quality?'. *Future Hosp Journal*, 3, 3, 191–194.

Exworthy, M., Gabe, J., Jones, I.R. and Smith, G. (2019) 'Professional autonomy and surveillance: The case of public reporting in cardiac surgery'. *Sociology of Health and Illness*, 41: 1040–1055.

Friedson, E. (1970) *The Profession of Medicine*. Chicago: University of Chicago Press.

Fulop, N. and Robert, G. (2015) *Context for Successful Quality Improvement*. London: The Health Foundation. https://www.health.org.uk/publicati ons/context-for-successful-quality-improvement

Fulop, N. and Ramsay. A. (2019) 'How organisations contribute to improving the quality of healthcare'. *BMJ*, 365, 1773.

Furnival, J., Boaden, R. and Walshe, K. (2018) 'Assessing improvement capability in healthcare organisations: A qualitative study of healthcare regulatory agencies in the UK'. *International Journal for Quality in Health Care* , 30, 9, 715–723.

Ham, C., Berwick, D. and Dixon, J. (2016) *Improving Quality in the English NHS: A Strategy for Action*. London: The King's Fund.

Harrison, S. and Pollitt, C. (1994) *Controlling Health Professionals: The Future of Work and Organisation in the NHS*. Buckingham: Open University Press.

Haslam, D. (2007) 'What is the Healthcare Commission trying to achieve?'. *Journal of the Royal Society of Medicine*, 100, 1, 15–18.

Health Foundation, The. (2021) *Quality Improvement Made Simple: What Everyone Should Know About Health Care Quality Improvement*. London: Health Foundation. https://www.health.org.uk/publications/quality-improvem ent-made-simple

Institute of Medicine. (2001) *Crossing the Quality Chasm: A New Health Care System for the 21st Century*. Washington, DC: National Academy Press.

Joss, R. and Kogan, M. (1995) *Advancing Quality: Total Quality Management in the National Health Service*. Buckingham: Open University Press.

Kings Fund, The. (2023) 'Leading through Covid-19: supporting health and care leaders in unprecedented times'. https://www.kingsfund.org.uk/ projects/leading-through-covid-19

Knight, M. and Stanford, S. (2022) 'Ockenden: Another shocking review of maternity services'. *BMJ*, 377, o898. DOI:10.1136/bmj.o898

Lalani, M. and Hogan H. (2021) 'A narrative account of the key drivers in the development of the Learning from Deaths policy'. *Journal of Health Services Research & Policy*, 26, 4, 263–271.

Lalani, M., Morgan, S., Basu, A. and Hogan, H. (2022) 'Understanding the factors influencing implementation of a new national patient safety policy in England: Lessons from "learning from deaths"'. *Journal of Health Services Research and Policy*, 28, 1, 50–57.

Leape, L.L. (1994) 'Error in medicine'. *JAMA*, 26, 4, 263–271.

Mannion, R., Blenkinsopp, J., Powell, M., McHale, J., Millar, R., Snowden, N. et al (2018) 'Understanding the knowledge gaps in whistleblowing and speaking up in health care: Narrative reviews of the research literature and formal inquiries, a legal analysis and stakeholder interviews'. *Health and Social Care Delivery Research* , 6, 30.

Mannion, R. and Braithwaite, J. (2017) 'False dawns and new horizons in patient safety research and practice'. *International Journal of Health Policy and Management*, 6, 12, 685–689.

Mannion, R., Goddard, M. and Bate, A. (2007) 'Aligning incentives and motivations in health care: The case of earned autonomy'. *Financial Accountability and Management*, 23, 4, 401–420.

Maxwell, R.J. (1992) 'Dimensions of quality revisited: From thought to action'. *Quality in Health Care*, 1, 3, 171–177. DOI: 10.1136/qshc.1.3.171

McDonald, R., Waring, J. and Harrison, S. (2006) 'Rules, safety and the narrativzation of identity: A hospital operating theatre case study'. *Sociology of Health and Illness*, 28, 2, 178–202.

McNulty, T. and Ferlie, E. (2002) *Reengineering Healthcare: The Complexities of Organisational Transformation*. Oxford: Oxford University Press.

McNulty, T. and Ferlie, E. (2004) 'Process transformation: Limitations to radical organizational change within public service organizations'. *Organization Studies*, 25, 8, 1389–1412.

Millar, R. (2013) 'Framing quality improvement tools and techniques in healthcare: The case of Improvement Leaders' Guides'. *Journal of Health Organization and Management*, 27, 2, 209–224.

Millar, R., Avery Aunger, J., Rafferty, A.M., Greenhalgh, J., Mannion, R., McLeod, H. and Faulks, D. (2023) 'Towards achieving interorganisational collaboration between health–care providers: A realist evidence synthesis'. *Health and Social Care Delivery Research*, 27, 2, 209–223.

Miller, R. and Millar, R. (2017) *Partnering for Improvement: Inter-organisational Developments in the NHS*. Birmingham: The Health Foundation & Health Services Management Centre, University of Birmingham.

Molloy, A., Martin, S. and Gardner, T. (2016) 'A clear road ahead: Creating a coherent quality strategy for the English NHS'. The Health Foundation.

Nadeem, E., Olin, S.S., Hill, L.C., Hoagwood, K.E. and Horwitz, S.M. (2013) 'Understanding the components of quality improvement collaboratives: A systematic literature review'. *Milbank Quarterly*, 91, 2, 354–394.

NHS Modernisation Agency. (2002) 'Managing the human dimensions of change'. https://www.england.nhs.uk/improvement-hub/wp-content/uploads/sites/44/2017/11/ILG-3.4-Managing-the-Human-Dimensions-of-Change.pdf

NHS Resolution. (2022) 'NHS Resolution, annual report, and accounts'. https://resolution.nhs.uk/wp-content/uploads/2022/07/NHS-Resolution-Annual-report-and-accounts-2021_22_Access.pdf

Pollitt, C. (1993) 'The struggle for quality: The case of the National Health Service'. *Policy and Politics*, 21, 3, 161–170.

Pollitt, C. (1996) 'Business approaches to quality improvement: Why they are hard for the NHS to swallow'. *Quality of Health Care*, 5, 2, 104–110.

Powell, M. (2019) 'Learning from NHS inquiries: Comparing the recommendations of the Ely, Bristol and Mid Staffordshire inquiries'. *The Political Quarterly*, 90, 229–237.

Public Health England. (2015) *The NHS Atlas of Variation in Healthcare: Reducing Unwarranted Variation to Increase Value and Improve Quality*. Public Health England.

Radnor, Z., Holweg, M. and Waring, J. (2012) 'Lean in healthcare: An unfulfilled promise'. *Social Science and Medicine*, 74, 3, 364–371.

Rosenthal, M. (1995) *The Incompetent Doctor: Behind Closed Doors*. Philadelphia: Open University Press.

Salyers, M.P., Bonfils, K.A., Luther, L., Firmin, R.L., White, D.A., Adams, E.L. et al (2017) 'The relationship between professional burnout and quality and safety in healthcare: A meta-analysis'. *Journal of General Internal Medicine*, 32, 4, 475–482. DOI: 10.1007/s11606-016-3886-9

Scally, G. and Donaldson, L.J. (1998) 'Clinical governance and the drive for quality improvement in the new NHS in England'. *BMJ*, 317, 61–65.

Shah, A. (2020) 'Emerging quality management system in the NHS: How to move beyond quality improvement projects'. *BMJ*, 370, m2319. DOI:10.1136/bmj.m2319

Shah, A. (2021) 'Quality in the design of integrated care systems, NHS Providers'. https://nhsproviders.org/news-blogs/blogs/quality-in-the-design-of-integrated-care-systems

Smith, J. (2004) *The Shipman Inquiry: Fifth Report: Safeguarding Patients: Lessons from the Past-Proposals for the Future*. Presented to Parliament by the Secretary of State for the Home Department and the Secretary of State for Health by Command of Her Majesty, December 2004. London: The Stationery Office.

Street, A. (2002) 'The resurrection of hospital mortality statistics in England'. *Journal of Health Services Research and Policy*, 7, 2, 104–110.

Vindrola-Padros, C., Ledger, J., Hill, M., Tomini, S., Spencer, J. and Fulop, N.J. (2022) 'The special measures for quality and challenged provider regimes in the English NHS: A rapid evaluation of a national improvement initiative for failing healthcare organisations'. *International Journal of Health Policy and Management*, 11, 12, 2917–2926.

van Dael, J., Reader, T.W., Gillespie, A.T., Freise, L., Darzi, A. and Mayer, E.K. (2022) 'Do national policies for complaint handling in English hospitals support quality improvement? Lessons from a case study'. *Journal of the Royal Society of Medicine*, 31 May (online ahead of print). DOI:1410768221098247

Wade, C., Malhotra, A.M., McGuire, P., Vincent, C. and Fowler, A. (2022) 'Action on patient safety can reduce health inequalities'. *BMJ*, 376, e067090.

Walshe, K. (1999) 'Improvement through inspection? The development of the new Commission for Health Improvement in England and Wales'. *Quality in Health Care*, 8, 3, 191–201.

Walshe, K. (2001) 'Offen NA very public failure: Lessons for quality improvement in healthcare organisations from the Bristol Royal Infirmary'. *BMJ Quality & Safety*, 10, 250–256.

Walshe, K., Boyd, A., Bryce, M., Luscombe, K., Tazzyman, A., Tredinnick-Rowe, J. et al (2017) 'Implementing medical revalidation in the United Kingdom: Findings about organisational changes and impacts from a survey of responsible officers'. *Journal of the Royal Society of Medicine*, 110, 1, 23–30.

Waring, J. (2005) 'Patient safety: New directions in the management of healthcare quality'. *Policy and Politics*, 33, 4, 675–692.

Waring, J. and Bishop, S. (2010) 'Lean healthcare: Rhetoric, ritual, resistance'. *Social Science and Medicine*, 71, 7, 1332–1340.

Waring, J. and Bishop, S. (2019) 'Safety and professions: Strange or natural bedfellows', in J. Le Coze (ed) *Safety Science Research*. London: Taylor & Francis and CRC Press, pp 133–149.

Waring, J., Bishop, S., Black, G., Clarke, G., Exworthy, M., Fulop, J. et al (2022) 'Understanding the political skills of leading the implementation of health services change: a qualitative interview study'. *International Journal of Health Policy and Management*, 11, 11, 2686–2697. DOI: 10.34172/ijhpm.2022.6564

Waring, J. and Crompton, A. (2017) 'A "movement for improvement"? A qualitative study of the adoption of social movement strategies in the implementation of a quality improvement campaign'. *Sociology of Health and Illness*, 39, 1083–1099.

Waring, J. and Currie, G. (2009) 'Managing expert knowledge: Organizational challenge and managerial futures for the UK medical profession'. *Organization Studies*, 30, 7, 755–778.

World Health Organization (WHO). (2022) WHO Quality Toolkit. https://qualityhealthservices.who.int/quality-toolkit/qt-

WHO. (2023) Quality of Care. https://www.who.int/health-topics/quality-of-care#tab=tab_1

8

Improving health and tackling health inequalities: what role for the NHS?

Martin Powell and Mark Exworthy

Introduction

Like many other health systems, the NHS has been regarded as more like a sickness than a health service, failing to place health before healthcare, and to focus 'upstream' on the 'social determinants of health' (SDH) (for example, Wanless 2002; Marmot and Wilkinson, 2005; Hunter 2016a). This has implications for both aggregate health and health inequalities. First, while life expectancy in the UK in the twentieth century increased 38 years for men and women, equivalent to an increase of 4½ months per year (ONS, 2015), much of this improvement in life expectancy and health status more generally, is associated with the SDH (Marmot, 2010). It has been estimated that only 10–25 per cent of the health of a developed population is attributable to the healthcare system (McGinnis, Williams-Russo and Knickman, 2002: 83; Harrison and McDonald, 2008: 165). However, only 'around 5% of the total UK government healthcare expenditure' is devoted to preventive healthcare, with about half of NHS staff not regarding prevention as a core part of the work of their organisation (Faculty of Public Health, 2019; see also Exworthy and Morcillo, 2019).

Second, the temporal pattern for health inequalities is more complex. There has long been a recognition of health inequalities in terms of geographical and social class differences in life expectancy since at least the Chadwick Report 1842 (for example, Bambra, 2016). However, while overall health, in terms of life expectancy, broadly increased for much of the twentieth and early twenty first century before stalling or reversing in recent years (Marmot et al 2020a), health inequalities have increased at some times and reduced at others. For example, according to Robinson et al (2019), absolute inequalities in the infant mortality rate (IMR) increased between the most deprived local authorities and the rest of England between 1983–1998, decreased during the period of the English health inequalities strategy (1999–2010), but increased again in the period 2011–2017.

This chapter will thus examine the ways in which the NHS has addressed the issue of health and health inequalities. First, it focuses on four chronological periods of policies on health and health inequalities in the 75 years of the NHS. Then, it explores health and health inequalities through the four analytical lenses introduced in Chapter 1, before moving to evaluate policies concerned with health and health inequalities.

Health and health inequalities in the NHS

This section examines health and health inequalities in the 75 years of the NHS, which for heuristic purposes is divided into four periods.

The 'classic' NHS (1948–1979)

The Coalition Government White Paper, *A National Health Service* (Ministry of Health 1944) advocated a comprehensive 'health' service, aiming to reduce ill-health and promote good health for all citizens (1944: 5). The NHS Act stated that: 'It shall be the duty of the Minister of Health … to promote the establishment … of a comprehensive health service designed to secure improvement in the physical and mental health of the people … and the prevention, diagnosis and treatment of illness' (quoted in Harrison and McDonald 2008: 15).

The structure of the 'classic' NHS was based on the 'tri-partite system' of hospitals under appointed boards, local practitioner services under Executive Councils, leaving public health as local authority responsibility. However, in the 1974 NHS Reorganisation Act, local public health responsibilities were given to the NHS (Powell, 1997).

It was hardly surprising that the 1948 reforms established a national hospital service or a national illness service rather than a national health service (Klein, 2013). The early years of the NHS saw a broad change from concerns about dealing with 'old' diseases (for example, infectious diseases such as TB) to 'new' or 'lifestyle' diseases such as those associated with smoking (Berridge, 2016), and latterly, obesity.

While the NHS inherited an unequal distribution of facilities and despite equity being a principle of the NHS (Powell, 1997), the early years saw few concrete policies to reduce inequalities. This may be partly because health inequalities were seen as less of a policy 'problem' at that time. One expression of this might be life expectancy, as Hiam, Dorling and McKee demonstrate: 'In 1952, when Queen Elizabeth II came to the throne, the UK had one of the longest life expectancies (as measured from birth) in the world' [namely 69.5 years for both sexes] (2023: 89).

Then, the UK ranked 7th in the world for life expectancy; by 2021, the UK ranked 29th (up from 36th the year before).

One major problem is that 'inequality' can mean many different things. Powell and Exworthy (2003) present an equality matrix. First, we need to differentiate between inequalities in health (outcome) and healthcare. Second, there are many different types of equality in healthcare such as equal provision (for example, beds per capita) and equal use (such as visits to GP). Third, it is possible to focus on different 'groups' such as social class or residents of geographical areas. Fourth, equality is different to equity, which involves taking need into account. For example, should provision in the form of beds per capita be the same across the country, or higher in areas of higher need? In short, there are many different aspects to 'equality' and the NHS has paid differential attention to these over different periods. Geographical inequality was perhaps the easiest type to recognise and to address (Powell and Exworthy, 2003). In primary care, the Designated Area Policy (DAP) was concerned with equalising the provision of general practitioners across the country through restricting entry to the 'over-doctored' areas and providing incentives to attract doctors to the 'under-doctored' areas. In secondary care, the 1962 Hospital Plan aimed to achieve geographical equality through a series of planning norms (such as 3.3 acute beds per 1,000 population) (Powell, 1997). The 1971 Crossman formula aimed to remove regional inequalities in the hospital service within 10 years. However, this was overtaken by the Resource Allocation Working Party (RAWP) (DHSS, 1976) which sought achieve 'equal access to health care for equal need' (that is, equity) by redistributing hospital resources from London to other parts of the country.

In terms of client groups, a series of scandals and inquiries led to a series of Green Papers promising 'better deals' for the 'Cinderella' groups such as 'the mentally ill' and 'the mentally handicapped' (Powell, 1997). Similarly, the 'Priorities' document of 1976 was largely 'a vocabulary of exhortation' (Klein, 2013: 92).

Finally, health inequalities (outcomes) between social classes were recognised with the Labour government setting up a committee under Sir Douglas Black. While the 'Black Report' (DHSS, 1980) led to significant academic attention, it resulted in little policy response. This was partly because it reported to the newly elected Thatcher Conservative government, which gave a cool reception to its call for government spending and redistribution. Black (1980) identified four potential explanations for health inequalities: artefactual explanations; natural or social selection; materialist or structuralist explanations; and cultural or behavioural explanations. It placed most weight on materialist or structural, which should be addressed by government intervention. This was largely to be echoed in a series of subsequent reports (for examle Acheson, 1998; Marmot, 2010; Marmot et al, 2020a).

Conservative governments (1979–1997)

The Thatcher Conservative governments (1979–1990) endorsed a range of screening, promotion and education measures, and commissioned an inquiry into public health that led to changed elements of public health administration, including the appointment of directors of public health in each Health Authority who were required to produce an annual report on public health. The Major Conservative Government (1990–1997) produced 'The Health of the Nation' strategy (DH, 1992) with targets for coronary heart disease and stroke, cancer, mental illness, accidents, HIV/AIDS and sexual health (Hunter, Fulop and Warner, 2000).

Klein (2013: 166) regarded this as a 'new health policy paradigm which … had its roots in the nineteenth century'. In short, the government acknowledged that it had responsibilities for the health of the population that went beyond the provision of a healthcare system. It set out 25 specific policy targets: for example, by the year 2000, the death rate for coronary heart disease and stroke in people under 65 was to be reduced by at least 40 per cent. However, it did not discuss structural factors such as income inequality and unemployment, and the targets appeared to be largely based on an extrapolation of past trends, designed to make sure that the Government would be able to congratulate itself on progress made. Significantly, it did not mention health inequalities, or 'health variations' as they were termed (Graham, 2000).

Labour governments (1997–2010)

The 'New' Labour government introduced a range of policy initiatives were introduced with the aim of improving health, preventing illness and reducing health inequalities (Hunter, 2003, 2016a). Among other initiatives, it implemented a series of Action Zones ('area-based initiatives to reduce the effects of persistent disadvantage' (Bauld et al, 2005), created the post of Minister of Public Health, introduced a new anti-smoking strategy (including a ban on tobacco advertising) and created an independent Food Standards Agency. Much of this policy direction was framed as 'joined-up government' (Exworthy and Hunter, 2011).

Soon after their election, the Labour government published green and white papers on public health (DH 1998, 1999) which set targets to reduce disease and illness in cancer, heart disease and stroke, mental illness and accidents. 'Our Healthier Nation' (DH, 1998) set out a 'third way' between the old extremes of individual victim blaming and 'nanny state' social engineering. While the green paper rejected health inequalities targets, the White Paper did set the first health inequalities targets for England. The government also commissioned the Acheson Report on Inequalities in

Health (Acheson, 1998; Exworthy, 2002), a successor to the Black Report two decades earlier. In keeping with the SDH perspective, only three of the 39 recommendations related to the NHS. In terms of the NHS itself, the NHS Plan (DH, 2000) focused on increasing capacity and tackling waiting lists. It also contained a chapter on improving health and reducing inequalities (Hunter, 2003: 64) which, *inter alia*, had the aim of 'reducing inequalities in access to NHS services'.

Public health continued to feature in Labour's second term. The Wanless Reports (2002, 2004), commissioned by the Treasury, argued that the future growth of health expenditure could be curbed through public health measures, particularly those aimed by changing individual lifestyles. They outlined three possible spending scenarios for healthcare up to 2022–2023: slow uptake, solid progress and fully engaged, depending on assumptions about the effectiveness of NHS performance and the health status of the population, with fully engaged the most ambitious and resource-efficient and slow uptake the least satisfactory and most expensive scenario. Yet, Wanless (2004) noted that, despite numerous policy statements and initiatives in the field of public health, they have not resulted in a rebalancing of policy away from healthcare ('a national sickness service') to health ('a national health service'). Timmin's (2021, p 90) argued that the Wanless report was the 'only serious attempt by any government since 1948 to make an independent assessment of the NHS's likely future needs, and likely cost, over the next 20 years'.

The White Paper, 'Choosing Health' (DH, 2004), focused on the causes of ill-health, although the key strategy stressed providing information and support to enable individuals to make healthy choices for themselves. Hunter (2016b) noted that the neo-liberal principles stressing individual lifestyle issues in 'Choosing Health' received further endorsement in July 2006 in a speech on public health delivered by Prime Minister Tony Blair, arguing that 'our public health problems are not, strictly speaking, public health questions at all. They are questions of individual lifestyles'.

In a systematic review of the effectiveness of the Labour's National Health Inequality Strategy, which was conducted in England between 1999 and 2010, Holroyd et al (2022) considered that it was broadly successful. They noted that the national targets were based on relative, rather than absolute, inequalities. They explain that absolute inequalities measure the numerical gap between groups, while relative inequalities measure the percentage difference between groups, and that there is a debate that exists as to which of these is the most appropriate measure of inequality. They concluded that the strategy met the infant mortality target, while the life expectancy target was reached for men but not women. Absolute health inequalities in life expectancy, mortality, infant mortality and multiple major causes of death reduced, but evidence there was less available for relative inequalities.

Similarly, Robinson et al (2019) concluded that the English health inequalities strategy period was associated with a decline in geographical inequalities in the IMR, which adds to the evidence base suggesting that it was at least partially effective in reducing health inequalities.

Coalition and Conservative governments (2010–2023)

This final period is marked by the Conservative/ Liberal Democrat Coalition and government (2010–2015) and Conservative governments (head by Cameron, May, Johnson, Truss and Sunak) (2015–2023). Across this period, three issues have dominated policy making: austerity policies (from 2010), the Brexit referendum (2016) and COVID-19 pandemic (from 2020). The cumulative effect is that, although only one of the three 'shocks' is external to government, politicians and policy makers have concluded that they afford limited scope to focus on health inequalities and public health.

The translation of the White Paper 'Equity into Excellence' (Secretary of State for Health, 2010a) into the Health and Social Care Act 2012 was one of the most controversial journeys in the history of the NHS (see Exworthy, Mannion and Powell, 2016). However, much less attention was paid to its public health elements. The Act devoted a chapter to 'improving healthcare outcomes'. In the name of 'Local democratic legitimacy' (Hunter, 2016b: 34), it transferred the public health functions to local authorities, essentially restoring the 1948 model. However, local authorities had seen their budgets halved between 2010 and 2017 (Lewer and Bibby, 2021).

The government proposed at the national level a dedicated new public health service (Public Health England (PHE)) that would support local innovation, help provide disease control and protection and spread information on the latest innovations from around the world. It was claimed by the government that the White Paper responded to Marmot (2010), adopting its life course framework for tackling the wider SDH.

Soon after his appointment as NHS Chief Executive, Simon Stevens introduced a plan for the future direction of the NHS – the 'NHS Five Year Forward View'. It estimated that the NHS was spending about £10 billion a year on diabetes. Yet again, it stressed the importance of moving the balance of the NHS away from the ill-health towards health improvement (NHS England, 2014: 9).

National policy was to be supported by work with industry and other partners to promote healthy lifestyles. However, concerns were expressed about this voluntary approach to health improvements, rather than a regulatory approach. This tension between state interventions (commonly referred to as the 'nanny state') and 'lifestyle drift'; regulation and taxation have often thus been avoided previously in favour of an emphasis on individual decision-making (Popay, Whitehead and Hunter, 2010). However, the government announced the soft drinks industry levy, often known as the sugar tax, in 2016, which was implemented in 2018. The recommendations of the Dimbleby review (2021) had initially been accepted by government but as of early 2023, there is little sign of action.

The Johnson government (2019–2022) emphasised an agenda of 'levelling up', an ill-defined set of strategies to address regional inequality, but this only generated a rather vague White Paper in April 2022 (Secretary of State for Levelling Up, Housing and Communities, 2022). To date, the rhetoric of addressing such inequality, with strong resonance in health inequalities, has not yet materialised into a comprehensive policy agenda, and was hampered by the political chaos of 2022.

In late 2021, following the government's criticisms of PHE's handling of aspects of the COVID-19 pandemic (Bambra, Lynch and Smith, 2021), the Secretary of State for Health decided, without consultation, to replace it with two new bodies – the UK Health Security Agency (UKHSA) and the Office for Health Improvement and Disparities (OHID). Among its responsibilities, OHID (which is located within the DHSC) will be expected to develop cross-government working to develop a 'health in all policies' approach in tackling the social determinants of health. A White Paper on tackling 'health disparities' had been promised but was been delayed a number of times. In January 2023, the government responded to a written question by announcing that it would not be 'As material for the Major Conditions Strategy will therefore cover many of the same areas as the Health Disparities White Paper, we will no longer be publishing it' (Neil O'Brien, 2023).

Nightingale and Merrifield (2023) bemoan this decision as it echoes similar developments in policy towards tackling smoking and obesity. 'While the content of the major conditions strategy is still taking shape, it does seem that action to reduce inequalities and improve long-term health has been sidelined for more visible, immediate outcomes.'

Specifically, it feeds an agenda which tends to favour treatment within the NHS (rather than public health measures).

Notwithstanding the fitful progress of policy, three policy developments might denote some positive signs for tackling inequalities. First, a series of city and regional mayors have given renewed impetus to regional devolution in England. This is perhaps most advanced in Greater Manchester where the so-called 'devo Manc' initiative has also included health and social care. Indeed, this was a stated aim of the policy in 2018, namely 'to improve health outcomes and reduce health inequalities both within Greater Manchester and between Greater Manchester and other areas of England' (Walshe et al, 2018: 18).

Second, there have been numerous local initiatives, partly inspired by the shift towards integration and Devo Manc, which have sought to inculcate health promoting agendas across local (statutory) agencies. Within a national framework of 'Core20Plus5' (indicating the most deprived 20 per cent of the population and five key areas), local agencies have been given autonomy to address local inequalities (Lewis, Buck and Wenzel, 2022). The Marmot reports (2010, 2020a, b) have also inspired cities such as Manchester and Coventry to address the SDH (Marmot, 2021).

Finally, in April 2022, the Health and Care Bill was enacted, leading to the introduction of 42 Integrated Care Systems (ICSs) in England in July 2022. The government claimed that such integration would enable 'greater ambition on tackling health inequalities and the wider determinants of health' (Department of Health & Social Care, 2021, para. 1.9, 9). Evidence of this remains illusory (Glasby and Miller, 2020).

Analytical lenses and health and health inequalities

Hierarchies, markets and networks

It has generally been claimed that the NHS has displayed features of (quasi) hierarchies, markets and networks (Chapter 1). It could be argued that all these have tended to marginalise the attention given to health and health inequalities. First, in a hierarchy, attention has tended to focus on 'P45 targets' (whereby failure to meet targets might mean job loss for senior NHS managers) such as waiting lists rather than long-term issues such as health and health inequalities (Exworthy, Berney and Powell, 2002). 'Policy making by exhortation' (Klein, 2013) produced few tangible outcomes. Put another way, the 'great expectations' of central policy documents were dashed with a weak transmission belt linking centre with periphery. To develop Bevan's phrase, dropped bedpans at local level associated with health and health inequalities made little noise in the Palace of Westminster.

While 'planning' led to some reduction of unequal healthcare in a geographical context (such as the Hospital Plan and RAWP), broader impacts on health and health inequalities were limited. Despite the rhetorical stress on networks (outlined next), it can be argued that the 'New Public Management' (NPM) variant of 'targets and terror' and performance indicators (for example, Ferlie) led to reductions in waiting times (Propper et al, 2008). However, the success of targets for health inequalities was less clear, partly because it was difficult to hold a single agency accountable for meeting them (Klein, 2013: 242–243; see next).

Second, networks offered more promise in theoretical terms as partners inside and outside the NHS could work together to improve health. Labour's 'Third Way' initially seemed to stress the NHS as network stressing collaboration and partnership. However, 'joined up government' has always remained elusive with problems of both horizontal (at central and local levels) and vertical coordination (Exworthy and Hunter, 2011).

A high-profile policy of the Labour government was Health Action Zones which were supposed to work across organisational boundaries in a defined geographical area for seven years in order to tackle engrained health inequalities. Sixty-four areas were given HAZ status (and about £4–5 million each) in 1998 and 1999 (Bauld et al, 2005). However, the HAZ scheme was no longer running by 2003, effectively only half way through their planned lifespan. Bauld et al (2005) conclude that HAZs had relatively limited impact, partly due to the 'difficult circumstances' into which they were implemented.

Finally, market competition was always unlikely to produce results as it was difficult to place health and health inequalities in 'contracts'. The Labour government moved from its earlier stress on networks towards markets. In terms of health and health inequalities, this was expressed in terms of 'choice' and an increasing focus on placing responsibilities on individuals, as suggested in the title of their 'Choosing Health' White Paper (DH, 2004). For the coalition government, the White Paper (Secretary of State for Health, 2010a) discussed the problem of poor health outcomes in a comparative sense, but did not state how the solution of greater competition would address the issue.

Public and private

While the 'curative' element of the NHS remains largely 'public', many of SDH are outside the NHS. This means that 'market power' and the level of de-commodification are important determinants of health (Maani, Petticrew and Galea, 2022). Put another way, the 'island of equality' of the NHS is set within a wider sea of inequality.

Nevertheless, the 'three-dimensional' approach (ownership, finance, and regulation) of the mixed economy of welfare literature may have some validity. First, it suggests the importance of regulation (or lack of regulation). Powerful vested interests such as food, alcohol and tobacco industries have often stymied policy to tackle public health. Many governments tend to stress 'self' regulation or voluntary codes of practice. However, some curbs have been apparent such as those on smoking, sugar tax and a minimum unit pricing for alcohol in Scotland (Hunter, 2016a; Chapter 4).

Centralisation and decentralisation

In the case of public health, issues of centralisation and decentralisation are most evident in relation to elected local authorities and appointed Health Authorities (and their successor organisations). Until 1974, public health was the remit of elected local authorities. The 1974 reorganisation transferred these functions to the appointed Health Authorities. Whereas the 1982 NHS reform stressed devolution, the 1991 quasi-market reforms stressed 'authority'.

There was some centralisation under New Labour, with new central institutions such as 'National Service Frameworks' and the 'National Institute of Clinical Excellence' and 'command and control' or 'targets and terror', but these were more concerned with secondary care than with public health. Political devolution in 1999 saw health becoming the responsibility of the nations of the UK, resulting in (more) 'intra-UK health system divergence' (Hunter, 2016a: 129).

The Lansley reforms (coalition government) effectively restored public health to its pre-1974 position. They aimed to 'liberate' the NHS from excessive central control. Critics wondered if devolving responsibility for public health to local authorities would undermine a national approach to improving health and tackling health inequalities. However, it has been argued that while the language and rhetoric was localist, proposals such as the national outcomes framework tended to be top-down and prescriptive (Hunter, 2016b). The same reforms created a new national agency of Public Health England. In 2015 Manchester was handed powers over its health and healthcare systems (Walshe et al, 2018). In short, Klein stated that 'successive Health Secretaries have adopted the rhetoric of decentralisation and localism' (2013: 312–313), which reached its highest pitch in 2010, but many have 'professed devolution while practising centralisation'.

Professional and managerial

At first glance, this professional-managerial axis has less relevance to public health and health inequalities. The government claimed that its reforms would: 'empower professionals and providers, giving them more autonomy and, in return, making them more accountable for the results they achieve, accountable to patients through choice and accountable to the public at local level' (Secretary of State for Health 2010a, para. 6.0).

Also, while individual clinician decisions need not be abstracted from the patient's social context, the inverse care law implies that those most in need are least likely to access care (Hart, 1971). However, clinicians are often faced with practical impediments in terms of addressing health inequalities when faced with patient need in their clinical consultations (Exworthy and Morcillo, 2019).

Organisationally, public health functions were, from 1974–2013, located in Health Authorities (and successors). While this gave public health an apparently pivotal role in the commissioning process (from 1991), it was also arguably detached from the main levers which influenced the SDH. This might be explained by the once-dominant position of the medical profession within public health (Evans, 2003). The transfer of public health functions to local authorities in 2013 disrupted this as (multidisciplinary) public health staff had to work within a non-medical, more political environment of local authorities (Brackley, Tuck and Exworthy, 2021; Evans, 2021).

Evaluation of health and health inequalities

There has been much debate on evaluating the performance of the NHS (for example, Dayan et al, 2018) and whether it is 'the best in the world' (for example, Marino and Papanicolas, forthcoming). Our three broad lenses are temporal, intrinsic and extrinsic evaluation (Chapter 1; Powell, 1997). Temporal evaluation focuses on changes over time: are health and health inequalities improving or deteriorating over time? Intrinsic evaluation compares the NHS to its stated objectives: for example, has it lived up to its founding principles associated with health and health inequalities? Extrinsic evaluation compares the NHS to other healthcare systems: for example, how do health and health inequalities diagnosis compare to other nations?

Temporal evaluation

It can be argued that 'health' certainly in terms of life expectancy and mortality rates (such as the infant mortality rate) have improved over the period of the NHS (see next). However, there are some caveats to this very broad conclusion. First, increases in life expectancy seem to have stalled at best and reversed at worst in recent years (see as follows). Second, while the length of life has increased, it is more difficult to come to clear conclusions about 'health' or the quality of life. Third, it is unclear how much of these changes can be attributed to the NHS in a narrow sense or public policy in a broader sense.

The picture is even less clear for health inequalities. As noted earlier (see Powell and Exworthy, 2003), both inequalities in healthcare and inequalities in outcomes are multifaceted. One of the arguments for the NHS in the 1940s was to reduce inequalities in healthcare. As argued earlier, there was limited progress on this until the 1970s when different types of healthcare inequalities were recognised, with some being addressed more successfully than others. Geographical inequalities were perhaps the easiest to recognise and address. However, while the post-RAWP geographical allocation has broadly decreased geographical inequality for secondary care, some primary care services, particularly GPs and dentists, still display significant geographical inequality.

Inequalities of outcome have proved to be intractable. Marmot et al (2020a) pointed out that ten years after the Marmot Review (2010) that life expectancy in England had stalled, years in ill-health had increased and inequalities in health had widened. The report continued that the social gradient in disability-free life expectancy is steeper than the gradient in life expectancy. They explained that the intervening period saw 'momentous social, economic and political changes' with ten years of austerity policies and rolling back the state resulting in widespread reductions in public spending and intervention in almost all areas that in turn impacted on the health of the population and on health inequalities in England; 'continued unchecked, they will have detrimental impacts in the future' (Marmot Review, 2010: 11).

Marmot et al (2020b: 13) argued that COVID-19 further revealed and amplified inequalities in health. They pointed out that there was a clear pattern to COVID-19 in terms of deprivation at regional and local authority levels, occupation (being in a key worker role, unable to work from home and being in close proximity to others), living conditions (for example, overcrowded living conditions and poor quality housing) and ethnicity (Black, Asian and Minority Ethnic (BAME) groups higher than White persons). Moreover, risks of mortality were cumulative: being male, older, and BAME with an underlying health condition, working in a higher risk occupation and living in deprived area in overcrowded housing led to much higher rates of mortality and reflect lifetime experience.

Intrinsic evaluation

Intrinsic evaluation is problematic as the NHS has rather vague and unclear aims and objectives regarding health and health inequalities. According to Klein (1982), in so far as there has any clearly stated objectives which might be used as NHS criteria of performance they are 'to secure improvement in the physical and mental health of the people' and 'in the prevention, diagnosis and treatment of illness' in the words of the 1946 Act creating the Service. However, the Royal Commission on the NHS (1979) was forced to conclude that this question was strictly unanswerable. The Royal Commission then set out its own objectives (para. 2.6) which are arguably equally problematic.

While the 1944 White Paper and 1946 NHS Act broadly mentioned health, there is little in terms of health inequalities. Moreover, in addition to vague aims, means or mechanisms are also unclear. It was broadly considered that making services free at the point of delivery would make them equitable. While there were some fairly weak mechanisms such as the Designated Area Policy for GPs, clearer and stronger mechanisms only really emerged from the 1970s onwards.

Extrinsic evaluation

Dayan et al (2018) set out to address their question of 'how good is the NHS' by comparing it with its peers of 18 healthcare systems in countries belonging to the same categories of high-income, industrialised countries as the UK. They found that its main weakness were healthcare outcomes, with the UK appearing to perform less well than similar countries on the overall rate at which people die when successful medical care could have saved their lives. They noted that while the gap closed over the last decade for stroke and several forms of cancer, the mortality rate in the UK among people treated for some of the biggest causes of death, including cancer, heart attacks and stroke, is higher than average among comparable countries. Moreover, the UK also had high rates of child mortality around birth.

Other studies broadly confirm that the UK tends to compare poorly to other healthcare systems in terms of outcomes such as mortality and life expectancy. For example, Papanicolas et al (2019) explored the healthcare systems of the UK and nine high-income comparator countries with 79 indicators across seven domains: population and healthcare coverage, healthcare and social spending, structural capacity, utilisation, access to care, quality of care, and population health. In terms of population health, life expectancy at birth in the UK was just below the average of the comparator countries (81.3 years versus study average of 81.7 years). Moreover, life expectancy in the UK had been below the average over the past 20 years, although the gap narrowed over the period 2008–2013 to a low of 0.3 years, increased over 2014–2015, before closing again in 2016–2017. Marmot et al (2020a) pointed out that between 2011 and 2017 the UK experienced lower rates of improvement annually than most high-income nations except the USA and Iceland.

However, the UK also appears to perform poorly on measures that may be more closely linked with healthcare services such as five-year survival rates and 'avoidable' mortality. Dayan et al (2018) stated that survival rates after a particular period of time are a widely recognised measure for comparing the quality of cancer care between countries.

For most of the cancers that were the highest mortality on wealthy nations within their comparison nations, the UK was the worst for pancreatic and colon cancer and the second-worst for lung cancer.

Papanicolas et al (2019) reported that, among the European countries where preventable deaths and treatable deaths are measured, the UK had greater than average rates of preventable deaths compared with the study average (154 versus 139 deaths/100,000 population), and the highest rates of amenable deaths (90 versus 72 deaths/100,000 population). However, the UK performed similarly to the EU average for preventable and treatable causes, but improvements in each of these measures over the previous five years in the UK were below the average improvement of the group. Maternal mortality in the UK was 7.8 deaths/100,000 live births, which was greater than the mean of the comparators (5.5 deaths/100,000 births) and above the OECD and EU averages (7.0 and 6.4 deaths/100,000 births, respectively). The UK had similar rates of infant mortality to other countries (3.9 versus study average 3.8; OECD, 3.7; EU, 3.2 deaths/1000 live births), and they are decreasing at a similar rate to the average. The UK had the lowest survival rates for breast cancer (UK, 85.6 per cent; study average, 87.4 per cent) and colon cancer (UK, 60 per cent; study average, 64.8 per cent), and the second lowest for rectal cancer (UK, 62.5 per cent; study average, 66.6 per cent) and cervical cancer (UK, 63.8 per cent; study average 66.6 per cent).

The Commonwealth Fund (Schneider et al, 2021) compared the performance of healthcare systems of 11 high-income countries by means of 71 performance measures across five domains (access to care, care process, administrative efficiency, equity, and healthcare outcomes). After some years as the best performing system, the NHS slipped to fourth place overall. The healthcare outcomes domain included ten measures of the health of populations selected to focus on outcomes that can be modified by healthcare (rather than public health measures such as life expectancy at birth, which may be affected more by social and economic conditions). The measures fall into three categories: population health outcomes; mortality amenable to healthcare; and condition-specific health outcomes measures. The NHS was ranked ninth in terms of healthcare outcomes.

The NHS generally rates more favourably in terms of equality of care (Dayan 2018). However, equality of (access to or provision of) care does not necessarily result in equality of outcomes. For example, Bambra (2016: 10–11) pointed out that geographical inequalities in mortality have varied over time, but in 2008–2010 the English health divide was the largest in Europe, with the gap between the most and least affluent regions greater than the gap in life expectancy between East and West Germany before reunification. She later explained that 'patterns of health and disease are produced by the structures, values and priorities of political and economic systems', pointing out that the UK was part of a 'Liberal regime' of nations, with less generous welfare states and higher levels of income inequality (Bambra, 2016: 139).

Greener (2021) examined SDH for the 11 'Commonwealth Fund' nations with Qualitative Comparative Analysis (QCA). He found that the UK had low health outcomes, but high health equity. Although the path to high health, equity seemed to be linked to low income inequality and high health expenditure, the 'deviant case' of the UK appeared to display a unique path due to the egalitarian NHS, which compensates to some extent for its poor SDH.

Conclusion

Given that estimates suggest that maybe as much as a quarter of the health of a developed population is attributable to the healthcare system, and that NHS rhetoric over many years has stressed the importance of prevention, re-focusing health policy to address upstream factors appears an obvious strategy. Yet, moving upstream may be as difficult as water defying gravity – a variant of Sisyphus' unending struggle (for example, Hunter, 2016b; Cairney and St Denny, 2020). Similarly, despite many reports focusing on health inequalities (see Black, 1980; Marmot, 2010), health inequalities have increased in recent years (Bambra, 2016; Marmot, 2020a).

Explaining the slow, patchy and intermittent progress of policy to tackle health inequalities can be partly interpreted with reference to the four axes which the editors framed in Chapter 1. The central–local axis is perhaps the most obvious frame for analysis, highlighting inter-area and intra-area inequalities. This needs to encompass devolution within the UK too. The modes of governance have relevance as well, with an oscillation between hierarchy and local network. Hierarchical strategies remain significant but networks have assumed more prominence recently. Implicit in much policy and analysis is a recognition that public sector approaches are most apt for tackling health inequalities and yet market-based solutions are coming to the fore with a growing recognition of the commercial determinants of health (Maani et al, 2022). This private axis might also include more individual solutions, associated with the lifestyle drift of policy. Finally, the professional-managerial axis might appear less pertinent but clinicians' understandings are crucial in how frontline staff address health inequalities.

Turning towards evaluation, life expectancy and mortality rates such as the infant mortality rate have improved over the period of the NHS, but it is unclear to what extent this is causally linked to the NHS, and there are indications of stalling or even reversing in recent years. In terms of intrinsic evaluation, the NHS has seen improvements in health over time (noting the caveat outlined), but NHS aims regarding health and healthcare inequalities are much more vague, and so difficult to evaluate. Finally, the UK seems to compare poorly to other nations in terms of healthcare outcomes.

Over the 75 years of the NHS, it has been claimed many times that the service has focused on improving health and reducing health inequalities. However, while there have been initiatives to increase healthcare equity in terms of provision, access, and use, its role in improving health outcomes and the wider SDH will inevitably be limited. The ability of the NHS to engage with relevant communities and agencies in addressing the SDH will be crucial in determining how well the UK can improve population health *and* tackle health inequalities.

References

Acheson, D. (chair) (1998) *Independent Inquiry into Inequalities in Health*. London: The Stationery Office.

Bambra, C. (2016) *Health Divides*. Bristol: Policy Press.

Bambra, C., Lynch, J. and Smith, K. (2021) *The Unequal Pandemic*. Bristol: Policy Press.

Bauld, L., Judge, K., Barnes, M., Benzeval, M., Mackenzie, M. and Sullivan, H. (2005) 'Promoting social change: The experience of Health Action Zones in England'. *Journal of Social Policy*, 34, 3, 427–445.

Berridge, V. (2016) *Public Health: A Very Short Introduction*. Oxford: Oxford University Press.

Black, D. (chair) (1980) *Inequalities in Health*. London: Penguin.

Brackley, J., Tuck, P. and Exworthy, M. (2021) 'Public Health interventions in English Local Authorities: Constructing the facts, (re)imagining the future'. *Accounting, Auditing and Accountability Journal*, 34, 7, 1664–1691.

Cairney, P. and St. Denny, E. (2020) *Why Isn't Government Policy More Preventive?* Oxford: Oxford University Press.

Checkland, K., Dam, R., Hammond, J., Coleman, A., Segar, J., Mays, N. and Allen, P. (2018) 'Being autonomy and having space in which to act: commissioning in the "new NHS" in England'. *Journal of Social Policy*, 47, 2, 377–395.

Dayan, N. Ward, D., Gardner, T. and Kelly, E. (2018) *How Good is the NHS?* The Health Foundation, the Institute for Fiscal Studies. London: The King's Fund and the Nuffield Trust.

Department of Health (DH). (1992) *The Health of the Nation: A Strategy for Health in England*. London: HMSO.

DH. (1998) *Our Healthier Nation*. London: The Stationery Office.

DH. (1999) *Saving Lives*. London: The Stationery Office.

DH. (2000) *The NHS Plan*. London: HMSO.

DH. (2004) *Choosing Health*. London: DH.

Department of Health and Social Care. (2021) *Integration and Innovation: Working Together to Improve Health and Social Care for All*. CP 381. London: DHSC.

Department of Health and Social Security (DHSS). (1976) *Sharing Resources for Health in England*. Report of RAWP. London: HMSO.

DHSS. (1980) *Report of the Working Group on Inequalities in Health* (The Black Report). London: DHSS.

Dimbleby, H. (2021) *National Food Strategy: An Independent Review for Government*. https://www.nationalfoodstrategy.org/the-report/

Evans, D. (2003) '"Taking public health out of the ghetto": The policy and practice of multi-disciplinary public health in the United Kingdom'. *Social Science & Medicine*, 57, 6, 959–967.

Evans, D. (2021) 'What price public health? Funding the local public health system in England post-2013'. *Critical Public Health*, 31, 4, 429–440.

Exworthy, M. (2002) 'The "second Black Report"? The Acheson Report as another opportunity to tackle health inequality'. *Contemporary British History*, special issue *Poor Health*, 16, 3, 175–197.

Exworthy, M., Berney, L. and Powell, M. (2002) '"How great expectations in Westminster may be dashed locally": The local implementation of national policy on health inequalities'. *Policy and Politics*, 30, 1, 79–96.

Exworthy, M., Blane, D. and Marmot, M. (2003) 'Tackling health inequalities in the UK: Progress and pitfalls of policy'. *Health Services Research*, special issue: *Social Determinants of Health*; part II, 38, 6, 1905–1921.

Exworthy, M. and Hunter, D.J. (2011) 'The challenge of joined-up government in tackling health inequalities'. *International Journal of Public Administration*, 34, 4, 201–212.

Exworthy, M., Mannion, R. and Powell, M. (eds) (2016) *Dismantling the NHS? Evaluating the Impact of Health Reforms*. Bristol: Policy Press.

Exworthy, M. and Morcillo, V. (2019) 'Primary care doctors' understandings of and strategies to tackle health inequalities: A qualitative study'. *Primary Health Care Research and Development*, 21, 20, e20. doi: 10.1017/S146342361800052X.

Exworthy, M. and Powell, M. (2004) 'Big windows and little windows: Implementation in the congested state'. *Public Administration*, 82, 2, 263–281.

Faculty of Public Health. (2019) *What the NHS Thinks About Prevention*. London: FPH.

Graham, H. (ed) (2000) *Understanding Health Inequalities*. Buckingham: Open University Press.

Glasby, J. and Miller, R. (2020) 'Ten lessons for integrated care research and policy – a personal reflection'. *Journal of Integrated Care*, 28, 1, 41–46.

Greener, I. (2021) *Comparing Health Systems*. Bristol: Policy Press.

Harrison, S. and McDonald, R. (2008) *The Politics of Healthcare in Britain*. London: Sage.

Hart, J.T. (1971) 'The inverse care law'. *Lancet*, 297, 7696, 405–412.

Hiam, L., Dorling, D. and McKee, M. (2023) 'Falling down the global ranks: Life expectancy in the UK, 1952–2021'. *Journal of the Royal Society of Medicine*, 116, 3, 89–92.

Holroyd, I., Vodden, A. and Srinivasan, A. Kuhn, I., Bambra, C. and Ford, J.A. (2022) 'Systematic review of the effectiveness of the health inequalities strategy in England between 1999 and 2010'. *BMJ Open*, 12: e063137.

Hunter, D.J., Fulop, N. and Warner, M. (2000) *From 'Health of the Nation' to 'Our Healthier Nation'*. Report. Copenhagen: WHO Regional Office for Europe.

Hunter, D.J. (2003) *Public Health Policy*. Cambridge: Polity.

Hunter, D.J. (2005) 'Choosing or losing health?'. *Journal of Epidemiology & Community Health*, 59, 1010–1013.

Hunter, D.J. (2016a) *The Health Debate* (2nd ed). Bristol: Policy Press.

Hunter, D.J. (2016b) 'Public health: Unchained or shackled?', in M. Exworthy, R. Mannion and M. Powell (eds) (2016) *Dismantling the NHS? Evaluating the impact of health reforms*. Bristol: Policy Press, pp 191–210.

Klein, R. (1982) 'Performance, evaluation and the NHS'. *Public Administration*, 60, 385–407.

Klein, R. (2013) *The New Politics of the NHS* (7th ed). Abingdon: Radcliffe Medical.

Lewer, D. and Bibby, J. (2021) 'Cuts to local government funding and stalling life expectancy'. *The Lancet*, 6, e623–624.

Lewis, T., Buck, D. and Wenzel, L. (2022) *Equity and endurance: How Can We Tackle Health Inequalities this Time?* 16 March 2022. London: King's Fund. https://www.kingsfund.org.uk/publications/how-can-we-tackle-health-inequalities

Maani, N., Petticrew, M. and Galea, S. (eds) (2022) *The Commercial Determinants of Health*. Oxford: Oxford University Press.

Marino, A. and Papanicolas, I. (forthcoming) 'The best in the world?', in M. Powell, D. Beland and T. Agaratan (eds) *The Elgar Handbook of Health Care Policy*. Cheltenham: Elgar.

Marmot, M.G. (chair) (2010) *Fair Society, Healthy Lives: Strategic Review of Health Inequalities in England Post-2010*. London: Department of Health.

Marmot, M.G., Allen, J., Boyce, T., Goldblatt, P. and Morrison, J. (2020a) *Health Equity in England: The Marmot Review 10 Years On*. London: Health Foundation.

Marmot, M. Allen, J., Goldblatt, P., Herd, E. and Morrison, J. (2020b) *Build Back Fairer: The COVID-19 Marmot Review. The Pandemic, Socioeconomic and Health Inequalities in England*. London: Institute of Health Equity.

Marmot, M., Allen, J., Goldblatt, P., Herd, E. and Morrison, J. (2021) *Build Back Fairer in Greater Manchester: Health Equity and Dignified Lives*. London: Institute of Health Equity.

Marmot, M. and Wilkinson, R. (eds) (2005) *The Social Determinants of Health* (2nd ed). Oxford: Oxford University Press.

McGinnis, J.M., Williams-Russo, P. and Knickman, J.R. (2002) 'The case for more active policy attention to health promotion'. *Health Affairs*, 21, 2, 78–93.

Ministry of Health. (1944) *A National Health Service*. London: Ministry of Health.

NHS England. (2014) *Five Year Forward View*. London: NHSE.

NHS England. (2019) *NHS Long Term Plan*. London: NHSE.

Nightingale, G. and Merrifield, K. (2023) 'The health disparities white paper disappearing shows a dangerous pattern for action on health'. Health Foundation blog, 27 January. https://www.health.org.uk/news-and-comment/blogs/the-health-disparities-white-paper-disappearing-shows-a-dangerous-pattern

O'Brien, N. (2023) 'Health: Disadvantaged. Question for Department of Health and Social Care'. UIN 128715, tabled on 20 January. https://questions-statements.parliament.uk/written-questions/detail/2023-01-20/128715#

Office for National Statistics (ONS). (2015) 'How has life expectancy changed over time?'. www.ons.gov.uk/peoplepopulationandcommunity/ birthsdeathsandmarriages/lifeexpectancies/articles/howhaslifeexpectancy changedovertime/2015-09-09

ONS. (2022) *Health State Life Expectancies by National Deprivation Deciles, England: 2018–2020*. 25 April. https://www.ons.gov.uk/peoplepop ulationandcommunity/healthandsocialcare/healthinequalities/bulletins/ healthstatelifeexpectanciesbyindexofmultipledeprivationimd/2018to2020

Papanicolas, I., Mossialos, E., Gundersen, A., Woskie, L. and Jha, A. (2019) 'Performance of UK National Health Service compared with other high income countries: Observational study'. *British Medical Journal*, 367, l6326. doi: 10.1136/bmj.l6326

Popay, J., Whitehead, M. and Hunter, D.J. (2010) 'Editorial: Injustice is killing people on a large scale – but what is to be done about it?'. *Journal of Public Health*, 32, 2, 148–149.

Powell, M. (1997) *Evaluating the National Health Service*. Buckingham: Open University Press.

Powell, M. and Exworthy, M. (2003) 'Equal access to health-care and the British NHS'. *Policy Studies*, 24, 1, 51–64.

Propper, C., Sutton, M., Whitnall, C. and Windmeijer, F. (2008) 'Did "Targets and Terror" reduce waiting times in England for hospital care?'. *B.E. Journal of Economic Analysis & Policy*, 8, 2. https://doi.org/10.2202/ 1935–1682.1863

Robinson, T., Brown, H., Norman, P. Fraser, L.K., Barr, B. and Bambra, C. (2019) 'The impact of New Labour's English health inequalities strategy on geographical inequalities in infant mortality: a time-trend analysis'. *Journal of Epidemiology and Community Health*, 73, 564–568.

Royal Commission on the National Health Service. (1979) *Report*. London: HMSO.

Schneider, E.C., Shah, A., Doty, M.M., Tikkanen, R., Fields, K. and Williams II, R.D. (2021) *Mirror, Mirror 2021: Reflecting Badly*. New York: The Commonwealth Fund.

Secretary of State for Health. (1989) *Working for Patients*, Cm 555. London: HSMO.

Secretary of State for Health. (2010a) *Equity and Excellence: Liberating the NHS*, cm 7881. London: The Stationery Office.

Secretary of State for Health. (2010b) *Healthy Lives, Healthy People: Our Strategy for Public Health in England*, Cm 7985. London: The Stationery Office.

Secretary of State for Levelling Up, Housing and Communities. (2022) *Levelling Up the UK*, CP 604, London: HMSO.

Timmins, N. (2021) *The Most Expensive Breakfast in History: Revisiting the Wanless Review 20 Years On*. London: Health Foundation. https://www. health.org.uk/publications/reports/revisiting-the-Wanless-review

Walshe, K., Lorne, C., Coleman, A., McDonald, R. and Turner, A. (2018) *Devolving Health and Social Care: Learning from Greater Manchester.* Manchester: University of Manchester. https://www.alliancembs.manchester.ac.uk/media/ambs/content-assets/documents/news/devolving-health-and-social-care-learning-from-greater-manchester.pdf

Wanless, D. (2002) *Securing Our Future Health: Taking a Long-Term View: Final Report.* London: HM Treasury.

Wanless, D. (2004) *Securing Good Health for the Whole Population.* London: HM Treasury.

9

NHS managers at a crossroads: part of the problem or the solution?

Ian Kirkpatrick

As the NHS celebrates its 75th anniversary, all is not well. Alongside the familiar list of ailments – chronic staff shortages, decaying infrastructure and waiting lists longer than the average lifespan – are doubts about the spiralling costs of managers. As the Tory MP, Philip Davies, glibly informed one of his constituents: 'The problem is that the NHS is appallingly run with far too many overpaid and utterly useless senior managers who wouldn't be able to get a similar job in the private sector' (McKay, 2023). Such claims are a recurring and depressing theme in contemporary public debate (Kirkpatrick, Veronesi and Altanlar, 2017a; Kings Fund, 2011) and, if anything, seem to have become increasingly common. Most recently, with great fanfare, the *Daily Mail* heralded a 'Bonfire of the pen pushers', reporting plans by Health Secretary Steve Barclay to 'Crackdown on NHS bureaucrats costing taxpayers £2.8 billion a year'. The government will 'root out waste, wokery and deadwood to cut costs and free doctors from red tape amid backlog crisis' (Huskisson, 2022). Even the political opposition are getting in on the act, with Kier Starmer, leader of the Labour party, pledging to slash 'nonsense bureaucracy in [the] NHS' (Turner, 2023).

Hence, for many concerned observers, NHS managers have become part of the problem. The dominant view is that the NHS employs too many managers and back room administrators, soaking up resources, stifling creativity and interfering with the work of frontline clinicians. Of course, some have challenged this view. According to Managers in Partnership (2015), '[NHS] Managers make a distinct contribution as the people who organise care, fix problems and ultimately take responsibility for the services people depend on'. Ultimately, 'Managers are the people who keep the show on the road, day-in day-out'. Claims about unsustainable management costs have also been subject to critical scrutiny by researchers (Kings Fund, 2011) as has the very idea that an organisation as large and complex as the NHS could ever function without managers to coordinate things (Mintzberg, 2017). This is especially in light of current plans to re-organise around integrated care and continuing problems associated with workforce planning, unequal access to services and 'unwarranted variation'. When looked at this way, it might seem perverse for so much attention to be focused on managers as the source of all evil and yet, here we are.

In this chapter, my aim is to review and critically assess these claims and counter claims about managers in the NHS. As many readers will be aware, debates about management are not new. In fact, attempts to reform the management and governance of the NHS, as the world's fifth largest organisation, have been ongoing almost from its inception. In more recent times, the NHS has been a trailblazer of what has come to be known as the New Public Management (NPM) (Kirkpatrick, Ackroyd and Walker, 2005; Exworthy, Mannion and Powell, 2016), with politicians on both sides of the political spectrum seeking to reform the way the service is organised and run. The medical profession itself has also embraced the importance of leadership, which has apparently moved from the 'dark side to centre stage' (Ham, Clark and Spurgeon, 2011). Nevertheless, despite these efforts, we find ourselves in a situation today where managers are viewed with suspicion, as either irrelevant or a costly and unproductive overhead. As such, a key question is: how did we get to this point? And, what is the substance (if any) of these criticisms and doubts about managers?

To address these concerns, I will start with the basics of how we should define and understand terms such as 'managers', 'management', 'leadership', 'administration' and 'bureaucracy'. Gaining conceptual clarity in terminology is crucial and often missing from recent debates. I then consider, albeit briefly, the history of management reforms in the NHS to date. This story has been told many times already, including the Introduction of this volume, so my own treatment of it will be relatively brief, focusing primarily on the development of managers as a *discrete occupation* in the NHS. I will then return to contemporary debates to understand the nature of critiques of NHS managers, highlighting some deeper ideological roots. A key argument I will develop, here, is in relation to the pervasive legacy of public choice theory (PCT) in shaping contemporary debates and policy (Veronesi, Kirkpatrick and Altanlar, 2019). This approach encourages us to question all forms of bureaucracy (including public services such as the NHS) and portrays managers (whose role is to help coordinate bureaucracy) as essentially self-interested.

Last, I will review the growing evidence base relating to the nature, antecedents and impact of NHS managers, some of it linked to my own ongoing research. In doing so my aim is to provide a sober analysis that dispels some of the myths about NHS managers. I will also reflect on future directions for research and policy. Crucially, I propose that, after many decades of reform, it is necessary, finally, to take seriously the need to develop managers and their capabilities as an occupation in the NHS. While there is scope to enhance management capabilities, it is wrong, as a starting point, to view managers as a wasteful and unproductive overhead. On the contrary, managers are essential for running (and maybe even helping to transform) the NHS as a *public* service in the *public* interest.

Managers and management: definitions

Starting with definitions, an important distinction is between 'management' *and* 'managers' (Diefenbach, 2009: 894), or between 'management' as a general process *and* 'management as a distinctive occupation' (Grey, 1999: 562). The former (management as an activity) relates to the work involved in the process of managing people and/or resources, essentially about planning, control and coordination (Fayol, 2013). In practice, anyone might perform this work: even when they do not hold a formal job title of 'manager'. As Alvesson and Willmott (1996: 9) explain:

> In all societies, people are involved in the complex and demanding business of organising their everyday lives. Each of us engages in a daily struggle to accomplish ordinary tasks and maintain normal routines. This management of routines is something we all contribute to, and are knowledgeable about – it is 'second nature'.

Hence, in the NHS, hospital consultants and senior nurses often engage in 'managerial' work such as the supervision or mentoring of junior colleagues or leading clinical improvement projects. They are, in effect, 'quasi managerial practitioners' (Exworthy and Halford, 1999).

In recent years, the volume and complexity of this hidden management work in the NHS has undoubtedly increased. This is partly due to the regulatory context (discussed next) and volume of top-down performance management demands and monitoring requirements (Verbeeten and Speklé, 2015: 955). One study, funded by the National Institute for Health Research, found that more than one in three clinical professionals spent time on these hidden management (or leadership) activities (Buchanan et al, 2013). The focus on 'managing things' has also been exaggerated by the growing emphasis on leadership in health systems and in particular the concept of 'shared' or 'distributed' leadership (Fitzgerald et al, 2013). This highlights the role that all clinical professionals (and non-clinicians) might play in the ongoing quality improvement and redesign of health services (O'Reilly and Reed, 2011). While the term 'leadership' has now become the preferred nomenclature in the NHS (Learmonth and Morrell, 2019), it is arguably just another way of describing this hidden management work.

By contrast, 'management as a distinct occupation' (Grey, 1999) is a narrower category, referring to people who occupy job roles with the title of 'manager'. As an occupation or function, specialist managers became increasingly important as organisations (including those in healthcare) grew in size and complexity. Accordingly, 'in modern societies, responsibility for the management of everyday tasks, routines and identities increasingly has become the preserve and monopoly of experts, including managers, who are trained and employed to shape, organise and regulate so many aspects of our lives' (Alvesson and Willmott, 1996: 9).

Historically, because the NHS tended to be 'bureaucracy-lite' (Hales, 2002), managers, as a distinct occupation, were initially less visible. However, from the mid-1980s onwards, there has been a growing focus on recruiting general (or 'pure play') managers to run NHS organisations, including hospitals and bodies responsible for commissioning and regulation (see as follows). The Binleys Database of NHS Management supplied by Wilmington Healthcare Ltd (collected and published since 1991) records over 100 management roles with 'decision making power'. These roles include operational (clinical directors and business managers) staff support functions (finance, procurement and HR) and roles that are strategic in nature, such as managers who sit on boards of acute trusts or regulatory bodies (executive and non-executive directors).

At the time of writing, the Binleys database recorded 27,484 managers in the NHS as a whole, with over 80 per cent employed in England. Women made up a majority (around 57 per cent) of managers and just under 50 per cent of strategic roles (including board membership) (Kirkpatrick, Altanler and Veronesi, 2021). Some of these managers have progressed through the NHS Graduate Management Training Scheme, which recruits 300 new trainees annually, while others have commercial backgrounds. Kirkpatrick, Veronesi and Vallascas (2017b), for instance, note that 51 per cent of board members of English NHS trusts (executive and non-executive) had previously worked in the private sector. It is also notable that, despite the media and political hype about managers as outsiders, a significant proportion of them have clinical backgrounds (doctors, nurses and AHPs). These are essentially part-time, or 'hybrid' roles (see Kirkpatrick, 2016 for an overview) such as Clinical Leads, Clinical Directors and Medical Directors. In 2018, one study recorded 6,090 doctors involved in these hybrid management roles, representing 3.2 per cent of the medical workforce and 22 per cent of the management workforce (Kirkpatrick, Altanler and Veronesi, 2021).

A final distinction is between managers and administrators mainly employed on clerical grades, who do not exercise management authority or control significant resources. The broader category of administrators also includes specialist staff in support roles, such as estates management, central functions, data analysis and scientists. When combined, the number of managers and administrators gives an indication of the 'administrative intensity' of the NHS, defined as the 'resources that organizations spend on administrative support functions rather than primary service and production processes' (Elston and Dixon, 2020: 113). Given its size, the NHS understandably employs a large number of administrators in non-clinical roles, although perhaps not as many as is often assumed. Most recently, the *Daily Mail* claimed that: 'The number of backroom staff and managers in the health service has been creeping up over the past decade', implying that because 'only 52.5 per cent are clinically trained staff', the remainder were 'bureaucrats' (Haywood, 2021). In fact, if one looks at acute NHS trusts (the largest area of employment) the actual administrative overhead is closer to 26.6 per cent of the workforce (Veronesi et al, 2022).

Management reform in the NHS: a brief history

Almost since the inception of the NHS, policy-makers and politicians have been concerned with the need to strengthen management to ensure 'control over input mix and level, outputs and scope of activities' (McKee and Healy, 2002). Taking a big picture view, one might understand this in terms of the interplay between the interests of 'corporate rationalizers' and 'professional monopolisers' (Alford, 1975). The former include civil servants, public health doctors and, crucially, managers and administrators directed to ensure cost-effective use of resources, standardisation, predictability, regulation, audit and control. These imperatives are present in any healthcare system given spiralling costs associated with population ageing and multi-morbidity, but are arguably harder to deal with in systems (such as the NHS) where the bulk of funding comes from direct taxation which creates additional political sensitivity (Kirkpatrick, Ackroyd and Walker, 2005). By contrast, 'professional monopolizers', who are dominated by the interests of the medical profession, emphasise the need for clinical autonomy and relative freedom to regulate themselves in the interests and assumed wellbeing of individual patients (Friedson, 1988).

This tension between the 'worlds' of care, cure and control has been played out at every level in the NHS, both in policy arenas and organisational settings (such as hospitals) (Glouberman and Mintzberg, 2001). In practice, the power of clinical professionals to define the meanings of disease and healthcare and to veto other interest holders' policies ensures that managers face an uphill battle in asserting control. Indeed, as Klein (2014: 222–223) suggests, '[NHS management] exercises least control over those who, in theory at least, exercise the greatest influence in determining demand for health care'. While much has changed over the past three decades, arguably this remains true today.

Turning to the specifics of how UK governments have sought to address this challenge of control, an initial phase of reform began in the 1960s. In 1967, for example, the Cogwheel Report raised concerns about efficiency, asking 'What contributions can practicing clinicians make to the management and administrative arrangements of the hospital complex?' (Ministry of

Health, 1967). A further major reorganisation of the NHS followed in 1974, focused on establishing a more hierarchical structure of regional and district authorities. This reform, however, did not introduce managers as a specialist function. Rather, it sought to formalise a team or consensus-based approach towards management and administration as a mechanism for controlling resources and addressing concerns about poor integration and unwarranted variation. However, in practice, the result was a form of diplomatic (Harrison et al, 1992) or 'custodial' management, which for the most part failed to challenge clinical autonomy (Ackroyd, Kirkpatrick and Walker, 2007).

By contrast, a far more significant break with the past came in 1983 with the publication of the Griffiths report (Griffiths, 1983). Taking an unusual step, the then Conservative government commissioned Sir Roy Griffiths, the Chief Executive of a large supermarket chain, to review management arrangements in the NHS. A key conclusion of this review was that the NHS lacked any system of individual management accountability for decisions, or indeed any effective framework for implementing policies and evaluating performance. Half-jokingly, Griffiths noted that 'if Florence Nightingale were carrying her lamp through the corridors of the NHS today, she would almost certainly be searching for the people in charge' (1983: 12).

As a solution, Griffiths called for greater accountability at all levels for the management of budgets and performance. His report also emphasised the need to strengthen management as a 'discrete activity' in the NHS, by creating 'an active managerial function' that would specialise in 'the organisation and co-ordination of services and the consideration of efficiency in service delivery' (Ackroyd, 1992: 342). Essentially the argument was that in order to achieve more effective management, the NHS needed agents who were fully committed to this task. Accordingly, the decision was taken to recruit a cadre or occupation of 'general managers' with their own professional identity and mission (Ackroyd, Kirkpatrick and Walker, 2007).

Initially, old style administrators and managers recruited from the private sector filled the majority of the new general management posts in the NHS (Kirkpatrick et al, 2009). This, however, was to change in subsequent years, as further policy initiatives sought to co-opt doctors and nurses into management, and later, leadership roles. From 1991 onwards, this saw the introduction of clinical directorates and boards, which included medical and nursing directors (Kirkpatrick et al, 2013).

Importantly, these reforms - kick-started by the Griffiths report - were (and remain) heavily influenced by a broader set of ideas linked to the NPM (Pollitt and Boukaert, 2011). In crude terms, the NPM refers to a cluster of doctrines and practices that are held to constitute a paradigm of management distinct from 'traditional modes of public administration' (Hood, 1995).

Implied by the NPM is the need to empower managers and stress their 'right to manage' with fewer constraints imposed by rules and bureaucracy. The NPM is also sympathetic to the idea of drawing on knowledge and expertise from the corporate sector.

In addition, the NPM has emphasises the need to re-configure the organisational landscape and modes of governance of public services. In the NHS, this saw a shift away from vertically integrated hierarchies and top-down planning and towards a looser structure where provider organisations (such as Foundation Trust hospitals) remain publicly owned, but have their own distinct identities, with governing boards and formal autonomy (see Kirkpatrick et al, 2016; Kirkpatrick, Veronesi and Altanlar, 2017a). This more devolved model aims to make public organisations more 'business like' and raise their performance. However, at the same time, a devolved model has also served a political purpose of helping to blur the lines of accountability. While in the past, government ministers and civil servants had no way of shirking responsibility for failures in the health system, now when things go wrong, it is easier to blame CEOs and other managers who run public hospitals that are formally autonomous.

Finally, and related to the introduction of the NPM, is the goal of using quasi-markets and competition for resources as a mechanism for driving improvements in efficiency and innovation. As noted in the Introduction, NPM reforms have led to a variety of policy experiments and re-organisations over the years under both Conservative and New Labour governments aimed at separating purchaser (and commissioner) and provider roles. At different points, this marketisation process also stimulated the outsourcing of services and the greater use of the private sector, although the extent of this has been greatly exaggerated (Kings Fund, 2021a). As the NHS reached its 75th anniversary, these reforms are still ongoing with policy fluctuating between different models of governance, which emphasise either markets, hierarchies or networks (or all three).

Reflections: mounting criticisms about the value of managers

Returning to the concerns raised earlier, despite the aforementioned reforms, significant doubts remain about the role and purpose of NHS managers. Most recently, in October 2021, the Secretary of State for Health and Social Care commissioned General Sir Gordon Messenger to lead a review of leadership in health and social care. This review, labelled 'the most far-reaching' in 40 years, is premised on the assumption that the NHS is poorly managed and possibly over-managed (NHS Confederation, 2022). Opposition politicians seem to agree. Shadow Health Secretary Wes Streeting, for example, recently complained about 'NHS bosses leeching cash away from frontline medical staff' (Nelson, 2021).

These doubts about managers in the NHS, which form part of the political and media zeitgeist in the UK, originate from many different sources. However, for the sake of simplicity, I will try to focus here only on two dominant perspectives. First is the view that, given the organisational and regulatory context, NHS managers have simply been too constrained to achieve their goals. Second – and even more damming – is the view that recruiting more managers and administrators in the NHS is essentially wasteful and perhaps even counter-productive.

The former perspective builds on many of the points already made about the ongoing struggles of managers, as 'corporate rationalisers' to assert their authority over powerful clinical (notably) medical interests (Glouberman and Mintzberg, 2001). Furthermore, unlike their counterparts in the private sector, NHS managers are also too constrained by bureaucracy to make any real difference. Asaria, McGuire and Street (2022: 6), for example, suggest that, 'it may be that NHS management is largely confined to … administrative roles, ensuring regulatory standards and requirements are met rather than inherently improving performance'.

For many, exacerbating this situation are relentless top-down targets and performance demands from central government, which have rendered managers powerless and ineffective (Exworthy, Mannion and Powell, 2016). According to one recent study, the chief executives of NHS trusts have been charged with '[d]elivering the impossible' (Kings Fund, 2018) and have become 'little more than conduits for the policies of the centre', fixated on 'saving the hierarchy' (Blackler, 2006). The fact that managers' jobs are on the line further complicates this picture. As Ed Smith, former chair of NHS Improvement, lamented, 'If you live in a country where the firing squad is the basis of encouraging people to step up and take risk you're not going to get people appearing to innovate, wanting to improve because they know what's coming' (Kings Fund, 2016). This is also borne out by the fact that the average tenure of chief executives in English acute trusts is 4.5 years, compared with 7.2 years for large private firms (Townsend et al, 2022).

In the worst cases, overbearing regulation could lead to bullying and 'hierarchical cultures' in NHS organisations that are narrowly focused on financial viability (Jacobs et al, 2013). Indeed, it is notable that the 2013 Francis report into failures of care at Mid-Staffordshire NHS Foundation Trust cited cost-cutting by management as a significant cause, alongside poor collaboration. Senior managers were accused of being preoccupied with 'targets and processes' and losing sight of their 'fundamental responsibility to provide safe care' (GovUK, 2013).

Hence, there is a view that while managers are probably necessary in the NHS given its size and complexity, they are unlikely to be able to make much difference. By contrast, the second perspective noted earlier goes a step further in questioning the very need for managers. As we saw before, the current government is calling for a root and branch review of NHS management, and indeed it would seem they have public support. An opinion poll published in January 2015, for example, found that 'too much being spent on management and bureaucracy' ranked first among public concerns, ahead of (arguably more pressing) issues such as hospital closures, staff shortages and access to drugs and treatments (Lord Ashcroft KCMG, 2015).

These attacks on NHS management have deeper ideological roots (Veronesi, Kirkpatrick and Altanlar, 2019). Critical, in this regard, is 'the extensive acceptance of public choice reasoning and conclusions by ... policy-relevant professions and some politicians' (Dunleavy, 1991: 3). Emerging from classical economics, Public Choice Theory (PCT) (Niskansen, 1971) sees public officials (referred to generically as 'bureaucrats') as rational decision-makers who act as self-interested, rent-seeking individuals who aim to maximise their personal utilities (salary, perquisites of the office, power and so on). This behaviour ultimately leads to the costly expansion of administrative hierarchies – sometimes referred to as 'bureaucratic bloat' – and to sub-optimal outcomes for service users. Following the predictions of Parkinson's Law (Parkinson and Osborn, 1957), it is argued that managers will seek to push up their own budgets and numbers regardless of the quantity of work that needs to be undertaken (Veronesi, Kirkpatrick and Altanlar, 2019).

Of course, one might query why the same, right-leaning politicians, who originally championed NPM reforms, are now so concerned about the risks of employing managers. To some extent, this reflects a degree of opportunism. However, it also highlights a deeper rift within the NPM project itself, between what Alford (1975), writing almost half a century ago, termed 'market reformers' (keen to break up and privatise public services) and 'bureaucratic reformers' (seeking improved coordination and integration). Aucoin (1990: 121) notes how PCT-driven ideas, emphasising 'distrust of the permanent bureaucracy', have sat uncomfortably with the objectives of managerialism. While the latter stresses the need to re-structure bureaucracy to 'empower' managers (Hood, 1995), when looked at through the lens of PCT, managers are simply rent-seeking 'bureaucrats'. As we saw, the neo-liberal remedy is to reign back the state and the power of these bureaucrats (including managers) to allocate resources by using private organisations incentivised to make profits. Following this logic, in the long-term competition and privatisation are the answer, not investments in more managers to run a public service bureaucracy that was always bound to fail.

Assessing the evidence base

In this section, I now turn to assessing the evidence base for NHS management and to what extent, if at all, it supports the attacks being made against it. In doing so, my approach will not be uncritical of managers. Nor do I wish to dismiss concerns raised about 'evidence based management' (Learmonth and Morrell, 2019). Rather my aim is to look more closely at what the available data and analysis are telling us about NHS managers and whether this supports the idea that managers are part of the problem. Specifically, I address three questions: Is the NHS over-managed? Are managers essentially self-serving? And, what do managers contribute to performance?

Is the NHS over-managed?

First, it is necessary to question the assumption that the NHS is over-managed and is suffering from 'bureaucratic bloat'. There can be no doubt that over the past 30 years the resources allocated to managers and the activity of managing have grown substantially. While in the early 1980s there were fewer than 1,000 managers employed in the NHS, by 2005 numbers had risen to a peak of 34,000 (Walshe and Smith, 2011). Administrative overheads have also increased, in large part due to transaction costs associated with quasi-markets, contracts and commissioning (Paton, 2014).

Nevertheless, while these trends imply bureaucratic bloat – especially with the growth of central functions (such as NHS England) – it is easy to over-exaggerate. At the system level, it is notable that the UK actually spends considerably less on 'central departmental governance' and 'regulatory activities' (including bodies as the Care Quality Commission) than many of its OECD counterparts (including France, Germany and the Netherlands), who fund healthcare through private or social insurance. In 2017, for example, the UK spent the equivalent of £53 per person on healthcare governance, compared with £639 in the US: effectively 12 times the amount (ONS, 2021).

The NHS also performs well in terms of overall efficacy and productivity. For example, between 2004–2005 and 2016–2017, NHS productivity increased by 16.5 per cent between compared to a growth rate of only 6.7 per cent in the economy as a whole (Kings Fund, 2022). Partly for this reason, the NHS has consistently ranked highly in Commonwealth Fund reports which compare 11 OECD health systems; the NHS is currently in 4th place for 'administrative efficiency' (Commonwealth Fund, 2021).

With regard to the management and administration of provider organisations (such as acute trusts), it is also hard to argue that the NHS is 'over managed' (Kings Fund, 2011). Based on the figures discussed earlier (for 2018) the number of managers in the NHS represents less than two percent of the workforce. By comparison, 'Managers, Directors and Senior Officials' in the UK as a whole make up 9.5 per cent of the workforce, falling to 8.3 per cent if the 'other' category – comprising managers employed in small medium sized enterprises – are excluded (Kirkpatrick, Veronesi and

Altanlar, 2017a). In reality, this means that, far from being over-burdened with managers and bureaucrats, the NHS is possibly 'one of the most undermanaged organisations on the planet' (Black, 2018).

Exacerbating this problem is the fact that in recent years the number of managers in the NHS has actually fallen. This process began with the Lansley reforms after 2010, which promised to direct 'more money to the front line' (Kirkpatrick and McCabe, 2011). Since then, the downward trend has continued. For the NHS as a whole, the figure of 25,119 managers reported earlier (for 2018) compares with 29,940 in 2007: a 16 per cent drop. Moreover, within acute trusts in England, as organisations have grown in size over the past decade, the proportion of managers has not kept pace with the rising staff numbers (Kirkpatrick, Altanler and Veronesi, 2021). This is especially in Foundation Trusts, which have opted for 'leaner administration' (Veronesi et al, 2022; Kirkpatrick, Veronesi and Vallascas, 2017b). In primary care, a trend towards work intensification is even more pronounced: with less than 1 per cent of costs relating to management (NHS Confederation, 2022).

Managers: a self-serving elite?

As we saw before, many contemporary observers view NHS managers as essentially self-interested and unaccountable. However, analysis by Veronesi, Kirkpatrick and Altanlar (2019), focusing on acute trusts over six years, finds no evidence to show that high numbers of managers employed lead to rises in employment of managers in future years. Other studies highlight the strong public service ethos that motivates NHS managers and their deep commitment to enhancing quality and patient care (Crilly and LeGrand, 2004). Recent ethnographic work also notes the unwavering commitment of managers to quality and the 'difficult dilemmas' they face to 'balance patient safety with limited available resources' (Hyde et al, 2016: 179).

These observations are especially significant given the low pay and remuneration of NHS managers compared to the private sector. Contrary to popular belief, this also applies at senior levels. For example, the majority of NHS trust chief executives are paid under £200,000, with only a minority paid £250,000 per annum or more (NHS Confederation, 2022). These salaries, however, compare unfavourably with the salaries of chief executives running FT 100 companies of a similar scale, where the demands of managing are arguably a lot less challenging. As Glouberman and Mintzberg (2001: 56–84) suggest: 'Running even the most complicated corporation must sometimes seem like child's play compared to trying to manage almost any hospital'. Studies focusing on the experiences of NHS CEOs, who are subject to a 'blame culture' and high levels of turnover and burnout, further reinforce this impression (Kings Fund, 2018).

The contribution of NHS managers

Last, what about the view that NHS managers are essentially an unproductive overhead? Here again, the evidence highlights the gap between myth and reality. While some studies find no evidence of an association between the quality and quality of managers and various measures of NHS hospital performance (Asaria, McGuire and Street, 2022), others reach starkly different conclusions. A much-publicised example is the work of Bloom and Van Reenen (2010). Applying a 20-point scale of management practices to over 2,000 hospitals (public and private) in nine countries (including the NHS), this study found that high management scores correlate strongly with clinical and financial outcomes.

Similarly, Veronesi, Kirkpatrick and Altanlar (2019), focusing on 150 NHS acute hospital trusts, find that even a small increase in the proportion of managers employed (from 2 to 3 per cent of the workforce in an average acute trust) can have a marked impact. Up to a certain point, larger management functions in trusts were associated with higher patient satisfaction scores, a 5 per cent rise in hospital efficiency and a 15 per cent reduction in infection rates. This work has also raised questions about the value of outsourcing management to external consultants – which generates inefficiency (Kirkpatrick et al, 2019) – and points to the performance benefits of relying more on in-house managers to deliver consulting projects (Sturdy et al, 2023).

Related to this are performance benefits associated with increasing the number of clinical professionals in management and leadership roles (Clay-Williams et al, 2017). These benefits are especially apparent in situations where doctors take on senior management roles, such as CEOs or membership of boards. Focusing on the top 100 hospitals in the US, Goodall (2011) found that having a chief executive with a medical background generates greater quality improvements and results in higher hospital rankings. Similarly, in the NHS, Veronesi, Kirkpatrick and Vallascas (2013) report that NHS hospital trusts achieving the highest quality ratings (level 4) had a higher proportion of directors with a medical background (15.01 per cent) than those achieving the lowest ratings (11.09 per cent). This research also noted positive outcomes for hospital mortality rates, patient experience scores, and efficiency (Kirkpatrick and Vallascas, 2014; Veronesi Kirkpatrick and Altanlar, 2015).

To be sure, these findings merit further work to understand why clinical leaders at board level have these effects. It is unclear, for example, whether the positive impact arises from having a greater critical mass of doctors on boards, or from the prior management experience of these doctors (in clinical leader and director roles). Nevertheless, it seems that involving clinicians in management work is not a wasteful activity or a distraction. As 'expert leaders' (Goodall, 2023), clinical professionals bring with them considerable knowledge and credibility to the task of managing health services, which might ultimately have wider benefits for patients and taxpayers.

Hence, there are compelling reasons to question some of the prevailing myths about managers and management in the NHS. Far from representing an unproductive overhead, managers can, up to a certain point, help to improve outcomes. And it is not hard to understand why. Theoretically, the literature on 'administrative intensity' notes the critical coordinating role that managers play, especially in large and complex organisations such as the NHS (Veronesi et al, 2022). As Andrews et al (2017: 116) suggest: 'organizations with a strong administrative component may ... be better placed to synchronize the many moving parts'. Given growing staff shortages and rising patient demand in the NHS (post-COVID-19), this coordinating role is perhaps more important than ever, simply to avoid the delegation of this work to busy (and increasingly stressed) clinicians. Indeed, when looked at in this way, failure to invest in managers could *reduce* productivity and further exaggerate problems of clinical staff turnover and retention in the longer term (NHS Confederation, 2022).

None of this, of course, is to deny that NHS managers are more constrained by regulation and have less autonomy than their counterparts in the business world. This is understandable given the publicly funded nature of the NHS. Nor is the raw number of managers employed a good proxy for their quality and the level of training and capabilities (Asaria, McGuire and Street, 2022). However, there is enough to indicate that managers are not simply glorified administrators with no scope to affect change. When managers are doing their job properly, they can take a system-wide view and provide the analysis that drives and sustains improvement in ways that are beneficial to patients and taxpayers. For example, managers contribute directly to 'high-quality administration' in the NHS, which 'has the potential to improve patient experience, reduce inequalities, and promote better care'. (Kings Fund, 2021b). By supporting clinical leaders, managers are also an essential part of what Richard Bohmer (2016) describes as 'the hard work of healthcare transformation'. As the NHS struggles to stay afloat, this additional management capacity to plan and coordinate improvement work will be critical in future. Therefore, far from being powerless, managers help to keep the 'show on the road' and, with the right mix of technical skills, could make a real difference.

Conclusion

In this chapter, I have sought to provide a balanced appraisal of NHS managers and management, and challenge some prevailing myths. In some ways, this supports earlier calls to avoid 'denigration of managers and the role they play in delivering high-quality health care' (Kings Fund, 2011), while going further by reviewing the latest evidence. In summary, this evidence tells us that the NHS is not, and nor has it ever been, 'over managed'. Furthermore, it suggests that, under certain conditions, managers can add significant value to the NHS. While there is considerable scope to improve management practice and skills, my argument is that it is fundamentally wrong to conceive of NHS managers as an 'unproductive overhead'.

These conclusions are theoretically interesting, but also have a number of policy implications. First, they highlight a pressing need to change the narrative about managers, as the NHS enters the deepest crisis in its history. For politicians and the media, this requires an end to the popular but ultimately destructive pastime of manager-bashing and blame culture. Clinical professionals also need to buy into this exercise, as do academics and other commentators. In some parts of the academic community, especially left-leaning, there is still an association made between managers and the 'creeping privatisation' of the NHS, threatening to alter its nature and fundamental values (Krachler, Greer and Umney, 2022). However, as I have tried to show, this view is mistaken and possibly ideologically driven. Crucially it ignores the distinction between what are essentially neo-liberal policy solutions, focusing on marketisation and downsizing the state, and the more practical and longstanding need to ensure that public services are managed effectively. While the NPM implies greater attention to learning from the corporate sector, this is not necessarily a slippery slope towards privatisation. Accordingly, a greater focus on management is not about dismantling the NHS, but could be about strengthening and preserving it. Furthermore, it is clear that self-regulating clinical professions, alone, will be unable to perform this task (Mintzberg, 2017). While it is naïve to assume that the tensions between the interests of 'corporate rationalizers' and 'professional monopolizers' will ever disappear completely, these relationships might be framed in a more productive way in future (see for example, Edwards et al, (2002)).

A second and related implication is simply the need to invest in NHS managers. For example, as part of any national workforce (or 'People Plan'), the NHS could increase spending on managers to a level that is closer to the national average for other UK organisations (Alderwick and Charlesworth, 2022). To date, while some attention has focused on CEO succession planning (Kings Fund, 2018), planning management staff numbers has been largely ad hoc. In future, it would be useful to focus on *all* managers (including clinical leaders and data analysts) as an occupational group. Allocating more resources in this way will free up clinical time and provide much-needed support for planning and improvement work.

Last, and more controversial, there might be scope in future to increase the autonomy of NHS managers, with longer planning horizons to deliver meaningful improvements. During the pandemic, it seems that this occurred in some parts of the NHS. For example, a study by Malby and Hufflett (2020) notes how 'CQC disappeared the minute the pandemic started' with more scope to introduce changes without the 'usual red tape'. In a report commissioned by the NHS Confederation, Ham (2022) has also argued that the time is now ripe for the NHS to reassess its operating model, shifting the balance from top-down control to local autonomy. Such a move, of course, would not be without risk. Nevertheless, greater delegation with less regulatory oversight might just help deliver better results. In the best case, this might lead to a virtuous circle whereby moves to strengthen management capabilities, generate improvements in the NHS which further increase both the ability and willingness of policy-makers to relax control.

Looking ahead, it is open to question whether UK governments will reassess their stance towards NHS managers. In all likelihood, the embattled Cinderella status of managers will remain unchanged, not least because it is politically expedient to have someone to blame. Nevertheless, at this important juncture in the history of the NHS, it is useful to reflect on the possibilities for a different compact. While managers may never become the most popular kids on the block, the hope is that there will at least be a greater acknowledgement of their critical role and contribution

References

Ackroyd, S. (1992) 'Traditional and new management in the NHS hospital service and their effects on nursing,' in Soothill, K.L., Henry, C. and Kendrick, K. (eds) *Themes and Perspectives in Nursing*. London: Chapman and Hall.

Ackroyd, S., Kirkpatrick, I. and Walker, R. (2007) 'Public management reform and its consequences for professional organisation: A comparative analysis'. *Public Administration*. 85, 1, 9–26.

Alderwick, H. and Charlesworth, A. (2022) 'A long term workforce plan for the English NHS', *BMJ*, 377. DOI: https://doi.org/10.1136/bmj.o1047

Alford, R. (1975) *Health Care Politics*. Chicago: University of Chicago Press.

Alvesson, M. and Willmott, H. (1996) *Making Sense of Management: A Critical Introduction*. London: Sage.

Andrews, R., Boyne, G. and Mostafa, A.M.S. (2017) 'When bureaucracy matters for organizational performance: Exploring the benefits of administrative intensity in big and complex organizations'. *Public Administration*, 95: 115–1139.

Asaria, M., McGuire, A. and Street, A. (2022) 'The impact of management on hospital performance'. *Fiscal Studies*, 1–17.

Aucoin, P. (1990) 'Administrative reform in public management: Paradigms, principles, paradoxes and pendulums'. *Governance*, 3, 115–137.

Black, S. (2018) *The NHS isn't Overmanaged*. https://www.linkedin.com/pulse/nhs-isnt-overmanaged-stephen-black/

Blackler, F. (2006) 'Chief executives and the modernisation of the English National Health Service'. *Leadership*, 2, 1, 5–30.

Bloom, N. and Van Reenen, J. (2010) 'Measuring and explaining management practises across firms and countries', *Quarterly Journal of Economics*, 122, 4, 1351–1408.

Bohmer, R.M.J. (2016) 'The hard work of health care transformation', *New England Journal of Medicine*, 375, 8, 709–711.

Buchanan, D.A., Denyer, D., Jaina, J., Kelliher, C. Moore, C., Parry, E. and Pilbeam, C. (2013) *How Do They Manage? The Realities of Middle and Front Line Management Work in Healthcare*. Southampton, UK: NIHR HS&DR (Project Ref: 08/1808/238).

Clay-Williams, R., Ludlow, K., Testa, L. Li, Z. and Braithwaite, J. et al (2017) 'Medical leadership, a systematic narrative review: Do hospitals and healthcare organisations perform better when led by doctors?'. *BMJ open*, 7, e014474., pp 1-11

Commonwealth Fund. (2021) *Mirror Mirror 2021: Reflecting Badly*. Commonwealth Fund Report.

Crilly, T. and LeGrand, J. (2004) 'The motivation and behaviour of hospital Trusts'. *Social Science and Medicine*, 58, 1809–1823.

Diefenbach, T. (2009) 'New Public Management in public sector organizations: The dark sides of managerialistic "enlightenment"'. *Public Administration*, 87, 892–909.

Dunleavy, P (1991) *Bureaucracy, Democracy and Public Choice*. Hemel Hempstead, UK: Harvester Wheatsheaf.

Edwards, N., Kornacki, M.J. and Silversin, J. (2002) 'Unhappy doctors: What are the causes and what can be done?'. *British Medical Journal*, 324, 835. doi:10.1136/bmj.324.7341.835

Elston, T. and Dixon, R. (2020) 'The effect of shared service centers on administrative intensity in English local government: A longitudinal evaluation'. *Journal of Public Administration Research and Theory*, 30, 113–129.

Exworthy, M. and Halford, S. (eds) (1999) *Professionals and the New Managerialism Across the Public Sector*. Buckingham, UK: Open University Press.

Exworthy, M., Mannion, R. and Powell, M. (2016) *Dismantling the NHS?* Bristol: Policy Press.

Fayol, S. (2013) *General and Industrial Management*. London: Martino Fine Books.

Fitzgerald, L. Ferlie, E., McGivern, J. and Buchanan, D. (2013) 'Distributed leadership patterns and service improvement: Evidence and argument from English healthcare'. *The Leadership Quarterly*, 24, 1, 227–239.

Freidson, E. (1988) *Profession of Medicine: A Study of the Sociology of Applied Knowledge*. Chicago: University of Chicago Press.

Glouberman, S. and H. Mintzberg (2001) 'Managing the care of health and the cure of disease. Part I: Differentiation and Part II: Integration'. *Health Care Management Review*, 26, 1, 56–84.

Goodall, A. (2011) 'Physician-leaders and hospital performance: Is there an association?', *Social Science & Medicine*, 73, 535–539.

Goodall, A. (2023) *Credible: The Power of Expert Leaders*. London: Basic Books.

Gov.UK. (2013) *Report of the Mid Staffordshire NHS Foundation Trust Public Inquiry*. https://www.gov.uk/government/publications/report-of-the-mid-staffordshire-nhs-foundation-trust-public-inquiry

Glouberman, S. and Mintzberg, H. (2001) 'Managing the care of health and the cure of disease. Part I: Differentiation and Part II: Integration', *Health Care Management Review*, 26, 1, 56–84.

Grey, C. (1999) '"We are all managers now", "we always were": On the development and demise of management'. *Journal of Management Studies*, 36, 5, 561–585.

Griffiths, E.R. (1983) *NHS Management Inquiry: Griffiths Report on NHS*. October. SHA.

Hales, C., Doherty, C. and Gatenby, M. (2012) *Continuity and Tension in the Definition, Perception and Enactment of First Line Management Role in Healthcare*. London: NIHR.

Ham, C. (2022) *Governing the Health and Care System in England: Creating the Conditions for Success*. NHS Confederation. https://www.nhsconfed.org/publications/governing-health-and-care-system-england

Ham, C., Clark, J. and Spurgeon, J. (2011) *Medical Leadership: From Dark Side to Centre Stage*. London: The King's Fund.

Harrison, S., Hunter, D.J., Marnoch, G. and Pollitt, C. (1992) *Just Managing: Power and Culture in the National Health Service*. London: Macmillan.

Hayward, E. (2021) 'General who led the Royal Marines' invasion of Iraq is appointed to lead the biggest shake-up of NHS management in 40 years'. *Mail online*. https://www.dailymail.co.uk/news/article-10051241/general-appointed-lead-biggest-shake-NHS-management-40-years.html

Hood, C. (1995) 'The "New Public Management" in the 1980s: Variations on a theme'. *Accounting, Organizations and Society*, 20, 93–109.

Huskisson, S. (2022) 'Crackdown on NHS bureaucrats costing taxpayers £2.8billion a year: Health Secretary Steve Barclay launches plan to root out waste, wokery and deadwood to cut costs and free doctors from red tape amid backlog crisis'. *Daily Mail*, 1 September.

Hyde, P., Granter, E., Hassard, J. and McCann, L. (2016). *Deconstructing the Welfare State: Managing Healthcare in the Age of Reform*. Oxon: Routledge.

Jacobs, R., Russell, M., Davies, HTO., Harrison, S., Konteh, F. and Walshe, K. (2013) 'The relationship between organizational culture and performance in acute hospitals'. *Social Science & Medicine*, 76, 115–125.

King's Fund, The. (2011) *The Future of Leadership and Management in the NHS: No More Heroes.* https://www.kingsfund.org.uk/sites/default/files/future-of-leadership-and-management-nhs-may-2011-kings-fund.pdf

King's Fund, The. (2016) *Ed Smith: How Should Quality Improvement Be Taken Forward?* Podcast. https://www.kingsfund.org.uk/audio-video/ed-smith-quality-improvement

King's Fund, The (2018) *Leadership in Today's NHS: Delivering the Impossible.* https://www.kingsfund.org.uk/publications/leadership-todays-nhs

King's Fund, The (2021a) *Is the NHS being Privatized?* https://www.kingsfund.org.uk/publications/articles/big-election-questions-nhs-privatised-2021

King's Fund, The (2021b) *Admin Matters: The Impact of NHS Administration on Patient Care.* https://www.kingsfund.org.uk/publications/admin-matters-nhs-patient-care

King's Fund, The (2022) *Health and Social Care in England: Tackling the Myths.* https://www.kingsfund.org.uk/publications/health-and-social-care-england-myths).

Kirkpatrick, I. (2016) 'Hybrid Managers and Professional Leadership', in J-L Denis, and M. Dent (eds) *The Routledge Companion to the Professions and Professionalism.* London: Routledge.

Kirkpatrick, I., Ackroyd, S. and Walker, R. (2005) *The New Managerialism and Public Service Professions.* London: Palgrave.

Kirkpatrick, I., Altanler, A. and Veronesi, G. (2021) 'Hybrid professional managers in healthcare: An expanding or thwarted occupational interest?'. *Public Management Review*, online ready.

Kirkpatrick, I., Bullinger, B., Lega, F. and Dent, M. (2013) 'The translation of hospital management reforms in European health systems: A framework for comparison.' *British Journal of Management*, 24, S48–61.

Kirkpatrick, I., Kragh Jespersen, P., Dent, M. and Neogy, I. (2009) 'Medicine and management in a comparative perspective: The cases of England and Denmark'. *Sociology of Health and Illness*, 31, 5, 642–658.

Kirkpatrick, I., Kuhlmann, E., Hartley, K. and Lega, F. (2016) 'Medicine and management in European hospitals'. *BMC Health.* https://bmchealthservres.biomedcentral.com/articles/supplements/volume-16-supplement-2

Kirkpatrick, I. and McCabe, C. (2011) 'A full blooded market system: at what cost to the NHS?'. *British Medical Journal*, 343,13 July. DOI: 10.1136.

Kirkpatrick, I., Sturdy, A., Reguera, N. and Blanco-Oliver, A. and Veronesi, G., (2019) 'The impact of management consultants on public service efficiency'. *Policy and Politics*, 47, 1, 77–95.

Kirkpatrick, I., Veronesi, G. and Altanlar, A. (2017a) 'Corporatisation and the emergence of (*under managed*) managed organizations: The case of English public hospitals.' *Organization Studies*, 38, 12, 1687–1708.

Kirkpatrick, I., Veronesi, G. and Vallascas, F. (2017b) 'Business experts on public sector boards: What do they contribute?'. *Public Administration Review*, 77, 754–765.

Klein, R. (2014) *The New Politics of the NHS*. London: Radcliffe.

Krachler, N., Greer, I. and Umney, C. (2022) 'Can public healthcare afford marketization? Market principles, mechanisms, and effects in five health systems'. *Public Administration Review*, 82, 876–886.

Learmonth, M. and Morrell, K. (2019) *Critical Perspectives on Leadership: The Language of Corporate Power*. London: Routledge.

Lord Ashcroft KCMG. (2015) 'The people, the parties and the NHS', in *Book The People, the Parties and the NHS* (ed). City: Lord Ashcroft KCMG PC.

Malby, R. and Hufflett, T. (2020) '10 Leaps Forward – Innovation in the Pandemic'. London South Bank University. https://openresearch.lsbu.ac.uk/item/8qq2w

McKay, J. (2023) 'Tory MP claims "overpaid and utterly useless" managers not Government to blame for "shambles of the NHS"'. *Nursing Notes*, 10 January.

McKee, M. and Healy, J. (2002) *Hospitals in a Changing Europe*, European Observatory on Health Care Systems series. Buckingham: Open University Press.

Managers in Partnership. (2015) *NHS Managers and the 2015 General Election: A Briefing for MiP Members*. London: MiP.

Ministry of Health. (1967) *First Report of the Joint Working Party on the Organisation of Medical Work in Hospitals*. London: Her Majesty's Stationary Office.

Mintzberg, H. (2017) *Managing the Myths of Health Care*. Oakland: Brent-Koehler.

Nelson, N. (2021) EXCLUSIVE: Tories 'leeching cash from frontline medics to fund NHS bosses' massive salaries'. *The Mirror*. https://www.mirror.co.uk/news/politics/tories-leeching-cash-frontline-medics-25786041

Niskanen, W.A. (1971) *Bureaucracy and Representative Government*. Chicago: Aldine-Atherton.

NHS Confederation. (2022) *Is the NHS Over-managed?* NHS Confederation. https://www.nhsconfed.org/long-reads/nhs-overmanaged

Office for National Statistics (ONS) (2021) *How Does UK Healthcare Spending Compare with Other Countries?* https://www.ons.gov.uk/peoplepopulationandcommunity/healthandsocialcare/healthcaresystem/articles/howdoesukhealthcarespendingcomparewithothercountries/2019-08-29

O'Reilly, D. and Reed, M. (2011) 'The grit in the oyster: Professionalism, managerialism and leaderism as discourses of UK public services modernization'. *Organization Studies*, 32, 8, 1079–1101.

Parkinson, C.N. and Osborn, R.C. (1957) *Parkinson's Law, and Other Studies in Administration*. Boston: Houghton Mifflin.

Paton, C. (2014) *At What Cost? Paying the Price for the Market in the English NHS*. London: CHPI.

Pollitt, C. and Bouckaert, G. (2011) *Public Management Reform: A Comparative Analysis-New Public Management, Governance, and the Neo-Weberian State*. Oxford: Oxford University Press.

Sturdy, A., Kirkpatrick, I., Blanco-Oliver, A. and Veronesi, G. (2023) 'The relative (in)efficiency of external private sector management consultancy expertise', Paper presented at 39th EGOS Colloquium, Cagliari, July.

Townsend, X., Kirkpatrick, I., Altanlar, A. and Veronesi, G. (2022) ' "Strong in the saddle": The effect of social capital on CEO exit'. Paper presented at OBHC conference, Birmingham, September.

Turner, C. (2023) 'Sir Keir Starmer: I will slash "nonsense" bureaucracy in the NHS', *The Telegraph*, 15 January. https://www.telegraph.co.uk/polit ics/2023/01/14/sir-keir-starmer-will-slash-nonsense-bureaucracy-nhs/

Verbeeten, F.H.M., and Speklé, R.F. (2015) 'Management control, results-oriented culture and public sector performance: Empirical evidence on new public management'. *Organization Studies*, 36/7, 953–978.

Veronesi, G., Kirkpatrick, I. and Vallascas, F. (2013) 'Clinicians on the board: What difference does it make?'. *Social Science and Medicine*, 77, 147–155.

Veronesi, G., Kirkpatrick, I. and Vallascas, F. (2014) 'Does clinical management improve efficiency? Evidence from the English NHS'. *Public Money and Management*, January, 1–8.

Veronesi, G., Kirkpatrick, I. and Altanlar, A. (2015) 'Clinical leadership and the changing governance of public hospitals: Implications for patient experience'. *Public Administration*, 93, 4, 1031–1048.

Veronesi, G., Kirkpatrick, I. and Altanlar, A. (2019) 'Are public managers a bureaucratic burden? The case of English public hospitals'. *Journal of Public Administration Research and Theory*, 29, 2, 193–209.

Veronesi, G., Sarto, F., Kirkpatrick, I. and Altanler, A. (2022) 'Corporatization, administrative intensity and the performance of public sector organizations'. *Journal of Public Administration Research and Theory*, online ready.

Walshe, K. and Smith, L. (2011) *The NHS Management Workforce*. London: Kings Fund.

10

Forgotten, neglected and a poor relation? Reflecting on the 75th anniversary of adult social care

Catherine Needham and Jon Glasby

Introduction: social care anniversaries

Although NHS anniversaries have been widely celebrated and form the basis of a number of detailed histories, adult social care has tended not to receive the same attention and focus. The National Assistance Act – the piece of legislation which many see as leading to the creation of the modern adult social care system – received Royal Assent on 13 May 1948, just weeks before the launch of the new National Health Service. In one sense, therefore, all the anniversaries set out in the opening chapter to this book could also be seen as joint anniversaries of both health and social care. This is very fitting, as health and social care have been so inextricably linked ever since – with a series of attempts to break people's lives down into separate 'health' and 'social care' needs proving increasingly meaningless over time. However, the vast majority of previous accounts have focused solely on the NHS, and adult social care is rarely mentioned, even in passing. As a result, the history of adult social care is largely overlooked – and even people working in adult social care may know little about the origins and evolution of their current services and roles.

In many ways, the current adult social care system is based on the legacy of the Poor Law, with frail older people, disabled people and people with learning disabilities or with mental health problems initially supported within local communities, and then – as problems of poverty and rapid industrialisation and urbanisation increased – in infamous institutions known as 'workhouses' (see Payne, 2005; Means, Richards and Smith, 2008; Pierson, 2011; Glasby, 2017; Humphries, 2022; for an overview of the history and development of adult social care and of the social work profession). Faced with more need that they could ever possibly meet, workhouses were deliberately designed to be as a harsh as possible so that only people who were absolutely desperate would seek support, with everyone else doing all they could to remain as independent as possible (a principle known as 'less eligibility'). After the Second World

War, an attempt was made to distance modern adult social care from this controversial and unfortunate legacy, with a clear separation between national financial support for those on low incomes or unable to work ('social security') and practical care and support for people who are frail or disabled ('adult social care'). Overseen by local rather than national government, the latter system grew up piecemeal over several decades, and new legislation tended to be discretionary (that is, giving powers to local councils to do certain things, rather than creating a duty to do so or a sense of clear entitlements for people drawing on care and support). As Humphries (2022: 21–23) explains:

> [I]f the NHS was a bright new dawn for health care, it was a different story for people with non-medical care and support needs – what today we call social care. In the same year as the NHS began to great fanfare, its sister legislation, the National Assistance Act quietly slid onto the statute book and was to serve as the legal cornerstone of social care for the next 66 years. ... From the outset, social care was never intended to be a universal service meeting a wide range of needs like the NHS. It offered only a safety net, with councils having very limited powers.

Following reforms in the late 1960s/early 1970s, local authority 'Social Services Departments' worked with both children and families and with adults (often known as a 'generic' approach). However, following a series of high-profile child protection scandals over time (in particular, the tragic death of Victoria Climbié in 2000), more recent changes have created increasingly separate systems (one overseen in England by the Department for Education, and the other by the Department of Health and Social Care – with local authorities often having very separate directorates for adult social care and for children's services). However, throughout these different configurations, adult social care has usually been the poor relation of other areas of the welfare state. While services such as the NHS and the education system are universal and free at the point of delivery, adult social care is targeted on people with very significant needs and subject to increasingly stringent means-testing. Simon Bottery, the social care lead at the King's Fund thinktank, has described this in terms of having to be both a 'pole vaulter' and a 'limbo dancer' (personal communication) in order to qualify for support – getting over very high eligibility thresholds at the same time as getting under a very stringent means-test. Hardly surprisingly, therefore, adult social care tends to be a lot less visible than the NHS, is less popular and is less well understood by policy-makers, the media and the general public (House of Lords Adult Social Care Committee, 2022).

Analysis of adult social care policy and practice

Using the four analytical axes set out in the first chapter of this book, we explore the different forms of governance (hierarchies, markets and networks) which co-exist within adult social care; the mixed economy of care; relationships between the centre and localities; and relationships between the state and professionals (including the position of the bulk of the workforce, who might not meet standard definitions of a 'profession'). In each case, adult social care is very different to the NHS, and so some of the concepts and ideas from earlier chapters are applied in a different context and taken in slightly different directions. Such difference also make attempts to integrate care – while laudable – extremely difficult to achieve in practice, which may account for such a longstanding failure to develop more joined-up services to people with multiple or complex needs.

Hierarchies, markets and networks

Other chapters in this collection review the different ways in which the NHS has shifted over time between different blends of hierarchy, markets and networks. In many accounts, this is portrayed as a largely linear/chronology journey from a traditional hierarchical approach to 1980s/1990s markets and to post-1997 networks (Glasby, 2017) – perhaps with a resurgence of markets at various stages since. However, as different contributors here outline, the reality has tended to be a situation where all three forms of governance have co-existed at the same time. Moreover, Glasby (2017) has previously argued that some of these changes may be more cyclical than linear (see also Exworthy, Powell and Mohan, 1999) – with an in-built tendency for health and social care to look first to hierarchy; then to open things out to markets to break up and encourage competition; then to look to networks as a way of reducing fragmentation – but then to resort to hierarchy again when an issue becomes politically important.

In adult social care, the interplay of these different modes of governance is complex, with the social work profession (which often prides itself on a non-hierarchical culture) employed by historically very hierarchical, bureaucratic local councils. Following the community care reforms of the early 1990s (overseen by the same Roy Griffiths who introduced general management within the NHS), social workers became 'care managers', assessing people's needs and securing a subsequent 'care package' from a mixed economy of private, voluntary and public services (see later for further discussion). They are now also meant to oversee a situation in which people who draw on care and support receive a 'personal budget'. This is a clear upfront sense of the money available to spend on meeting their needs, which can be structured in various ways – including the option of a 'direct payment' in order to purchase care direct or for people to hire their own personal assistants (see Needham and Glasby, 2014; Glasby and Littlechild, 2016). At the same time, local authority managers increasingly became 'strategic commissioners', responsible for identifying the needs of the local area and shaping the nature of the local care market to ensure that services are in place to respond (see Needham et al, 2022 for a discussion of local authorities' role in terms of 'market shaping').

Over time – and under New Labour (1997–2010) in particular – social care was increasingly encouraged to work in partnership with the NHS, but also with partners in housing and the voluntary and community sector. However, this was within the context in which the relationship between commissioners and providers remained essentially competitive (for example, governed by formal procurement codes and underpinning legislation). Moreover, the nature of this mixed economy is very different in adult social care to that in the NHS, making joint working more difficult. As an example, one former Director of Adult Social Services (in England), in a national policy workshop, expressed frustration with NHS colleagues extolling the virtues of partnership working, asking everyone if they realised that around 90 per cent of his budget was spent in the private sector (personal communication). This was at a time when many commentators were opposing the 2012 Lansley reforms as potentially leading to greater 'privatisation' of the health service. Perhaps not unreasonably, the director asked: 'When you say you want to join your services up with mine, do you mean with the 90% that are in the private sector?' The only answer was dead silence, as no-one previously seemed to have fully appreciated the different mixes of hierarchy, markets and networks at play in their respective sectors – and the director's question was never answered.

A mixed economy of care

With the passage of the NHS and Community Care Act in 1990, local authorities became responsible for arranging and funding the care of people in independent sector care homes (who had previously been able to access various forms of social security to fund their care). This was seen by many as an attempt to transfer responsibility for bringing a rapidly escalating budget under control from national government to local councils, and was perceived at the time as 'the only thing Thatcher ever gave local government' (popular saying). That local government has successfully managed these financial tensions for so many decades is arguably a major unsung achievement, albeit the funding pressures inherent in the 1990 reforms have since intensified into a major and arguably existential crisis (see Glasby et al, 2021 for an overview of social care spending from 2010–2020, and a series of projections as to future spending, depending on a series of different reform scenarios).

While local government received a transfer of funding from the social security budget to help with its new responsibilities (known as 'the Special Transitional Grant'), 85 per cent of this money was to be spent in the independent sector (that is, either private or voluntary sector services – not in the public sector). Despite ongoing debates about the most appropriate mix of public and private healthcare provision, it remains politically untenable that any government could make such a stipulation with NHS funding. The result of these reforms was a situation in which 'care managers' (social workers) assess people's needs and design a 'care package' for people who qualify for publicly funded support. This might be made up of a mix of services from the private, voluntary or public sectors – although over time, the private sector has become by far the largest player. As Bob Hudson (2016: 8 – see also Hudson, 2021) explains:

> Since then [the 1990 Act] the transformation towards a market in adult social care has progressed steadily, with no attempt by any government to halt or reverse the trend. Early talk of a 'mixed economy of care', with local authorities, private companies and the voluntary sector competing on a 'level playing field', soon evaporated. In 1979 64% of residential and nursing home beds were still provided by local authorities or the National Health Service; by 2012 the local authority share was 6%; in the case of domiciliary care, 95% was directly provided by local authorities as late as 1993; by 2012 it was just 11%. This also means the bulk of the adult social care workforce – around 72% – is now employed in the private and voluntary sectors, along with another 14% employed by individual service users making use of 'personal budgets', leaving just 14% employed by local authorities.

These changes have been particularly prominent in terms of care homes, where over 90 per cent of residential care (in England) is now provided via the independent sector (and mainly by the private sector) (Institute of Public Care (IPC), 2014; Competition and Markets Authority (CMA, 2017). There has also been a very clear trend towards a smaller number of very large providers (often national/multinational companies which have merged with/bought up others – some funded by private equity) (CQC, 2017). Although this might provide economies of scale for cash-strapped local authorities, there is a major risk should one of the large providers fail. This became very real in 2012 when Southern Cross, the largest provider with 31,000 beds, ceased to trade (IPC, 2014). More recently, there have been significant financial challenges for other providers and warnings of a potential 'care collapse' (Crawford and Read, 2015). Indeed, such has been the level of concern that there has been a major review by the Competition and Markets Authority (2017) – itself an indication of the extent to which the provision of adult social care is essentially privatised.

It should also be noted that many of these figures and trends are for people who receive publicly funded care and support, with many people who are not eligible for such support having no choice but to arrange and pay for their own care (Henwood et al, 2022). By 2016–2017, the National Audit Office (2018) estimated that such 'self-funders' were purchasing care worth some £10.9 billion per year. This compares to a total value of care arranged by local authorities of £20.4 billion (albeit £2.7 billion of this came from charges which people paid themselves towards the cost of their care). Moreover, whereas the wealthier can sometimes navigate various public services better than those on lower incomes, the situation in adult social care is the opposite: people in residential care who fund their own care tend to pay just over 40 per cent more for the same services as people whose care is arranged by the local authority (CMA, 2017), effectively cross-subsidising publicly funded residents.

All this is very different to healthcare, where the 'mixed economy of care' has traditionally been much more weighted towards the public sector. Moreover, NHS policies such as 'payment by results' set out very clear tariffs for different types of service, with competition meant to be based on quality and responsiveness rather than on price (Mannion, Marini and Street, 2008). Such safeguards simply do not exist in adult social care, with increasingly financially desperate local authorities having little choice but to participate in a race to the bottom, where quality often seems to come a long way behind price in dictating what happens next (see, for example, Fotaki, Ruane and Leys, 2013). As a result of all this, the government has exhorted councils to pay a 'fair cost' for care – but the policy has been seemingly kicked into the long grass following very contentious debates about what this means and whether it is even possible in the current climate. This is really well illustrated by the annual budget survey produced by the Association of Directors of Adult Social Services (ADASS, 2022), in which only 12 per cent of Directors were confident that they have the resources to deliver on all of their responsibilities this year (and just 3 per cent next year); 54 per cent of Directors overspent on their budgets last year, with a strong reliance on drawing on reserves; and 67 per cent of Directors reported that providers in their area had closed, ceased trading or handed back local authority contracts during the course of the year.

Another key difference with the NHS is that people who draw on care and support can receive 'direct payments' (the cash equivalent of services, with which to employ their own personal assistants or to pay for an independent sector agency to provide their care). Introduced after a longstanding campaign by disabled people's organisations to give people greater choice and control over their services and hence over their lives, such models have since been hotly debated (see Needham and Glasby, 2014 for examples of a series of different perspectives and for the background debates relating to the different world views discussed in this paragraph). Whereas some people see direct payments as the product of a civil rights campaign and as a very powerful mechanism for achieving greater citizenship and social justice, others see them as a form of 'privatisation by the backdoor' and the product of a neo-liberal attempt to 'roll back the boundaries of the welfare state'. Leaving aside the details of these debates, the key issue here is that such ways of working make adult social care very different to the NHS, where (despite recent initiatives such as personal health budgets) such developments remain limited and can often be bitterly resisted by health professionals. Whereas the NHS has undergone a series of reforms in terms of different approaches to 'commissioning', many disabled and older people receiving adult social care are effectively the 'micro-commissioners' of their own services, yet struggle to given the same opportunities when it comes to their healthcare (Musekiwa and Needham, 2021).

Centralisation versus decentralisation

One of the distinguishing characteristics of social care, in comparison to the NHS, is that it is run by local government rather than by the central state. Although eligibility criteria and means-testing thresholds are set centrally, each 'higher tier' local authority (city or county) can decide how it arranges care for people and 'shapes' its care market (Needham et al, 2022). Hence in England alone we could point to 152 distinct local social care systems, with different arrangements for care.

The balance of responsibility between the national and the local in relation to social care has been a cause of contention. As we discussed earlier, local authorities were given key powers by the National Assistance Act 1948 and further powers by the NHS and Community Care Act 1990. However, over time they have become increasingly financially dependent on the central state, and have struggled to meet their statutory duties on a shrinking base of central funding. Hudson notes the extent to which English local government is 'now largely marginalised as an independent source of power and authority' (Hudson, 2021: 77). A decade of austerity, at the same time as rising demand, has left local authorities in a perilous financial position. The Care Act 2014 provided a vision of a more preventative and personalised approach to care, with a focus on wellbeing, but a lack of funding has made many parts of it impossible to implement (Burn and Needham, 2020). One of the plans from central government to reform social care funding is to collect more of it from local council tax, a proposal that risks further worsening the gap between rich and poor areas (HM Treasury, 2022). This financial precarity has created a paradox for local authorities, which sees them calling for reform but then pressing for delays to new approaches because the funding is not there for local implementation (for example, County Councils Network, 2022).

Increasingly there have been calls for a national (or at least England-wide) solution to the underfunding of social care (see also what follows for further discussion of a 'National Care Service' in Scotland and Wales). A cap on private care spending has twice been passed into law – in the Care Act in 2014 and then again (following abandonment of the original plan) in the Health and Care Act 2022. In both cases, with minor differences in the rules, the plan was to put a ceiling on how much a private individual would have to pay for care. This would limit personal liability for care costs in situations where people had long-term and complex conditions. The 2022 Act also proposed to make the means-test more generous with a sliding scale of help for anyone with assets less than £100,000 (compared to the current means-test level of £23,250). By the end of 2022, however, the cap, the means-test change and associated reforms to help self-funders had been postponed, with the government citing cost of living pressures (HM Treasury, 2022). The cycle of overdue legislation, welcomed reform, postponement and eventual abandonment that began with the Care Act 2014 looks to be happening again. As one of the editors of this book suggests (and as Oscar Wilde might have said): to abandon a cap once might be a misfortune, to abandon a cap twice begins to look like carelessness (personal communication).

The relationship between the local and the national is rendered more complex as localised social care nudges up against the centrally-led NHS at various points of interface. Efforts to increase joint working between health and social care have taken different forms over time. The current incarnation are Integrated Care Systems (ICSs) within localities which bring together the NHS, local government and other partner organisations to plan and deliver 'joined up' health and care services. However, a 2022 House of Lords Adult Social Care Committee report noted that 'Integration is an elusive grail' (2022: 68). It went on:

> ICSs are one in a long line of attempts to integrate health and social care, for instance through the 2010 Spending Review, the Better Care Fund (2013), the Integrated Care and Support Pioneers Programme (2013) and NHS England's Five Year Forward View (2014).368 Further back, we have had Care Trusts, the Health Act flexibilities, Local Area Agreements, Local Strategic Partnerships, Health Action Zones, the New Deal for Communities and many, many more initiatives and mechanisms. (House of Lords, 2022: 68)

In many of these integration initiatives attention has been focused on the point where the NHS and social care interface most closely: when someone needs a care package in place before they can leave hospital. However, too much focus on this has led to an approach in which social care is often positioned as solving the problems of the NHS rather than as important in its own right. There is a fear that ICSs will be just another attempt at solving the problems of the NHS, rather than an opportunity for a genuine partnership of equals between the NHS, local authorities and other partners in the local health and care landscape (Humphries, 2022).

Central-local relations have been further complicated by the emergence of combined authorities in many parts of England (Shutt and Liddle, 2019). These are regional bodies, bringing together local government on a city-region footprint such as Greater Manchester. Many of these new bodies are led by elected mayors, with a mandate to address strategic issues such as transport, homelessness and public health. In Greater Manchester in particular, there have been efforts to bring together health and social care systems within the city region, with a commitment to investing in prevention and better coordination of services (Alderwick, 2022). Early evaluation of this has indicated some potential health benefits (for example, increases in life expectancy) (Britteon et al, 2022), but the impact on social care is unclear and the health benefits themselves are hard to attribute to the structural reforms.

This complex landscape of local government, combined authorities and Integrated Care Systems may be making it more rather than less difficult to identify a shared vision of how to reform adult social care in a way that is sustainable for the future. One strategy would be to centralise provision through a National Care Service, a type of NHS for social care. This was proposed by the Labour Party under Gordon Brown in 2010, but the party lost the election that year. A National Care Service is currently being developed in Scotland, with plans to remove local authority powers over social care and give them to care boards (Feeley, 2021). The current Labour administration in Wales also plans to develop a National Care Service (Welsh Government, 2021). Quite what is meant by a National Care Service is unclear, however. There seems to be an assumption that borrowing the branding of the NHS might build public support for social care in a way that has been lacking to date. However, none of the variants of the National Care Service proposed so far mirror the NHS: there are no proposals to bring care provision back in-house nor to make social care predominantly state funded. In the Scottish case, it is not clear as yet why moving responsibility for care commissioning from local authorities to care boards will deal with key issues such as underfunding and workforce shortages.

Professionals versus the state

The state-professional relationship in social care is notably different to that in the medical profession.

While the profession of social work is well established in the UK, historically social workers have lacked the status of their medical counterparts (Cootes, Heinsch and Brosnan, 2022) – similar in many ways to ongoing debates about the status of the nursing profession in relation to medicine. In recent years 'fast track' university training courses have undermined the extent to which qualifying social workers can draw on a distinct and critical knowledge base (Tunstill, 2019). As discussed before, the 1990 reforms changed the role of social workers to that of care managers and gatekeepers, reducing the scope for holistic and preventative types of support (Hudson, 2021).

Evans' (2010) work on managerialism in social work highlights that – like clinicians – many social workers in managerial posts retain a dual identify. Their professional identify remains important and may be their primary identifier, particularly for junior managers with a caseload. The dominant forms of knowledge may be those of resource allocation and risk assessment (managerial) or they may be about professional insights into family dynamics, strengths-based practice and person-centred planning (Needham, 2020). In the last 20 years, a third locus of knowledge has disrupted this binary: the choices of people who use social care and those who support them. Such approaches prioritise the authority of the person using service over that of the professional (Mansell and Beadle-Brown, 2005). This may involve devolving funds directly to the person using services or their family, through a direct payment as discussed earlier (Glasby and Littlechild, 2016). It may involve the co-design and co-production of support, with professionals working in partnership with people with lived experience of services (Needham and Carr, 2009).

The personalisation and co-production agendas have influenced social work much more than the medical professional, where claims to specialist knowledge continue to dominate (Vennik et al, 2015; McMullin and Needham, 2020). Given that much social care is about the activities of daily living (getting up and dressed, eating and activities), it is harder to retain the line that professionals know more about this than people themselves. Even in social care, however, people's claims to be 'experts by experience' is contested, requiring continued efforts to remake the case for why it is important and how to do it well (Beresford, 2020; Luff, 2022).

As discussed in Chapter 1 in the context of the NHS, there has been an increased interest in leadership in social work in recent years, with the emergence of leadership programmes and the embedding of the Principal Social Worker in each authority. However Miller, Schaub and Howarth (2019) argue that social work still doesn't accord sufficient attention to leadership as an integral part of people's professional identity, lagging behind other sectors such as health. The underdevelopment of leadership for social workers is part of a broader ambivalence about where leadership lies in the sector. In a COVID-era report from the King's Fund – 'Stories from social care leadership: Progress amid pestilence and penury' – Humphries and Timmins (2021) draw attention to the dispersed nature of leadership in social care. It is shared between central and local government, as discussed before, but also between local authorities, providers and communities. When the COVID-19 pandemic hit, and actions had to be taken rapidly on infection control, access to personal protective equipment and discharge from hospital, it was hard to make authoritative decisions.

Care work itself increasingly has parallels with the work of an NHS healthcare assistant – for example, catheter care, medication management – but the pay and terms and conditions are far worse. The pandemic also drew attention to the marginal and precarious position of frontline care workers, who lack status, job security, adequate pay or training. The toll of the pandemic on these staff was particularly high, in terms of death rates and also experiences of trauma and burnout (House of Lords, 2022). Vacancy rates for 2021 in England were at their highest ever, at around 105,000, with the greatest rates of turnover being for people on zero hour contracts (Skills for Care, 2021). By 2022, these figures had jumped over 50 per cent to over 165,000 vacancies, out of a total adult social care workforce of 1.79 million (Skills for Care, 2022). Most of these are women (82 per cent), with 23 per cent being of a Black, Asian or Minority ethnicity and 16 per cent being non-British (Skills for Care, 2022). An All-Party Parliamentary Group (APPG, 2019) report on social care highlighted that half of care workers leave their job within the first year. The King's Fund notes in 2012–2013 care workers were paid more than cleaners and sales assistants but this is no longer the case (King's Fund, 2022). The simultaneous pressures on staff numbers of Brexit and COVID-19 has further worsened worker shortages (Turnpenny and Hussein, 2022).

There have been proposals to professionalise care workers through a registration process and required set of qualifications. Scotland, Wales and Northern Ireland already have some variant of care worker registration. In a report for the APPG, Hayes et al (2019) note that care worker registration is likely to lead to improved retention and recognition for staff, as well as better quality and safer care. In England, the 2021 White Paper, 'People at the Heart of Care', included proposals for a voluntary 'skills passport' which was described as providing a foundation for registration of staff in the future (DHSC, 2021: 76).

The professionalisation of care work is not without its critics. If care is framed as an adjunct to health, undertaking medical tasks such as wound dressing, then it makes sense to ally it more closely to nursing. However, if it is about helping people get out in their communities and have a life then there has been resistance to making this a professional role with all the embedded assumptions about power inequalities. Securing a more professionalised care workforce is resisted by some people receiving care because of the way it limits their choice and control (see the debate in Gerlich and Farquharson, 2020). Many people with a direct payment choose to appoint personal assistants to provide support and have been critical of suggestions that they only be able to appoint people from an approved register or with a formal set of skills.

Certainly what is untenable is a continuation of the current arrangements where care workers can move to the NHS to do a very similar job and get much better pay – or indeed move to a supermarket to get similar/bettter pay. As demand for care rises with an ageing population, the availability of care workers is going in the wrong direction. Each of the socio-economic upheavals of recent years – Brexit, the COVID-19 pandemic and the cost of living crisis – has made care work less viable and appealing (Turnpenny and Hussein; House of Lords, 2022). In its damning report on the state of adult social care in England, the House of Lords Adult Social Care Committee concluded: 'What is certain is that nothing strategic can be achieved without an equivalent to the NHS "People Plan", which sets out its workforce strategy and is key to delivering its objectives over the next 10 years' (2022: 56).

The failure of successive governments to take a strategic approach to the care workforce in the way that they have to health constitutes one of the major missed opportunities of the last decade.

Evaluating success in social care

To take stock of social care requires attention to the question of 'whose success' as Chapter 1 highlights. While the sense of crisis in social care is pervasive, different stakeholders have distinctive views on the key problems and how they should be solved. The King's Fund identified a range of 'personas' in social care – including the homeowner objecting to selling their house to pay for care, the NHS defender who is only interested in the impact of social care on the NHS, the overwhelmed carer needing more support and the beleaguered provider desperate for a more sustainable cashflow (Bottery, 2020). Recent political priorities from the Conservative government have been focused on the homeowner – protecting people's housing wealth in old age – with much less to say about improving the quality of social care or enhancing the life experiences of working age people with disabilities (Powell and Hall, 2020).

A variety of social care reform proposals have been brought forward in the last two decades to address the multiple challenges facing the sector. Taking a temporal perspective on reform, Compton and 't Hart's book on *Great Policy Successes* draws attention to the criteria of policy endurance: 'the extent to which the achievements and success of a policy are maintained' (2019: 4). Within the recent history of social care we would have to say that there has been a very poor record of endurance (Burn and Needham, 2022). New Labour undertook an extensive consultation process on care reform in 2009 and came into the 2010 election with detailed proposals for a National Care Service. Defeat in that election killed off that phase of reform. Under the Conservative and Liberal Democrat coalition government of 2010–2015, a broad coalition of care stakeholders worked together to develop a white paper that led to the Care Act 2014. A well-regarded and wide-ranging piece of legislation, it has been poorly implemented. Moreover, the austerity context into which it was introduced has made it very difficult to deliver on its promises of enhancing individual wellbeing, investing in prevention and supporting carers (Burn and Needham, 2020). The proposals for a cap on private care costs were delayed and then abandoned. More recently these were revived and again passed into law in the Health and Care Act 2022, but have again been delayed.

If we look at intrinsic measures of success, it is hard to argue that social care has succeeded on its own terms. There are high levels of unmet need, unsustainable pressures on carers, record vacancies and high rates of provider exit (Hudson, 2021; Humphries, 2022). Hudson (2021) notes that it has become a truism that local authorities are faced with an impossible challenge. Reform initiatives have come and gone, but as the 2011 Dilnot report put it, 'Care is the one major area of our lives where, at the moment, there is no way for people to protect themselves against the risk of high costs ' (2011: 2). We are still a long way off a political or public consensus on how we should collectively protect ourselves from the risks of disability and frailty.

It is clear also that levels of public satisfaction with social care are extremely low. British Social Attitudes data for 2021 show that only 15 per cent of those surveyed were satisfied with social care, compared to 36 per cent for health (Curtice et al, 2022). It is notable also that both of these figures have fallen sharply since the pandemic, with the equivalent 2018 data showing 26 per cent of respondents satisfied with social care compared to 53 per cent satisfied with health (Robertson et al, 2019). Even before the pandemic, research on kindness in public services found that in England, of those with direct and close experience of using the service, only 23 per cent strongly agreed that people are treated with kindness when using social care (compared to 40 per cent for GP's surgeries (Unwin, 2018: 16).

In terms of extrinsic measures of success, it is important to note that there is wide variance in what people want social care to be and do. Social care can be a list of tasks on a care plan, but increasingly it is recognised to be a route to wellbeing in a much broader sense (Hamblin, 2020). The social movement Social Care Future (https://socialcarefuture.org.uk) has developed the following statement as a guiding principle for social care: 'we want to live in the place we call home with the people and things that we love, in communities where we look out for one another, doing the things that matter to us'. If achieving this is the measure of success in social care, which we believe it should be, then the current social care system has a very long way to go to achieving this.

Conclusion

In this chapter we have considered the history and current provision of social care. Parts of social care engage directly with the NHS, particularly around hospital discharge. For people needing some kinds of support the distinction between health and social care is paper thin, such that it feels like a 'lottery' whether people are assigned to (free) universal health services or (expensive) means-tested social care (Barker, 2014: 18). But other elements of social care are about living a good life as someone who needs additional long-term support – accessing education, employment and socialising. This kind of social care is a long way from the medical model and is often poorly understood by those who see social care as an extension of health.

We have also looked at how the organisation of social care differs from the NHS: in being more privatised and fragmented; less professionalised; less centralised; and more poorly staffed and funded. The mixed economy of care is very different to that in health: most social care provision is in the private sector and a substantial proportion is purchased by private payers outside the purview of the state. There is no coherent national workforce strategy. Social care is a local government responsibility making it hard to generalise about how care is designed and delivered. All of these distinctive features make it difficult to pursue an integrated approach across health and social care, although efforts to bring them together into integrated systems continue.

Assessing the future, the challenge which looms largest is that of workforce. The demographic changes which will increase demand will further worsen the shortfall in recruitment unless a new approach is taken. Sector leaders have been calling for a national workforce strategy, akin to that in the NHS, but successive governments have failed to act. It remains unclear whether the best way to address workforce shortages is to make the sector more professional and regulated (akin to nursing) or whether this only increases the barriers to entry. All four nations of the UK have workforce shortages despite trying different approaches to care worker regulation (Needham and Hall, 2023).

A further challenge is that of political stagnation as yet another attempt at reform – the care cap – is delayed and may be abandoned. It is dismaying to find that the political will required to address care funding reform dissipated so quickly. Overall, it is perhaps fitting that the 75th anniversary of the National Assistance Act 1948 will pass off with much less fanfare than the anniversary of the NHS. Whereas the 75 year anniversary of the NHS gives us something to celebrate in the ongoing commitment to universal and tax-funded healthcare, the National Assistance Act provides a much more ambiguous legacy.

References

Alderwick, H. (2022) *Understanding the Impact of Devolution in Greater Manchester on Health*. London: Health Foundation, https://www.health. org.uk/news-and-comment/blogs/understanding-the-impact-of-devolut ion-in-greater-manchester-on-health

All Party Parliamentary Group (APPG) on Adult Social Care. (2019) *The Future of Adult Social Care*. London: APPG on Adult Social Care.

Association of Directors of Adult Social Services (ADASS). (2022) *Spring Budget Survey 2022*. https://www.adass.org.uk/media/9390/adass-spring-budget-survey-2022-pdf-final-no-embargo.pdf

Barker, K. (2014) *A New Settlement for Health and Social Care*. London: The King's Fund.

Beresford, P. (2020) 'PPI or user involvement: Taking stock from a service user perspective in the twenty first century'. *Research Involvement and Engagement*, 6, 1, 1–5.

Bottery, S. (2020) 'Twelve social care personas: which one(s) are you?', The Kings Fund, 23 November. https://www.kingsfund.org.uk/blog/2020/ 11/twelve-social-care-personas

Britteon, P., Fatimah, A., Lau, Y.S., Anselmi, L., Turner, A.J., Gillibrand, S. et al (2022) 'The effect of devolution on health: A generalised synthetic control analysis of Greater Manchester, England'. *The Lancet Public Health*, 7, 10, e844–e852.

Burn, E. and Needham, C. (2020) 'Implementing the Care Act, 2014: A synthesis of project reports on the Care Act commissioned by the National Institute for Health Research'. Birmingham: University of Birmingham. https://www.birmingham.ac.uk/documents/college-social-sciences/soc ial-policy/publications/implementing-the-care-act-2014.pdf

Care Quality Commission (CQC). (2017) *The State of Health Care and Adult Social Care in England*. London: CQC. https://www.cqc.org.uk/sites/defa ult/files/20171123_stateofcare1617_report.pdf

Competition and Markets Authority (CMA). (2017) *Care Homes Market Study: Final Report*. London: CMA.

Compton, M.E. and 't Hart, P. (2019) 'How to "see" great policy successes. A field guide to spotting policy successes in the wild', in M.E. Compton and P. 't Hart (eds) *Great Policy Successes*. Oxford: Oxford University Press, pp 1–20.

Cootes, H., Heinsch, M. and Brosnan, C. (2022) '"Jack of all trades and master of none"? Exploring social work's epistemic contribution to team-based health care'. *The British Journal of Social Work*, 52, 1, 256–273.

County Councils Network (CCN). (2022) 'New analysis warns government has "seriously underestimated" the costs of adult social care charging reforms', CNN News, 18 March. https://www.countycouncilsnetwork. org.uk/new-analysis-warns-government-has-seriously-underestimated-the-costs-of-adult-social-care-charging-reforms/

Crawford, E. and Read, C. (2015) *The Care Collapse: The Imminent Crisis in Residential Care and its Impact on the NHS*. London: ResPublica.

Curtice, J., Scholes, A., Ratti, V., Cant, J., Bennett, M., Hinchcliffe, S. et al (2022) *British Social Attitudes Survey 39*, London: NatCen, https://www.bsa.natcen.ac.uk/media/39485/bsa39_nhs-and-social-care.pdf

Department of Health and Social Care (DHSS). (2021) *People at the Heart of Care: Adult Social Care reform White Paper*. London, HMSO.

Dilnot, A. (2011) *Fairer Care Funding: The Report of the Commission on Funding of Care and Support*. London: The Stationery Office.

Exworthy, M., Powell, M. and Mohan, J. (1999) 'Markets, bureaucracy and public management: the NHS – quasi-market, quasi-hierarchy and quasi-network?'. *Public Money and Management*, 19, 4, 15–22.

Evans, T. (2010) 'Professionals, managers and discretion: Critiquing street-level bureaucracy'. *The British Journal of Social Work*, 41, 2, 368–386.

Feeley, D. (2021) *Independent Review of Adult Social Care in Scotland*. Scottish Government: Edinburgh.

Fotaki, M., Ruane, S. and Leys, C. (2013) *The Future of the NHS? Lessons from the Market in Social Care in England*. London: Centre for Health and the Public Interest.

Gerlich, K. and Farquharson, C. (2020) 'Experts' debate: Will registering care workers reduce risk or reduce choice?'. *The Guardian*, 27 February. http://www.theguardian.com/society/2020/feb/27/experts-debate-registering-care-workers

Glasby, J. (2017) *Understanding Health and Social Care* (3rd ed). Bristol: Policy Press.

Glasby, J. and Littlechild, R. (2016) *Direct Payments And Personal Budgets: Putting Personalisation into Practice* (3rd ed). Bristol: Policy Press.

Glasby, J., Zhang, Y., Bennett, M. and Hall, P. (2021) 'A lost decade? A renewed case for adult social care reform in England'. *Journal of Social Policy*, 50, 2, 406–437.

Hamblin, K. (2019) *Adult Social Care and Wellbeing Policy in the Four Nations of the UK*. Sheffield: University of Sheffield. http://circle.group.shef.ac.uk/wp-content/uploads/2019/12/WPO_final-v2.pdf

Hayes, L., Johnson, E. and Tarrant, A. (2019) *Elevation, Registration and Standardisation: The Professionalisation of Social Care Workers*. London: APPG on Adult Social Care.

Henwood, M., Glasby, J., McKay, S. and Needham, C. (2022) 'Self-funders: Still by-standers in the English social care market?'. *Social Policy and Society*, 21, 2, 227–241.

HM Treasury. (2022) Autumn Statement. London: HM Treasury. https://www.gov.uk/government/publications/autumn-statement-2022-documents/autumn-statement-2022-html#:~:text=The%20Autumn%20Statement%20sets%20out%20a%20package%20of%20targeted%20support,bill%20increases%20following%20the%20revaluatio

House of Lords Adult Social Care Committee. (2022) *A 'gloriously ordinary life': Spotlight on Social Care.* https://committees.parliament.uk/publications/31917/documents/179266/default/

Hudson, B. (2016) *The Failure of Privatised Adult Social Care in England: What Is to Be Done?* London: Centre for Health and the Public Interest.

Hudson, B. (2021) *Clients, Consumers or Citizens? The Privatisation of Adult Social Care in England.* Bristol: Policy Press.

Humphries, R. (2022) *Ending the Social Care Crisis: A New Road to Reform.* Bristol: Policy Press.

Humphries, R. and Timmins, N. (2021) Stories from *Social Care Leadership*: Progress amid *Pestilence* and *Penury*. London: The King's Fund. https://www.kingsfund.org.uk/publications/social-care-leadership

Institute of Public Care (IPC). (2014) *The Stability of the Care Market and Market Oversight in England* (on behalf of the Care Quality Commission). Oxford: IPC. www.cqc.org.uk/sites/default/files/201402-market-stability-report.pdf

King's Fund, The. (2022) *Social Care 360*. London: The King's Fund. https://www.kingsfund.org.uk/publications/social-care-360

Luff, R. (2022) 'What more can we do to understand the difference that co-production makes in social care?'. Blog. Centre for Care Commentary. https://centreforcare.ac.uk/commentary/2022/10/co-production-in-social-care/

Mannion, R., Marini, G. and Street, A. (2008) 'Implementing payment by results in the NHS'. *Journal of Health Organisation and Management*, 22, 1, 79–88.

Mansell, J. and Beadle-Brown, J. (2005) 'Person centred planning and person-centred action: A critical perspective', in P. Cambridge and S. Carnaby (eds) *Person Centred Planning and Care Management with People with Learning Disabilities*. London: Jessica Kingsley Publishers, pp 19–33.

McMullin, C. and Needham, C. (2018) 'Co-production and healthcare', in T. Brandsen, T. Steen, and B. Verschuere (eds) *Co-production and Co-creation: Engaging Citizens in Public Service Delivery*. New York: Routledge, pp 151–160.

Means, R., Richards, S. and Smith, R. (2008). *Community Care: Policy and Practice* (4th ed). Basingstoke: Palgrave.

Miller, R., Schaub. J. and Howarth, S. (2019) 'Does social work have a problem with leadership?'. Blog. University of Birmingham. https://www.birmingham.ac.uk/news/2019/does-social-work-have-a-problem-with-leadership

Musekiwa, E. and Needham, C. (2021) 'Co-commissioning at the micro-level: personalized budgets in health and social care', in E. Loeffler and T. Bovaird (ed) *The Palgrave Handbook of Co-production of Public Services and Outcomes*. Palgrave Macmillan, Cham, pp 249–263.

National Audit Office. (2018) *Adult Social Care at a Glance*. London: NAO.

Needham, C. (2020) 'Managerial discretion', in T. Evans and P. Hupe (eds) *Discretion and the Quest for Controlled Freedom*. Cham: Palgrave Macmillan, pp 295–312.

Needham, C. and Carr, S. (2009) *Co-production and Social Care*. London: Social Care Institute for Excellence.

Needham, C. and Glasby, J. (eds) (2014) *Debates in Personalisation*. Bristol: Policy Press.

Needham, C. and Hall, P. (2023) *Social Care in the UK's Four Nations: Between Two Paradigms*. Bristol: Policy Press.

Needham, C., Allen, K., Burn, E., Hall, C., Mangan, C., Al-Janabi, H. et al (2022) 'How do you shape a market? Explaining local state practices in adult social care'. *Journal of Social Policy*, 1–21. doi:10.1017/S0047279421000805

Payne, M. (2005) *The Origins of Social Work: Continuity and Change*. Basingstoke: Palgrave.

Pierson, J. (2011) *Understanding Social Work: History and Context*. Maidenhead: Open University Press.

Powell, M. and Hall, P. (2020) 'An idea whose time has not yet come: Government positions on longterm care funding in England since 1999'. *Research, Policy and Planning*, 33, 3–4, 137–149.

Robertson, R., Appleby, J. and Evans, H. (2019) *Public Satisfaction with the NHS and Social Care in 2018: Results from the British Social Attitudes Survey*. London: King's Fund and Nuffield Trust.

Shutt, J. and Liddle, J. (2019) 'Are combined authorities in England strategic and fit for purpose?'. *Local Economy*, 34, 2, 196–207.

Social Care Future. (2019) *Talking about a Brighter Social Care Future*. www.camphillvillagetrust.org.uk/wp-content/uploads/2019/10/iC-SCF-report-2019-d-1.pdf

Skills for Care. (2021) *The State of the Adult Social Care Sector and Workforce in England, 2020–21*. London: Skills for Care.

Skills for Care. (2022) *The State of the Adult Social Care Sector and Workforce in England, 2021–22*. London: Skills for Care.

Tunstill, J. (2018) 'Pruned, policed and privatised: The knowledge base for children and families social work in England and Wales in 2019'. *Social Work and Social Sciences Review*, 20, 2, 57–76.

Turnpenny, A. and Husssein, S. (2022) 'Migrant home care workers in the UK: A scoping review of outcomes and sustainability and implications in the context of Brexit'. *Journal of International Migration and Integration*, 23, 23–42.

Unwin, J. (2018) *Kindness, Emotions and Human Relationships*. Dunfermline: Carnegie UK Trust.

Vennik, F.D., van de Bovenkamp, H.M., Putters, K. and Grit, K.J. (2015) 'Co-production in healthcare: Rhetoric and practice'. *International Review of Administrative Sciences*, 82, 1, 150–168.

Welsh Government. (2021) *The Cooperation Agreement*. Cardiff: Welsh Government.

11

The NHS at 75
in comparative perspective

Ian Greener

Introduction

This chapter will aim to answer the question 'What kind of health system is the NHS, on how does it compare to others?'. It aims to do this through an examination of a range of different health statistics from the OECD, G7 and Commonwealth Fund and by locating the NHS in relation to a recent typology of health systems. The strategy is to consider the NHS in 2019 (the last year pre-COVID-19), and compare statistics for total spend, funding sources, capacity (doctors, nurses, beds, scanners) and health outcomes at that date as a means of exploring changes during the pandemic and to try and see its effects. These three elements cannot capture all the dimensions of health systems (and measures of care will also be introduced), but they do cover many of the most distinctive dimensions of differences between such systems. Having explored changes during the pandemic in terms of the UK in relation to other countries in the OECD, it then performs further comparisons with the G7 group of nations and the 11 countries included in the Commonwealth Fund's most recent reports, and which it argues reflect better comparisons as they are made up of advanced industrial nations which the UK would more often regard as its peers, and so are likely to be facing more similar challenges in relation to healthcare than countries that less obviously fit into that category.

The chapter then performs two further comparisons – with the situation in 2000 (broadly 20 years ago, and at the beginning of the period in which the NHS Plan was meant to expand resources for the health service) and 2009 (the end of the funding expansion under the NHS Plan, and after which there was a change in government) to consider whether the position of the NHS in comparative context has improved or worsened since. This date was chosen to get some sense of how the NHS has changed over the last 20 years under governments of different political parties, but also with a pragmatic eye in that good comparative data often becomes much harder to come by prior to that date. The chapter then considers how its analysis fits with a key typology of health systems presented by Reibling, Ariaans and Wendt (2019), and what gaps the chapter highlights in that typology. Finally, it utilises data from the Commonwealth Fund in 2017 and 2021 to try and understand if the UK's relatively poor health outcomes are due to problems with its healthcare systems, or possibly wider societal challenges, before presenting its conclusion.

The NHS in comparative context in 2019

The OECD's health statistics for the NHS (at the time of writing in November 2022) show it spent just under 9.9 per cent of GDP on healthcare in 2019 – the last year pre-pandemic (we will return to the effects of the pandemic later), and which equates to $4,385 per person (purchasing power parity) (see also Chapter 3). Although we can track these figures over time, showing their rise over several decades, it is hard to categorise the NHS without comparing those figures (and others) to different health systems.

The OECD mean spend on healthcare in 2019 was 8.8 per cent, with a spend per person of $4,002, with the UK 14th ranked in terms of GDP expenditure and 16th on purchasing power parity (PPP) (out of 38 nations). In these terms, the NHS spent slightly higher than the OECD average, giving some fuel to those on the political right to claim that healthcare in the UK is too expensive. However, a key question is whether OECD averages are a sensible benchmark. While the UK is a member of the OECD, so are Columbia, Costa Rica, the Czech Republic, Estonia, Hungary, Lithuania, Mexico, the Slovak Republic, Slovenia and Turkey. It is not entirely clear what the UK has in common with those countries other than that they are also members of the OECD. Perhaps we need to consider some alternative benchmarks.

The UK is also a member of the G7 – the group of advanced economies which regularly meet to discuss global challenges (including health and wellbeing). How does it compare to those countries? The mean spend in the G7 in 2019 was 11.4 per cent of GDP, or $5,740 PPP. These figures are a little distorted because of the very large spend of the USA, but the UK was ranked sixth (out of seven) on both expenditure as a proportion of GDP and expenditure PPP, with only Italy spending less on both measures.

If we broaden the list of countries we compare to, a useful sample which allows further comparisons comes from the Commonwealth Fund (Schneider et al, 2017, 2021), which uses 11 countries in its most recent international healthcare rankings, all from highly developed nations and so being sensible comparators for the UK. These countries also provide diversity of comparison, including all three of Esping-Andersen's 'Worlds of Welfare' types (liberal, conservative and social democratic). In that list the mean spend in 2019 was 11.1 per cent of GDP (so slightly lower than the G7) but $5,986 PPP, so slightly higher. The UK ranked 10 out of 11 on both measures, with only New Zealand spending less.

In all then, despite the UK spending above average compared to OECD countries, perhaps a more sensible comparison is with the G7 and Commonwealth Fund sample, which ranked the UK in 2019 as near the bottom, suggesting that, among closer peers, the UK was not a comparatively big spender on healthcare.

If we now turn to how that spending was funded, then the OECD present three broad categories, government and compulsory insurance, out-of-pocket payments and voluntary health insurance. In 2019 the UK funded 79.4 per cent of its healthcare spending from government and compulsory insurance, and 15.3 per cent from out-of-pocket payments. That leaves 5.4 per cent for voluntary health insurance. Again, though, we need to compare these numbers to other healthcare systems to better understand what they mean.

The OECD mean funding from government and compulsory insurance in 2019 was 74.2 per cent, with 19.9 per cent from out-of-pocket spending and 6 per cent from voluntary health insurance. As such, the UK appears high on government and compulsory health insurance, a little low on out-of-pocket spending, and just below the average on voluntary health insurance, with the UK ranked 14th, 22nd and 12th against other OECD nations on these measures. These numbers often suggest to those on the political right that the NHS should make greater use of private sources for health funding.

If we compare to the G7, the mean government and compulsory funding in 2019 was 79.6 per cent, with out-of-pocket payments being 14.4 per cent and voluntary health insurance just under 6 per cent. In these terms, the NHS does not appear to be an outlier, being ranked 5th for the first two categories and 4th for voluntary health insurance. When comparing to the Commonwealth Fund 11 countries, the mean government and compulsory insurance was 79.2 per cent, with out-of-pocket spending at 14.25 per cent and voluntary health insurance at 6.6 per cent (excluding NZ for the last two figures, for which no figures were available). This ranks the UK 8th out of 11 for government and compulsory insurance, 2nd out of ten for out-of-pocket payments, and 7th out of ten for voluntary health insurance.

What all this suggests is that the UK's extensive use of government and compulsory insurance is not untypical of similar countries, but with the UK being an outlier because it does not have compulsory insurance in the same way as many European countries (and with a very different system to the USA). In terms of OECD and G7 it is mid-table in terms of its use of out-of-pocket payments, but higher in terms of the Commonwealth Fund, suggesting there is little traction in debates around making use of additional charges to see doctors or increasing charges further for prescription medications (and where there are differences in the UK's home nations approach). The UK has low funding from voluntary health insurance, but a warning note to increasing this aspect of funding comes from research showing the strong link between a range of negative health system outcomes and high use of voluntary health insurance (Greener, 2021).

As well as comparing expenditure levels and funding sources, we can also look at what the NHS spends its money on, looking at numbers of doctors, numbers of hospital beds, numbers of nurses, and the availability of technology such as CT and MRI scanners. This is necessarily a little reductionist, but does give us an idea of the capacity of the healthcare system. Here we will use the most recently available numbers from the OECD as little has changed during the pandemic – which we might expect given the considerable training time needed to increase numbers (doctors and nurses), relatively tangential relationship to the pandemic (scanners), and lack of change in hospital bed numbers since 2019.

The UK has just over 3 doctors, 8.5 nurses and 2.4 hospital beds per 1,000 people, with 9 CT scanners and 7.8 MRI scanners per million people. On all these measures the UK is below the OECD average, which is 3.6 doctors, 8.9 nurses, 4.3 beds, 27.4 CT scanners and 17.3 MRI scanners. The UK is ranked 28 (out of 38) for doctors, 21st for nurses, 33rd for beds, 35th for CT scanners and 32nd for MRI scanners. The capacity of the NHS, by these measures, is not strong.

Comparing to the G7 we find an average of 3.2 doctors, 10.3 nurses, 5.3 beds, 39 CT scanners and 27 MRI scanners. The UK is ranked 4 (out of 7) for doctors, 6th for nurses, 7th for CT scanners, and 7th for MRI scanners. So despite a mid-table performance for doctors, the comparison elsewhere is not good.

Comparing to the Commonwealth Fund 11 nations, the mean doctor number is 3.7, nurses 12.3, beds 3.7, CT scanners 30, and MRI scanners 19. The UK ranks 9/11 for doctors, 11th for nurses, 10th for beds, 11th for CT scanners and 11th for MRI scanners.

In all then, the capacity of the NHS seems to be low on almost any measure and any comparison. Its doctor numbers are its strongest statistic where it appears mid-table for G7, but even then it is relatively poor by OECD and Commonwealth Fund measures.

How has the NHS changed?

We can make three additional comparisons. First, how has the NHS changed in terms of its expenditure and funding sources during the pandemic? Second, we might consider how the NHS has changed since 2000 – a gap of around 20 years, and chosen as being the beginning of Labour's 'NHS Plan' (Secretary of State for Health, 2000) in the 2000s, to get a sense of its development since then. Third, given allegations about the impact of the Conservative government on the NHS which has been in power since 2010, how has the NHS changed since 2009?

The pandemic response

The UK has seen a sharp rise in healthcare expenditure between 2019 and the most recent year, 2021, from 9.8 per cent of GDP to 12 per cent, along with a rise from $4,385 to $5,019.[1] It is unclear whether these increases will remain in place post–pandemic (when that time arrives), but the expectation is that the UK faces significant funding cuts across the board as soon as savings can be found.

In terms of the OECD, the UK moved from the 14th highest spend (measured as a proportion of per cent GDP) to 5th – a dramatic increase. However, in terms of $ PPP it moved from 16th to 15th only.

Within the G7, the UK rose from 6th to 5th in terms of both measures of health expenditure (per cent of GDP and expenditure $PPP). overtaking Japan, whose pandemic response appears to have been far more effective than the UK. Within the Commonwealth Fund, the significant rise in UK health expenditure lifted the UK from 10th to 5th in terms of health expenditure as a proportion of GDP, but made no difference at all in terms of PPP spend, remaining 10th.

These changes suggest that although it devoted a greater proportion of its national income to healthcare, that increase in spend was not disproportional in real spending terms compared to other nations, despite concerns about the ineffectiveness and cost of the pandemic response in the UK (Beaumont and Connolly, 2020; O'Donnell and Begg, 2020; King-Hill, Greener and Powell, 2021).

The UK saw a rise in government and compulsory funding from 79.3 per cent to 82.9 per cent during the pandemic, with a fall in out-of-pocket expenditure from 15.3 per cent to 12.5 per cent, and a fall in voluntary health insurance from 5.4 per cent to 4.6 per cent. On OECD measures, the rise in government and compulsory funding made little difference to the UK's ranking (a move from 14th to 12th), but the change in out-of-pocket ranking (22nd to 29th) being more significant (there was a move from 14th to 19th in voluntary health insurance). Within the G7, there was no change to the government and compulsory funding ranking (5th) but with a small change in terms of out-of-pocket spending (from 2nd to 3rd) and no change to its voluntary health insurance ranking (4th).

In relation to the Commonwealth Fund nations and its means of healthcare funding, the UK moved from 8th to 7th in terms of its increase in government and compulsory insurance, from 2nd to 6th in terms of its use of out-of-pocket funding, and from 7th to 8th in its voluntary health insurance ranking.

The pandemic response in the UK then, has seen a significant increase in total healthcare system spend, with a greater proportion of GDP going to healthcare. However, in terms of spend PPP, this has not made much of a difference to the UK's spend in relation to other nations, where it remains at the low end of comparable nations. During the pandemic there has been an increase in public sources of funding, with a decline in other types. However, there appears to be little scope in increasing either out-of-pocket or private health insurance to try and raise additional NHS funding, with the former not being significantly out of line with other countries at its pandemic levels, and the higher levels of the latter being associated with poor health outcomes across a range of different measures.

How does 2019 compare to 2000?

Comparing the NHS to itself and other health systems in 2000 provides a means of assessing how it has changed under both Labour and Conservative governments over the last 20 years, with good quality data available to compare it to other countries over the same period. It is important to be clear that debates around the funding and scope of the NHS did not begin in 2000 – they have existed since its creation (Klein, 2006; Greener, 2008). As far back as the 1950s there were concerns and complaints that the NHS was unaffordable, despite the government's own inquiry finding it to be remarkably cost-effective (Public Records Office, 1955). The NHS also exists in a particular political context – compared to other political systems the UK is highly centralised (Lijphart, 2012), and it is possible for a government with a majority in parliament to radically change the direction of policy and organisation in ways that are simply not possible in other countries (Steinmo and Watts, 1995). It is difficult in a chapter of this length to deal with all of this complexity. What it can do, however, is explore how the NHS has changed, both in terms of its own measures, but in relation to other health systems, over a reasonable period of time.

In 2000, the NHS spent 7.2 per cent of national income on healthcare, compared to 9.9 per cent in 2019. The OECD mean at that time was 7.14 per cent, so almost the same, but the mean for the G7 was 8.9 per cent, and for the Commonwealth Fund countries, 8.6 per cent, with the UK 11th out of 11 countries for spend. In terms of spend PPP, the UK was at $1,897, compared to an OECD average of $1,806, a G7 mean of $2,620 and a Commonwealth Fund mean of $2,658. The UK was ranked 6 out of 7 in the G7 (with only Japan spending less) and 10th out of 11 in the Commonwealth Fund, with only New Zealand spending less. As such, in 2000, the UK was not a high spender on healthcare.

The UK's health system was 76.1 per cent from public sources (effectively taxation and national insurance), 17.3 per cent from out-of-pocket expenditure, and 6.6 per cent from voluntary insurance, compared to 79.4 per cent, 15.3 per cent, and 5.4 per cent in 2019 – showing a rise in public spending as a source of funding by the latter date. This mix of funding put the UK middle-table in the G7 and Commonwealth Fund for public and compulsory insurance expenditure (4th and 6th respectively), with the second highest out-of-pocket expenditure (in terms of overall funding) in the G7, but ranked fourth in the 11 Commonwealth Fund countries. The NHS funding pattern, in these terms, does not appear untypical compared to its peer nations.

In 2000 the NHS had 2 doctors, 8.1 nurses and 4 hospital beds per 1,000 people, placing it 6 out of 7 in the G7 nations for doctors, and last place by the same measure in Commonwealth Fund countries (but with missing data for two countries). In terms of nurses, data is rather incomplete, but with the NHS lagging in second-last for the countries with data. In terms of beds, the NHS does a little better – being ranked 5th in both the G7 and Commonwealth Fund. Data for scanners (CT and MRI) is too incomplete to be meaningful in 2000, but in terms of preventable life years, the NHS ranks 6 out 7 in the G7, and 10th out of 11 in the Commonwealth Fund, suggesting its outcome measures are not strong.

In all then, in 2000, the NHS is at the lower end of overall funding, even if its sources of funding are not particularly distinctive. In common with 2019, it is middle-table in terms of doctor numbers it is mid-table, but at the low end in terms of both nurses and beds.

How did the NHS in 2009 compare to both 2000 and 2019?

Having gone back to 2000, we can then move the story of the last 20 years forward to consider the effects of Labour's NHS Plan. Did the NHS Plan make a difference to the trajectory of the NHS?

In 2009, health expenditure was 10 per cent of GDP, a figure broadly similar to that of 2019 (9.9 per cent) and a considerable rise from 2000 (7.2 per cent), but even after that increase was 5th in the G7 (ahead of Japan and Italy) and 6th in the Commonwealth Fund (ahead of the Netherlands, New Zealand, Norway, Sweden and Australia). In GDP terms, this was a significant change. Spending PPP showed less change, with the 2009 figure being $3335, compared to $1897 in 2000 and $4,385 in 2019. This spend ranked the NHS as 5th in the G7 nations (higher than Japan and Italy) but 10th of the Commonwealth Fund nations (with only New Zealand spending less).

Much of the increase in NHS expenditure came from public sources, with 80.6 per cent coming from public expenditure in 2009, a figure being similar to 2019 (79.3 per cent) and a rise from 2000 (76.1 per cent); 14.2 per cent of funding was from out-of-pocket expenditures, a fall from 17.3 per cent in 2000, and slightly lower than 15.3 per cent in 2019. The majority of NHS funding in the 2000s came from the public purse.

Having seen an increase in funding for the NHS in the 2000s, what difference did it make to NHS capacity? In 2009 there were 2.64 doctors, 8.5 nurses and 3.3 beds per 1,000 people, compared to 2 doctors, 8.1 nurses and 4 hospital beds in 2000. As such, there has been an increase in doctors, but a fall in nurses and beds in relation to the population. However, the figures in 2009 have the NHS ranked fourth in the G7 for doctors and nurses, and fifth for beds, a slight improvement compared to both 2000 and 2019. In the Commonwealth Fund rankings, the NHS is ranked 7th for doctors, 9th for nurses and 7th for beds, a slight improvement for nurses and beds, but a slight decline in rankings for doctors. In 2009 accurate data for scanners of both types is still not available, making comparisons not possible.

We can also see that the increased investment by 2009 led to some improvements in rankings over preventable years of life lost, with the UK being ranked 6th in the G7 for men and 4th for women, whereas it was 9th for men and 8th for women in the Commonwealth Fund – these rankings are still concerning, but there was cause for optimism at that point in seeing that increased investment could lead to health improvements for the country.

In all then, there was an increase in health expenditures in the 2000s, and although they did not translate in absolute terms into improvements in the measured elements of capacity outlined earlier, in relative terms, the NHS did seem to do better in international comparisons of them.

If we move the clock forward again to 2019, the NHS appears to be in a broadly similar situation (in absolute terms) in most of the measures considered here as in 2009. However, in international terms, this means that it had fallen behind other countries, and that increased demand for services in the UK were not being met. Equally, the improvements in the 2000s of the UK's position in terms of preventable years of life lost for both men and women have been lost and that has to be a significant source of concern.

The UK healthcare system in comparative perspective

From this, we can make some broad characterisations about the healthcare system in the UK. First, although health expenditure rose in the 2000s, and during the pandemic, the NHS has not historically received high levels of funding compared to either the G7 or Commonwealth Fund, both of which make more sensible comparators than the wider range of OECD nations, and which include countries which are less comparable to the UK as an advanced industrial nation.

Second, the NHS does not fund its health services from an especially unusual mix, at least in terms of the OECD's top-level measures. Below those measures there is something distinctive in that the NHS is primarily funded from public sources rather than making use of compulsory health insurance as many (but not all) European countries do. The main difference between paying for health services through general taxation and through compulsory insurance is a possible reason for the relative underfunding of the NHS, as the health service has to compete for resources with other public services in each spending round rather than receiving a longer-term settlement. It is also the case that the relative levels of out-of-pocket payments made in the NHS have historically been relatively high, although their proportion of overall funding has fallen during the pandemic.

Third, the capacity of the NHS appears, on most measures, to be lower than many other comparable health systems in terms of numbers of nurses, numbers of beds, and is a laggard in technological adoptions in terms of the availability of scanning technology. In terms of doctor numbers, the NHS is broadly mid-table, but the lack of capacity in other areas has to be an area of concern, and suggest an urgent need for additional investment.

Finally, in terms of the preventable life years lost measure, which is highly correlated with a range of other attempts to capture both health system and life expectancy measures, the UK does poorly in almost any sensible comparison to other countries. This is a topic worth discussing at greater length, and is an area to which the chapter will turn to after it has located the NHS further in typologies of international health systems.

How does the analysis here compare to typology-based approaches to healthcare systems?

There are a number of ways of comparing different health systems through the use of frameworks or typologies (Blank, Burau and Kuhlmann, 2018). Perhaps the most significant work has been conducted by Wendt, who has developed a distinctive approach to generating typologies of health systems alongside a range of collaborators (Wendt, 2009, 2015; Marmot and Wendt, 2012). In recent work (Reibling, Ariaans and Wendt, 2019), he has collaborated with others to present a typology of OECD healthcare systems, and it is useful to compare that analysis with the raw data produced earlier, while bearing in mind the caveats already expressed as to the extent that several of the nations in the OECD share the same advanced economy as the UK.

The typology presented in this work is based around a range of factors under the broad headings of supply (health expenditure, GP numbers), public private mix (public health expenditure levels, out-of-pocket expenditures, the way specialists are remunerated), access regulation (broadly the extent to which social rights are operationalised in health systems and based on whether individuals have to register to see a GP, operationalised in terms of the extent to which they make use of cost-sharing, and an attempt to measure the extent of patient choice within the system), primary care orientation (measured in terms of health expenditure on outpatient care and the ratio of GPs to specialists). In addition, there are a range of performance measures based on smoking rates, alcohol consumption rates and an overall quality index based on a range of routine health measures including readmission rates). Having gathered all the data, cluster analysis is then performed using a range of different algorithms and distance measures (so that 24 different analyses were conducted) and the links between countries assessed in terms of how often they appeared in the same cluster. As such, the approach is more comprehensive than the simple measures presented in this paper. How do its results compare?

After some debate and interpretation, the paper presents five clusters of countries within the OECD, with the UK appearing alongside Canada, Denmark, Estonia, Italy and the Netherlands, and characterised as being a regulation oriented public system, with medium supply, high to medium public private mix, maximum access regulation with no cost–costing and limited choice, medium primary care orientation and medium performance. The key factor in this cluster is 'its reliance on public regulation' (Reibling, Ariaans and Wendt, 2019, p 616). In broader terms, the characterisation of the NHS does not seem an unfair one. However, as we have just noted, there appear to be two differences between the analysis presented here and that in Reibling, Ariaans and Wendt.

First, the health outcomes of the NHS, compared to either G7 or Commonwealth Fund 11 nations, as outlined, are not good in terms of preventable mortality. These measures are highly correlated with the outcome measures presented in the Reibling, Ariaans and Wendt (2019) paper, and the characterisation of the NHS as having medium levels of performance appears to be skewed by the UK having reasonably good measures of tobacco and alcohol consumption, so presenting it as having medium performance when it is perhaps more accurately considered as being at the poor end.

Second, the Reibling, Ariaans and Wendt cluster analysis does exactly what it claims to – to put healthcare systems into clusters. There is no location of the healthcare systems in their political or social context, and this means that issues about the pressures that political decisions made about income and wealth distribution, and the different pressures they may place upon healthcare systems, are not included. This would seem to be an important omission – we need to consider healthcare systems in the wider social context in which they exist in order to understand the different challenges that they might face.

As well as considering the healthcare system and the social context within which it exists, it is also important, as noted, to explore the political system within which decisions about healthcare and key issues such as whether and how inequality will be addressed are made. One of the key explanations offered for the existence (or not) of healthcare reform in the 1990s and 2000s was attempted had been linked to the extent of centralisation of political decision-making (Wilsford, 1994, 1995; Steinmo and Watts, 1995; Spithoven, 2011) the existence of 'veto points' which prevent change from occurring (Immergut, 1992a, 1992b) and the extent to which interest groups are either isolated from policy making or included within it (Alford, 1972, 1975). All these factors are relevant in understanding not only the current form of policy making (more generally), but also of the political system within which healthcare specifically has to function. It does appear that political systems which are more inclusionary in terms of interest groups, while at the same time retaining sufficient central control to enforce national policy making, out-perform other healthcare systems in terms of the health outcome measures used in this chapter (Greener, 2021). There is clearly a complex chain of causation in the link between political systems and health outcomes, but one that makes theoretical sense – if a wider range of interests are being included in policy making, then this might lead to lower levels of inequality, and if the state is able to implement health reform (especially in a context where the views of different interests are sought first), then it might make healthcare more adaptable than in countries where political divisions make such changes all but impossible.

In the context of that discussion, the UK has a highly centralised political system (making significant reform more possible than in many other countries), but is also highly exclusionary in terms of incorporating a wide range of interests into policy making (Lijphart, 2012; Maleki and Hendriks, 2016), with its 'Westminster model' being fairly unusual in international comparative terms (especially among the G7 or Commonwealth Fund 11), and does not appear to lead to consistency or consensus-seeking in policy making, both of which might important to achieve long-term investment in the healthcare system, or to improve on the UK's relatively poor health outcomes. It is to these poor health outcomes that the chapter now turns.

Why does the UK have such poor health outcomes and such high preventable mortality?

A first possibility for the UK's poor preventable mortality measures might come from the under capacity of the NHS leading to poor care. Is this the case?

International measures of care quality are difficult to compile, but perhaps the most complete comes from the Commonwealth Fund. Looking at the two most recent versions of their 'Mirror, mirror' report comparing the health systems of 11 countries (Schneider et al, 2017, 2021), we can see a concerning fall in the UK's situation. In the 2017 report, the UK was ranked first of the 11 countries for care process, third in terms of care access, and first for care equity. Although the UK was ranked tenth out of 11 countries for health outcomes, it was still overall ranked first in terms of its overall ranking among the 11 countries. By 2021, however, things were not as good. In that year the UK was ranked fifth for care process, fourth for care access, and fourth for care equity. The UK's overall ranking moved from first to fourth as a result, with its health outcomes nineth out of the 11 countries. Although the UK has moved from an overall ranking of first to mid-table, its fall in the rankings is clearly a source of concern, but suggests that the care the NHS is offering does not really account for the relatively poor health of people in the UK.

If the care provided by the NHS is not the primary reason for the UK's poor premature mortality, what else could be the cause? An explanation advanced in a range of different research locates the UK's problems in its levels of inequality (Marmot, 2015; Bambra, Lynch and Smith, 2021). Amongst the 11 countries of the Commonwealth Fund, the UK has the second highest GINI coefficient (after taxes and transfers) among the countries with a measure of 0.35 (compared to the USA at 0.38, the highest score and the poorest preventable mortality, and Norway at 0.26).

The argument for the UK's poor preventable mortality being linked to its inequality levels can be explained in terms of higher levels of inequality leading to 'status syndrome' (Marmot, 2012) which leads to higher levels of strain not only for those in poor positions in terms of income and wealth, but for everyone in that society, because of the greater emphasis on material wealth rather than wider wellbeing. This, in turn, has been linked to other social 'bads' such as higher crime levels and family breakdown (Wilkinson and Pickett, 2010).

The importance of considering inequality as an explanation for the differences in outcomes for health systems is that it asks us to raise our eyes beyond healthcare institutions alone, and to consider the social context in which the healthcare system has to function. One reason for comparably higher preventable mortality in the UK might be that people more generally are sicker, so the NHS has to deal with greater need for its services (when, as we have seen, there may be significant issues in relation to its capacity to provide care), both in terms of the volume of need as well as to the extent of illness when people do require healthcare. In August 2020 there were over 4 million people in the UK claiming personal independence payments or incapacity benefits – which although exacerbated by the pandemic, seem to form a longer-term trend towards increasing numbers of people requiring state support because of their health.[2]

As such, we have some explanation of the NHS in terms of its level of funding, its pattern of funding, its capacity, and its relationship to the health outcomes in the UK. We can also look wider still to see how this characterisation fits with at least other major typology of healthcare, that of the work of Wendt and his collaborators.

Conclusion

In conclusion, comparing the NHS to other health systems and attempting to measure its individual performance, we can say that it rates strongly on equity, in that it does not discriminate between patients in terms of their ability to pay for care, and does not leave them with debt as a result of receiving its services. At the same time, its services are under severe pressure because of the effects of both the pandemic, but also because of a range of wider social inequalities which governments of the last decade have little to alleviate. There is clear and strong evidence of the relationship between these inequalities and the nation's health, putting increased burdens on the health system which, although it has received significant increases in funding during the pandemic, has, for most of its history, been funded at levels below other health systems which make sensible comparisons.

There is clear evidence of the impact of 'austerity' policy over the last ten years on the nation's health as well as its impact during the pandemic (Ruckers and Labonte, 2017; Williams, Rajan and Cylus, 2021). It is also evident that the significant waits for care people now experience in the NHS are part of a longer-term trend rather than being specific to the pandemic, and date back nearly a decade.[3] Health services in the UK were struggling before the pandemic. While it is laudable that the NHS scores strongly on equity in international rankings, giving everyone equitable access to services they all have to wait years to receive isn't going to help any of us. There is an urgent need to look at longstanding problems with doctor, nurse, bed and technology capacity if the NHS it going to be able to deal with the challenges ahead. There is also an urgent need to address the massive shortfalls in capacity in social care, and which lead to patients who could be better looked-after in non-NHS settings being stranded in hospitals rather than receiving the community-based services they really need.

There is an urgent need then to look beyond the NHS in itself in understanding and confronting the health challenges that the UK faces. The NHS is under such pressure due to the cumulative effects of inequalities, and its political systems have failed to put in place long-term plans to address medical and clinical training to provide adequate levels of workforce, or to plan adequately in terms of bed or technology capacity. Until social care capacity is also addressed, the NHS will be left trying to look after patients who could be cared for significantly better in other settings. What is urgently needed is a rigorous, cross-party plan to secure the future of the NHS, but it appears that in the fractured UK political system such a possibility is unlikely.

Notes

[1] Statistics, unless otherwise specified, are from the OECD are from https://www.oecd.org/els/health-systems/health-data.htm, with the G7 data comparison taken from countries in that data as well. Technically the EU is included as an honorary eighth member of the G7, but won't be included in comparisons here as it does not represent a single nation or healthcare system.

[2] See https://www.gov.uk/government/statistics/dwp-benefits-statistics-february-2021/dwp-benefits-statistics-february-2021

[3] See for example, https://www.kingsfund.org.uk/projects/urgent-emergency-care/urgent-and-emergency-care-mythbusters, https://www.kingsfund.org.uk/projects/positions/nhs-waiting-times

References

Alford, R. (1972) 'The political economy of health care: Dynamics without change'. *Politics and Society*, 12, 127–164.

Alford, R. (1975) *Health Care Politics*. Chicago: University of Chicago Press.

Bambra, C., Lynch, J. and Smith, K.E. (2021) *The Unequal Pandemic: COVID-19 and Health Inequalities*. Bristol: Policy press (Policy press shorts insights).

Beaumont, P. and Connolly, K. (2020) 'Covid-19 track and trace: What can UK learn from countries that got it right? Pledge of "world-beating" system will have to look to likes of South Korea and Germany'. *The Guardian*, 21 May.

Blank, R.H., Burau, V. and Kuhlmann, E. (2018) *Comparative Health Policy*. London: Palgrave.

Greener, I. (2008) *Healthcare in the UK: Understanding Continuity and Change*. Bristol: Policy Press.

Greener, I. (2021) *Comparing Health Systems*. Bristol: Policy Press.

Immergut, E. (1992a) *Health Politics: Interests and Institutions in Western Europe*. New York: Cambridge University Press.

Immergut, E. (1992b) 'The rules of the game: The logic of health policy-making in France, Switzerland and Sweden', in S. Steinmo, K. Thelen, and F. Longstreth (eds) *Structuring Politics: Historical Institutionalism in Comparative Analysis*. Cambridge: Cambridge University Press, pp 57–89.

King-Hill, S., Greener, I. and Powell, M. (2021) 'Lesson-drawing for the UK government during the COVID-19 Pandemic: A comparison of official, media and academic lenses', in M. Pomati, A. Jolly, and J. Rees (eds) *Social Policy Review 33: Analysis and Debate in Social Policy*. Bristol: Policy Press.

Klein, R. (2006) *The New Politics of the NHS: From Creation to Reinvention* (5th ed). Abingdon: Radcliffe Publishing.

Lijphart, A. (2012) *Patterns of Democracy: Government Forms and Performance in Thirty-Six countries*. London: Yale University Press.

Maleki, A. and Hendriks, F. (2016) 'Contestation and participation: Operationalising and mapping democratic models for 80 electoral democracies, 1990–2009'. *Acta Politica*, 51, 2, 237–272.

Marmot, M. (2012) *Status Syndrome: How Your Social Standing Directly Affects Your Health*. London: Bloomsbury.

Marmot, M. (2015) *The Health Gap: The Challenge of an Unequal World*. London: Bloomsbury.

Marmot, T. and Wendt, C. (2012) 'Conceptual frameworks for comparing healthcare politics and policy'. *Health Policy*, 107, 11–20.

O'Donnell, G. and Begg, H. (2020) 'Far from well: The UK since COVID-19 and learning to follow the science(s)'. *Fiscal Studies*, 41, 4, 761–804.

Public Records Office. (1955) 'Treasury Social Services Division File on the Guillebaud Report, T.227.424'.

Reibling, N., Ariaans, M. and Wendt, C. (2019) 'Worlds of healthcare: A healthcare system typology of OECD countries'. *Health Policy*, 123, 7, 611–620. https://doi.org/10.1016/j.healthpol.2019.05.001

Ruckers, A. and Labonte, R. (2017) 'Health inequities in the age of austerity: The need for social protection policies'. *Social Science & Medicine*, 187, 306–311. DOI: 10.1016/j.socscimed.2017.03.029

Schneider, E., Sarnak, D.O., Squires, D., Shah, A. and Doty, M.M. (2017) *Mirror Mirror 2017*. New York: Commonwealth Fund.

Schneider, E., Shah, A., Doty, M.M., Tikkanen, R., Fields, K. and Williams II, R.D. (2021) *Mirror, Mirror 2021*. New York: Commonwealth Fund.

Secretary of State for Health. (2000) *The NHS Plan: A Plan for Investment, A Plan for Reform*. London: HMSO.

Spithoven, A. (2011) 'It's the institutions, stupid! Why US health care expenditure is so different from Canada's'. *Journal of Economic Issues*, 45, 1, 75–95.

Steinmo, S. and Watts, J. (1995) 'It's the institutions, stupid! Why comprehensive National Health Insurance always fails in America'. *Journal of Health Politics, Policy and Law*, 20, 2, 329–372.

Wendt, C. (2009) 'Mapping European healthcare systems: A comparative analysis of financing, service provision and access to healthcare'. *Journal of European Social Policy*, 19, 5, 432–445. https://doi.org/10.1177/09589 28709344247

Wendt, C. (2015) 'Healthcare policy and finance', in E. Kuhlmann, R.H. Blank, I.L. Bourgeault and C. Wendt (eds) *The Palgrave International Handbook of Healthcare Policy and Governance*. London: Palgrave, pp 54–68.

Wilkinson, R. and Pickett, K. (2010) *The Spirit Level: Why Equality Is Better for Everyone*. London: Penguin.

Williams, G., Rajan, S. and Cylus, J. (2021) 'COVID-19 in the United Kingdom: How austerity and a loss of state capacity undermined the crisis response', in S. Greer, E.J. King, E. Massard da Fonseca and A. Peralta-Santos (eds) *Coronavirus Politics: The Comparative Politics and Policy of COVID-19*. Ann Arbor: University of Michigan Press, pp 215–234.

Wilsford, D. (1994) 'Path dependency, or why history makes it difficult, but not impossible, to reform health care services in a big way', *Journal of Public Policy*, 14, 251–283.

Wilsford, D. (1995) 'States facing interests: Struggles over health care policy in advanced industrial democracies', *Journal of Health Politics, Policy and Law*, 20, 571–613.

12

Our NHS? The changing involvement of patients and the public in England's health and care system

Ellen Stewart, Amit Desai and Giulia Zoccatelli

Introduction

This chapter focuses on the changing local structures of patient and public involvement (PPI) in the English NHS, and on their basis in health policy. Reforms to processes of PPI intersect with, and have co-existed alongside reforms to, all the key analytic axes highlighted in this volume: hierarchies, markets and networks; the public and the private; professionals and the state. However in this chapter, our focus is how PPI intersects with one of the axes identified by the editors: dynamics of centralisation and decentralisation in the NHS. At the core of this interest is something of a paradox. Greer et al have argued, with a focus on health governance during the pandemic, that political decisions about centralisation and decentralisation are a question of credit and blame: 'politicians who wish to be effective and elected seek credit and avoid blame' (Greer et al, 2021). In this view, decentralisations – especially those driven by New Public Management logics – are a route by which government ministers avoid public blame and muddy accountability. Thus we might assume that questions of *public* voice are better served by a centralised healthcare system with clean, direct lines of accountability. To draw on one of Bevan's ever-quotable speeches (discussed further in the next section), the 'slops bucket' is knocked over, and a patient's complaint will be heard in Whitehall. However, the English NHS, is, by the standards of similar health system types, far *too* large for this centralised vision of responsiveness to be viable via command and control. Substantive calls for greater democratic control of the NHS are invariably couched at the local, and not the national, level (Klein, 2010).

The NHS in England has seen repeated attempts to devise adequate local structures of patient and public voice over the decades, alongside repeated dynamics of decentralisation, and recentralisation, in broader structural change (Peckham et al, 2005). Within the reforms (listed in Table 12.1) we argue that there are at least two competing visions of effective PPI, reflecting a distinction Day and Klein (1987) posit between political and managerial accountability. The first is concerned with the population as a source of intelligence on whether the NHS is meeting acceptable standards of care, with the substance of what is acceptable understood as national and pre-defined. This is PPI as a mechanism of managerial accountability, and sits comfortably within consumerist or instrumental visions of participation in healthcare (Stewart, 2013). The second, which is much more at home in a genuinely decentralised healthcare system, is PPI as a mechanism of political accountability (Klein, 2010). In this model, PPI creates spaces within which dialogue and even deliberation about local public priorities takes place. This serves democratic ends, as the substance of how a local healthcare system should operate is subject to debate and contestation among the local population (Stewart, 2013). The realisation of either of these visions depends not only on the intent of those designing policy reforms, but also on the work of local actors and members of the public implementing them 'on the ground'. Political and managerial visions of PPI can co-exist in practice both across and even within specific locales. In this chapter, we offer them as lenses through which we might assess the evidence on PPI across the 75 years of the NHS in England.

We begin this chapter with a historical overview of how local structures of PPI within the NHS have developed and been reformed over the decades. We then focus on evidence on Healthwatch, which has been in place since 2012's Health and Social Care Act, and which, at time of writing, remain in place as Integrated Care Systems are established. We reflect on the way that Healthwatch responded, locally and nationally, to the health emergency of the COVID-19 pandemic. Given the complexity and dynamism of these structural arrangements, we do not attempt to fully review related mechanisms – including patient complaints mechanisms, ombudsman organisations and attempts to institute local authority oversight of NHS services – within this chapter. However, in a final section, we sketch an account of how the contemporary work of Healthwatch sits in this broader context of multiple modes of public input in the NHS, including online patient feedback, and public campaigning.

Overall, our assertion is that the landscape of PPI has become increasingly disaggregated and diffuse within the English NHS. This relates to the frequent reform of formal structures (both those designed to involve patients and the public, and the underlying organisational structure of the NHS itself). It can be seen in the current highly decentralised and variable structures of Healthwatch at local levels. And its effects can be seen in the multiplication of alternative routes for patient and public feedback in the NHS. These changes, we suggest, relate to fundamental tensions in the policy conceptualisation of how the NHS should respond to patient and public knowledge and perspectives, as the (always tenuous) idea of a single 'consumer' voice within the service becomes increasingly *un*tenable. While potentially better able to respond to diverse perspectives and experiences, the fragmentation of these routes (as compared, for example, to the rigid yet cohesive structures of Community Health Councils) also has risks for the overall picture of patient and public voice in the English NHS.

The historical development of patient and public involvement in the NHS in England

Although patient and public involvement (PPI) has become a capitalised acronym since the late 1990s (Department of Health, 1999), its antecedents are crucial to an understanding of questions of centralisation and decentralisation regarding contemporary policy debates. Concerns about the public accountability of the NHS can be traced back to its creation (Hunter and Harrison, 1997) but in the early years, emphasis was placed firmly on direct ministerial responsibility rather than local voice. The inclusion of lay members on Health Authorities, although offering both managerial and political influence, was considered to be tokenistic, lacking independence and legitimacy (Baggott, 2005). Bevan famously declared in 1946 that:

> The Minister of Health will be whipping-boy for the Health Service in Parliament. Every time a maid kicks over a bucket of slops in a ward an agonised wail will go through Whitehall. After the new Service is introduced there will be a cacophony of complaints. The newspapers will be full of them. ... For a while it will appear that everything is going wrong. As a matter of fact, everything will be going right, because people will be able effectively to complain. (Quoted in Foot, 1973: 192–193)

While often held up as an indicator of extreme centralisation, this quote's concern with uncontroversial service standards – the kicked-over slops bucket as the forerunner of contemporary anxieties about hospital cleanliness – are specifically about managerial accountability. Patient and public voice, here, can provide surveillance that things are as they should be in hospitals across the country. What is missing from this early understanding of NHS accountability is any notion that service users or publics might hold and wish to pursue distinctive preferences for their healthcare, requiring instead some measure of political accountability (Day and Klein, 1987), as might be provided by direct accountability to elected local authorities (see Hagen and Vrangbaek, 2009).

Community Health Councils (CHCs) were created in the 1974 reorganisation of the NHS in England, separating representation of patients and the public from managerial responsibilities. They were created: 'almost by accident because, when the plans for a reorganised NHS were almost complete, all those involved realised that something was missing: an element which ... could be seen as providing a degree of local democracy, consumer participation or public involvement' (Klein and Lewis, 1976: 11).

While CHCs formalised and expanded public representation, the key aim was 'to give the CHCs a constructive role to play, while keeping them out of the management structure of the NHS' (Klein and Lewis, 1976: 22; see also Mold, 2016). In this separation the basic format bore a close resemblance to structures which were to follow. However CHCs were additionally responsible for dealing with enquiries from the public (later carved out into separate services such as the Patient Advice and Liaison Service), had a more complex membership (Klein and Lewis, 1976: 20), and lacked any statutory right to be consulted except on major service changes (Baggott, 2005). One early assessment noted difficulties including gaining access to primary care facilities, early enough input into decision-making processes, and in hearing from a broad range of the local population (Levitt, 1980). CHCs were represented by a proactive and assertive national membership body: the Association of Community Health Councils of England and Wales (Alexander, 2003a).

Over the decades CHCs were perceived by some to have lost focus, described as 'just one of many voices representing the public' (Warwick, 2006: 2) and 'parochial, quirky and irrelevant' (Pickard, 1997: 278). Public and patient involvement in England had to this point been 'a policy of encouragement rather than central prescription' (Milewa et al, 2002: 42). However this was to change with New Labour. In 2001, two documents pushed patient and public involvement high on the policy agenda. First to be published was the Health and Social Care Act 2001, which placed a 'statutory duty' on NHS organisations to involve and consult patients and the public. Two months later, the Kennedy Report (The Report of the Public Inquiry into children's heart surgery at the Bristol Royal Infirmary 1984–1995) was published, which stated, based on the inquiry, 'For a healthcare service to be truly patient-centred it must be infused with the views and values of the public (as patients past, present or future). The public must be involved.' The report offered a searing critique of PPI structures at the time (implicitly, CHCs): 'A principal reason must be the lack of real power enjoyed by the bodies set up within the NHS to give the public their voice. Without power, such bodies swiftly become "talking shop"', attractive to those who like to talk but ineffective in terms of translating talk into action.'

The report additionally proposed a series of principles for how to involve the public and patients in the NHS. The abolition of the CHCs was acrimonious, with threats of legal action from the national association. People within the CHC community resisted the suggestion that their work had been ineffective. Speaking in the final meeting of the Association of

Community Health Councils of England and Wales, its director Malcolm Alexander praised the campaigning work of the CHCs:

> CHCs have jealously guarded their independence. You can't battle for patients' right with one hand tied behind your back. ... Of course it is important to be constructive and to have a good relationship with the DH and local trusts. But sometimes you need to have the courage to stand apart, to be independent. (Alexander, 2003b)

Tensions around the risk of a gap in patient representation after the abolition of the CHCs led to a massive rush to get new arrangements in place. This was described by one academic and erstwhile forum member as 'performance-management induced frenzy', and blamed for later problems (see also Baggott, 2005; Warwick, 2006: 4). PPI Forums were created by the NHS Reform and Healthcare Professions Act 2002 and two statutory instruments (HMSO, 2003a; 2003b), as one component of a statutory system of public and patient involvement. Individual complaints and support were to be handled by Patient Advice and Liaison Services (PALS) and the Independent Complaints Advisory Service (ICAS), leaving forums to the tasks of 'monitoring and reviewing services and influencing and informing management decision-making in their Trust' (Department of Health, 2001: 10). Specific Forum powers include the right to request information from the Trust and Strategic Health Authority and the right of entry to inspect facilities (HMSO, 2003a). Unlike CHCs, which were geographically-bounded, PPI Forums were specifically linked to a particular trust, and so there were far more of them across the country, supported by the national Commission for Patient and Public Involvement in Health (Hogg, 2007). Their role went no further than consultation: the duty placed upon Strategic Health Authorities, PCTs and NHS trusts by the 2001 Health and Social Care Act was only to 'to make arrangements to involve and consult patients and the public' (Department of Health, 2003). PPI Forums, as one example of such arrangements, had little clout: they had the right to speak on an issue, but not necessarily to be heard.

Reflecting longstanding concerns about CHCs' role in representing the public (Levitt, 1980), the question of whether members should, or could, be representative was an area of ambiguity in official documents about PPI Forums. One document, analysed by Martin (2008), answers criticism about unrepresentativeness by retorting 'Unrepresentative of who or what? Patients and members of the public bring their own experiences to the debate' while guidance for practitioners conflictingly instructs them to recruit a 'representative cross-section' (both quoted in Martin, 2008: 17). In a discourse analysis of central government and CPPIH documents on the 'multifaceted ideal-type individual sought by the state',

Martin characterises them as 'experts in laity': people who: 'know and can make knowable their constituencies ... aided by the combination of their ordinariness – their very laity – and their extraordinary enthusiasm and armoury of reflexive skills' (Martin, 2008). Members were self-selecting, with a check by the CPPIH to ensure members have sufficient time and interest, enthusiasm, team-working skills and an understanding of the health needs of the community (Martin, 2008). In practice, membership was essentially first-come-first-served, particularly as few areas have had enough volunteers to have scope for turnover (House of Commons – Health Committee, 2007).

PPI Forums, and their umbrella body the CPPIH were remarkably short-lived experiments. Created in 2003, abolition was discussed from 2004 onwards and actioned in 2006. This reflected broader shifts in health policy: Martin suggests that the replacement structures, Local Involvement Networks, were seen as backup for a system in which the key means of public and patient power was patient choice: 'collective input ... is thus to some extent seen as secondary to, or a substitute for, the direct choices made by individuals as consumers' (Martin, 2009). One key element of this choice-based model allowed hospitals to become autonomous Foundation Trusts, with a poorly defined 'membership' role available to local publics (Allen et al, 2012; Day and Klein, 2005).

Reverting to the CHC model of locality-based organisations, LINks were to be commissioned by local authorities, rather than the NHS, and the delivery of each one was to be led by a local 'host organisation'. Writing shortly after the announcement, Hogg emphasised the diminution of the PPI role that the plans represented:

> LINks were to have no statutory rights. CHCs and Forums had rights to information and to inspect NHS premises. CHCs also had the right to observer status on trust boards as well as to be consulted about changes of use and to appeal to the Secretary of State in a dispute, a right inherited by OSCs. Little further detail is given on how the LINks might operate and the intention is to leave local areas to decide how they should be set up and managed locally. (Hogg, 2007)

More positively, Tritter and Koivusalo argued that LINks were 'not an inspectorate but a source of intelligence about what the experience of service users, and what the priorities for health and social care services should be' (Tritter and Koivusalo, 2013). Studies suggested highly variable degrees of influence between different LINks, including some sites where they were 'just one of a wide range of community inputs' (Marks et al, 2011). Little matter, for, but six years later, the Health and Social Care Act – a reorganisation 'so big you could see it from space' (Nicholson, quoted in Greer, Jarman and

Azorsky, 2014) – abolished LINks and proposed broadly the structure that still exists at the 75th anniversary of the NHS: Healthwatch.

Contemporary PPI: Healthwatch

The creation of Healthwatch in the HSCA 2012 marked the latest phase in the transformation of legal PPI mechanisms over the last 50 years. From being principally directed by lay members of the community participating in local decision-making processes (as in the CHCs), through local Healthwatch, PPI is now officially provided by professional organisations which elicit, promote and convey public voice in local health and care systems.

Like LINks, each local Healthwatch is commissioned by and accountable to their local authority. However, in a departure from LINks, local Healthwatch were given functions directly by statute. These include obtaining the views of people about their health and care services and communicating those views to Clinical Commissioning Groups (CCGs), local Care Quality Commission (CQC) officers and local authorities, providing information to the public about accessing the range of health and care services available to them in their area. Local Healthwatch retain the power held by previous iterations of official PPI to monitor the quality of health and care services by conducting 'enter and view' visits. Importantly, they are also asked 'to promote public and patient involvement in health and care planning, service delivery and monitoring' (Healthwatch England, 2022a). In so doing, local Healthwatch are expected to be the formal champions of PPI in local systems. This formality is buttressed by their mandatory named seat on Health and Wellbeing Boards in each local authority, themselves created by the 2012 Act. The boards brought together key local stakeholders such as public health and social care, NHS trusts, CCGs, GP representatives, councillors, council officials, as well as Healthwatch. Sitting on Health and Wellbeing Boards was meant to more effectively embed PPI for the first time at a strategic and planning level.

However, local Healthwatch's role and position within local health and care systems is replete with tensions and contradictions (Gilburt, Dunn and Foot, 2015; Carter and Martin, 2016; Martin and Carter, 2017; Zoccatelli and Desai et al, 2022). Carter and Martin (2016) have identified the mismatch between Healthwatch's responsibilities and the accountability structures in which they operate, leading to what they term 'jurisdictional misalignment' (see also Coleman et al, 2014; Hunter et al, 2018). While Healthwatch is expected to monitor the quality of NHS services by visiting services and producing publicly available reports, there is no specific requirement for NHS organisations to consider or act on Healthwatch recommendations nor a formal mechanism to force local consideration of any resulting concerns. While formally empowered to escalate specific issues to Healthwatch

Table 12.1: Key legislative changes in PPI structures in England

Year	Act or regulation	Key initiatives
1948	National Health Service Act 1946	Limited role for lay members on Regional Hospital Boards.
1973	NHS Reorganisation Act 1973	Community Health Councils created.
2001	Health and Social Care Act 2001	Places statutory duty on NHS organisations to involve and consult patients and the public in the planning of service provision, the development of proposals for and decisions about how services operate.
2002	NHS Reform and Healthcare Professions Act 2002	CHCs abolished. Patient and Public Involvement Forums and PALS and ICAS created.
2003	Health and Social Care (Community Health and Standards) Act 2003	Foundation Trusts with public membership created.
2004	Department of Health Arms' Length Body Review	CPPIH abolition proposed.
2006	A Stronger Local Voice	PPI Forums abolished. Local Involvement Networks created.
2007	Local Government and Public Involvement in Health Act 2007	Strengthened Section 11 of the Health and Social Care Act for consultation and involvement of the public and patients in service planning and provision.
2012	Health and Social Care Act	Local Involvement Networks abolished and local Healthwatch created. Health and Wellbeing Boards created in each local authority, involving key stakeholders (including Healthwatch) to provide strategic direction for local health and care matters.
2019	NHS Long Term Plan	Proposes a National Assembly of 'national clinical, patient and staff organisations; the Voluntary, Community and Social Enterprise (VCSE) sector; the NHS Arm's Length Bodies (ALBs); and frontline leaders from ICSs, STPs, trusts, CCGs and local authorities.'
2022	Health and Care Act	Establishes Integrated Care Systems on legal footing. No significant change in local Healthwatch role specified.

England, their umbrella organisation and a subcommittee of England's regulator, the Care Quality Commission (CQC), such escalation powers are rarely used. The key obstacle is the risk of compromising much valued local relationships, by 'bit[ing] the hand that feeds them' (Carter and Martin, 2016). A national survey of local Healthwatch found that in 2018–2019 only eight Healthwatch out of 96 respondents had escalated an issue to Healthwatch England which was later actioned (Zoccatelli et al, 2020).

Other challenges include local Healthwatch's need to work in a sometimes-crowded local field of PPI organisations and structures within which they compete for attention. As discussed, Healthwatch operate in an environment in which health and care providers use a vast array of tools and processes for collecting patient and service user experience data. CCGs and trusts may maintain their own locally developed engagement processes that leave little space for Healthwatch to contribute. For instance, as reported in a recent study (Zoccatelli and Desai et al, 2022), a local Healthwatch in one part of England was often marginalised in attempting to influence the work of a local hospital Trust. The Trust had an active and well-resourced engagement and communications department, which from its perspective was equipped to collect a wide range of insight; Healthwatch's own reports on the Trust's hospital services were often responded to in a minimal way or ignored completely (Zoccatelli and Desai et al, 2022).

Local Healthwatch: between local responsiveness, and national inequalities

All local Healthwatch share the same legal functions but an emphasis on local control means that local Healthwatch are extremely variable one from the other, shaped by the different institutional landscapes in which they operate, including size and type of local authority, the funding they receive, and individual organisational arrangements. There is no standard national template for how they work. The only requirement is that they are set up as social enterprises which must involve local volunteers. This requirement preserves the lay element which dominated previous iterations of official PPI within a contemporary framework of PPI professionalism. The degree to which volunteers are involved in the work of local Healthwatch varies greatly. For instance, Desai and Zoccatelli found that in some Healthwatch, the organisation's board members represent the only voluntary element; in others, volunteers contributed substantially to operational activities such as liaising with health providers and writing reports on service quality (Zoccatelli and Desai et al, 2022). The formal organisational arrangements of Healthwatch are also very diverse. Organisations can be registered as charities, community interest companies or private limited companies. Furthermore, some local Healthwatch are 'standalone', which means that they are operated by an organisation which primarily exists to run Healthwatch in that specific area. For instance, Healthwatch Essex is currently provided by Healthwatch Essex Ltd. Other local Healthwatch are 'hosted', which means that the Healthwatch is run by an organisation which also holds other contracts, potentially including Healthwatch contracts for other areas. For example, at the time of writing, Engaging Communities Solutions (ECS) – a not-for-profit organisation that specialises in social research, community engagement and consultation, and advocacy – provides Healthwatch services in seven local authority areas (Bedford, Walsall, Warrington, Halton, Sandwell, Leicester and Leicestershire and Stoke-on-Trent). Some Healthwatch are hosted by social enterprises which have only one Healthwatch contract alongside contracts to deliver other services. For instance, the Healthwatch Northumberland contract is held by Adapt NE, which runs several projects to help people with disabilities in that area.

Local authorities receive a grant from the Department of Health and Social Care to fund a local Healthwatch service. This funding is not ring-fenced; moreover, the DHSC's expectation is that this money will also be topped up by funds from the general local government settlement (Healthwatch England, 2022b). Local Healthwatch have been operating during a period of falling local authority budgets which has exerted downward pressure on the value of awards they receive, and for which many Healthwatch re-bid every two or three years (Carter and Martin, 2016; Martin & Carter, 2017). Their total funding has fallen over the past ten years, posing challenges to local Healthwatch's ability to fulfil its statutory functions. Whereas Healthwatch received a total of £40.3 million in 2013–2014, by 2021–2022 this had fallen to an estimated £25.4 million (Healthwatch England, 2022b).

Differing levels of funding provide an instructive example of local Healthwatch variability which influences the way in which they represent patient and public voice locally. In 2020–2021, individual local Healthwatch awards ranged from around £50,000 to over £500,000. These differences might be explained by population size differences between local authority areas. However, as a recent study has shown, these larger absolute amounts of funding are not used by these better funded Healthwatch to provide the services of smaller Healthwatch on a larger scale. Rather, the larger award value enables such Healthwatch to recruit staff specialised in a greater range of skills and so can offer local people and system partners different services. For example, a large Healthwatch may be able to employ experienced staff with expertise in co-design or academic research to support patient and public involvement in the planning of new health services. Smaller Healthwatch, by way of comparison, may only be able to employ part-time generalist staff who perform a range of different tasks such as engagement or communication which in larger Healthwatch are allocated to specific job positions. Such smaller Healthwatch may need to rely on volunteers to keep the organisation running. This significant variability in Healthwatch's work 'raises questions about whether there is equitable treatment of people across England in their ability to participate effectively in local health and social care planning and provision' (Zoccatelli and Desai et al, 2022).

Healthwatch and the COVID-19 pandemic

The COVID-19 pandemic looms large in any sense of how the current system for PPI in England functions. The initial health emergency context of 2020 and 2021, and its longer drawn-out aftermath, have had a significant impact. NHS organisations made previously unthinkable service changes in tight timescales, generally bypassing normal consultative processes with local populations. This context provided both challenges and particular opportunities for local Healthwatch. There is some evidence that local health and care systems were often particularly keen to hear from Healthwatch, as their usual avenues of information-gathering and engagement became impossible (Zoccatelli et al, 2021; Zoccatelli and Desai et al, 2022). Some local Healthwatch were able to capitalise on this opportunity, becoming highly responsive as information-gatherers for insights on the experiences of different sectors of the local population (for example, pregnant women, local ethnic minorities). This sort of rapid, responsive work was generally praised by local partners, and Healthwatch England emphasised the potential for these new ways of working to boost Healthwatch's impact and relevance in local systems. However, such roles also posed crucial questions about the 'independence' of local Healthwatch. It left some local Healthwatch in the uncomfortable position of not having capacity to set their own priorities and seriously limited their ability to respond to spontaneous issues raised by local service users rather than the priorities of the system itself. In short, an enhanced role in managerial accountability (providing much-needed intelligence for managers to evaluate services and make decisions) risked crowding out scope for the more outward-facing work of Healthwatch as a potential space for more political forms of accountability. These tensions are, at the time of writing, unresolved: the long-term effects of the transformation wreaked by COVID-19, particularly when framed in the broader shifts of health and care commissioning and provision through ICSs, remain unclear.

Healthwatch and Integrated Care Systems

In 2022 the NHS in England developed the new Integrated Care Systems as an organisational form, and the emergent role of Healthwatch within this new structure, remains somewhat unclear (Petsoulas and Allen, 2021). Policy goals of giving autonomy to local systems to find their own paths create potential opportunities for creativity in involving patients and the public, with parallel risks that local systems overlook PPI entirely. Certainly, an article posted on the staff and volunteer resource website of the Healthwatch Network suggests that local Healthwatch will need to actively pursue a new role:

> It's essential that you understand how ICSs will affect the way you work locally, as well as the steps you'll need to take to be ready for this change. If we aren't prepared as a network, it will be harder for us to get NHS decision-makers to hear people's views and hold services to account moving forward. (Healthwatch Network, 2021)

The development of Integrated Care Systems, which shift NHS planning and provision from the local to the regional level, is only likely to increase variability of Healthwatch locally. ICSs mark a broader change from an emphasis on competitive commissioning (enshrined in the HSCA 2012) to an emphasis on collaboration across health and care stakeholders in a system, breaking down the distinction between 'commissioners' and 'providers' of services (and now given statutory force in the HCA 2022).

This change poses several challenges to the work of local Healthwatch and their ability to convey the voice of their local communities within these new structures. First, despite the changes in the NHS since 2012, Healthwatch's formal functions have not been reviewed. For instance, while local Healthwatch have a statutory right to sit on Health and Wellbeing Boards at the local authority level, they do not enjoy a corresponding right to sit on the new regional ICS Boards, although an 'expectation' is outlined in NHS England reports (NHS England & NHS Improvement, 2021). Therefore, the role of Healthwatch and the type of PPI they enact is dependent on the willingness of ICS organisations to engage with them. One implementation report from NHS England lists engaging with 'Healthwatch, and the voluntary, community and social enterprise sector' as one of ten core principles for working with people and communities (NHS England & NHS Improvement, 2021): Healthwatch's role is clearly not seen as primary. Second, since local Healthwatch are only funded to work at the local authority level, they may not have resources to adequately contribute to ICS work even if ICS show a willingness to engage with them. Guidance suggests that local Healthwatch must be 'involved' at the level of ICPs, but goes no further than that (Petsoulas and Allen, 2021). Third, guidance documents suggest that local Healthwatch may be required to collaborate more closely and coordinate their work more formally with neighbouring Healthwatch within the same ICS (NHS England & NHS Improvement, 2021). However, local Healthwatch still operate in a tendering environment in which they compete for renewing their Healthwatch contracts, often against potential rival bids from these very same neighbouring Healthwatch. The emerging role for local Healthwatch within this new health and care landscape reveals the tension between moving towards greater collaboration while elements of the system are still shackled to the framework of marketisation and competition.

Healthwatch in context: a more complex landscape of patient and public voice

Healthwatch, local and national, have therefore worked hard to establish a foothold within the complexities of contemporary NHS governance. However, especially when compared to the advent of PPI with Community Health Councils, they carry out their statutory roles within a much more crowded landscape of organisations and platforms who work outwith the structures of representative democracy, but claim to give voice to patients and the public. In this section we sketch out a selection of the most notable to illustrate some of the complexities of the current system.

First, at the same juncture as the creation of Healthwatch, NHS England created an ambitious plan for a national deliberative assembly around the NHS in England, in NHS Citizen. A research paper by Dean, Boswell and Smith (2019) describes the somewhat organic development of this plan, originating with the suggestion of a celebrity assembly to hold NHS England to account. As eventually operationalised, NHS Citizen was a remarkably ambitious plan inspired by systems thinking in deliberative democracy, including multiple strands of data gathering (known as 'Gather' and 'Discover') as well as a national Assembly Meeting of members of the public from across England (Bussu, 2014). Eventually falling victim to the sheer complexity of the health and social care system in England (Dean, Boswell and Smith, 2019), NHS Citizen seems at the time of writing depleted and perhaps even in abeyance, but its web presence remains (NHS England, 2022).

Another contemporary route for PPI, heavily referenced in ICS guidance as discussed earlier, is the voluntary, community and social enterprise sector. A key change in the early 2010s was the formation of National Voices, a coalition of health and social care charities which articulates a mission heavily grounded in patient voices: their tagline is 'Making what matters to people matter in health and care' and their mission 'inclusive and person-centred health and care, shaped by the people who use and need it the most' (National Voices, 2022). The key difference between National Voices and the rest of the voluntary sector is their very targeted potential to speak with one voice for a broad coalition of organisations who are relevant stakeholders in NHS decision-making (including organisations who otherwise compete for funding and donations). Their board includes an impressive combination of senior charity professionals and NHS 'insiders', and their advocacy and campaigning work is high-profile and slick. In autumn 2022 the organisation 'took over' the sector magazine *Health Service Journal* for a week, spotlighting issues of patient-centered care (Augst, 2022).

NHS organisations also have more, and more effective, routes to hear directly from patients than has ever been the case before. This is especially valuable in the search for examples of patient experience which might support managerial accountability, by identifying when standards have not been met at the local level. Digital communications have transformed the potential for individual patients or members of the public to voice their experiences or priorities, and indeed for organisations to aggregate them. Care Opinion is one example: a website where members of the public can submit 'stories' about their care, linking them to the different 'provider' organisations they interacted with during their care (Mazanderani et al, 2021). Created in 2005, Care Opinion was originally envisaged as part of the expansion of patient choice within the NHS in England (Appleby, Harrison and Devlin, 2003). However, over time, its role has evolved into a more collaborative focus on quality improvement: its founder describes its role as 'turn[ing] the moving, thoughtful and reflective stories that people share into better health and social care services' (Hodgkin, 2013). The key mechanism here is of provider organisations reading and responding to the stories patients share. As a non-profit-making Community Interest Company, Care Opinion finances its platform by selling subscriptions to health and social care organisations. In England these subscriptions are taken out by specific provider organisations (whereas in Scotland and in Northern Ireland, Care Opinion has been contracted by the Scottish Government and Public Health Agency respectively (Care Opinion, 2022)). The idea of Care Opinion as a useful broker between patient experience and organisational improvement has been supported by research which has found that staff value the learning (Baines et al, 2021) and that, when tapping into the potential of machine learning to elicit pertinent information from narratives, reviews might help identify safety incidents which have otherwise gone unreported through official channels (Gillespie and Reader, 2022).

A final, longstanding mode of public participation in the NHS which increasingly challenges the claim of statutory structures to be 'the' champion of the public, is public campaigning, often, but by no means exclusively, against service reconfiguration (Crane, 2022; Ocloo and Fulop, 2012; Ryan, 2019; Stewart, Dodworth and Ercia, 2022). New modalities of activism and mobilisation, not least online, offer rapid rebukes to decision-makers (Pushkar, 2018). Campaigning itself, is, of course, nothing new (Crane, 2019): as discussed earlier, harmed patient and carer campaigning in the wake of the Bristol scandal contributed to the abolition of CHCs. However as digital activism becomes increasingly intertwined with public discourse, formal PPI structures in the NHS have to be understood in interrelationship with more activist public campaigning.

Conclusion

The sheer frequency of structural reform in patient and public involvement in the last 25 years is not uncommon in England's fretful, oft-reformed NHS (Smith, Walshe and Hunter, 2001). The changes shown in Table 12.1 often reflect these broader structural changes, and not just dissatisfaction with current arrangements, let alone a fully worked through alternative strategy for how patient and public involvement *should* be delivered. By contrast, in Wales, Community Health Councils endured until 2019. In Scotland, arrangements continue to be supported by the work of national agency Scottish Health Council (now absorbed into Healthcare Improvement Scotland), and following abandoned pilots of directly electing non-executive members of Health Boards (Greer et al, 2014). In Northern Ireland, the Patient Client Council fulfils many of the functions of Healthwatch, often with a province-wide remit. The comparative instability of reforms in England have reflected the magnitude of the task at its much greater scale. However the repeated churn of organisational forms in the 2000s proved damaging for relationships, for trust, and for the important question of public visibility of these structures (Baggott, 2005; Warwick, 2006). Furthermore, as Newbigging noted in a review of reforms up until 2016, the legal powers enjoyed by the Community Health Councils have never been restored to any of their structural descendants: 'the power of the engine for PPI has been incrementally reduced' (Newbigging, 2016).

Already forced to compete with other potential organisations to deliver local Healthwatch, and working hard to achieve influence locally, Healthwatch also now finds itself one among many routes through which NHS organisations might hear from the population they serve. What can be pitched as appropriately responsive local variations can also be understood as a problematic 'postcode lottery' in how effectively local Healthwatch hears from and represents people in different areas of the country. What remains to be seen is whether a more diffuse landscape of PPI can *better* give voice to the range of experiences of healthcare within England's population, via engagement with 'much richer forms of participation and data about people's perspectives, priorities and reasoning' (Cribb, 2018). An alternative trajectory is that a plethora of weaker PPI structures simply renders decision-makers more able to pick and choose the messaging that fits their own priorities, evading accountability to the people they serve.

Patient and public involvement is one area of health policy where success is particularly difficult to define (Stewart, 2013; Martin and Carter, 2017).

In practice, evaluations tend to measure achievement intrinsically, by congruence with policy goals (see Levitt, 1980). However when it comes to PPI, this approach is limited by the relative vagueness of these goals. Especially if PPI is understood as a route to political, and not managerial accountability (that is, the influence of public views on the substantive structure of services, rather than only intelligence on the extent to which agreed managerial standards are met), any straightforward measure of success is likely to be both elusive, and dynamic, rather than measurably achieved. In this, a democratically-oriented understanding of PPI's role – the desire to create a healthcare system which meaningfully responds to collective population preferences – evades straightforward metrics of healthcare performance.

References

Alexander, M. (2003a) *ACHCEW and CHCs: A Short History*. London: Association of Community Health Councils for England and Wales. https://www.achcew.org/

Alexander, M. (2003b) *The Golden Age of Public Involvement*. London: Association of Community Health Councils for England and Wales Special General Meeting, 8 July. https://www.achcew.org/uploads/6/6/0/6/6606397/ma_speech.pdf

Allen, P., Keen, J., Wright, J., Dempster, P., Townsend, J., Hutchings, A. et al (2012) 'Investigating the governance of autonomous public hospitals in England: Multi-site case study of NHS foundation trusts'. *Journal of Health Services Research & Policy*, 17, 2, 94–100.

Appleby, J., Harrison, A. and Devlin, N. (2003) *What Is the Real Cost of More Patient Choice*? London: The King's Fund. https://www.kingsfund.org.uk/sites/default/files/field/field_publication_file/what–is–real–cost–more–patient–choice–john–appleby–tony–harrison–nancy–devlin–kings–fund–1–june–2003.pdf

Augst, C. (2022) *NHS Leaders* and *Patients Must Stand Together* to *Combat this Crisis*. Health Service Journal, 17 October. https://www.hsj.co.uk/service-design/nhs-leaders-and-patients-must-stand-together-to-combat-this-crisis/7033469.article

Baggott, R. (2005) 'A funny thing happened on the way to the forum? Reforming patient and public involvement in the NHS in England'. *Public Administration*, 83, 3, 533–551.

Baines, R., Underwood, F., O'Keeffe, K., Saunders, J. and Jones, R.B. (2021) 'Implementing online patient feedback in a "special measures" acute hospital: A case study using Normalisation Process Theory'. *Digital Health*, 7. https://doi.org/10.1177/20552076211005962

Bussu, S. (2014) 'Citizen engagement and the NHS: Time to move from many deliberative forums to one deliberative system? NHS Citizen could be the answer'. *Involve*, 23 April. https://involve.org.uk/resources/blog/opinion/citizen-engagement-and-nhs-time-move-many-deliberative-forums-one

Care Opinion. (2022) *How is Care Opinion funded?* [Online]. Care Opinion. https://www.careopinion.org.uk/info/funding

Carter, P. and Martin, G. (2016) 'Challenges facing Healthwatch, a new consumer champion in England'. *International Journal of Health Policy and Management*, 5, 4, 259–263. https://doi.org/10.15171/ijhpm.2016.07

Coleman, A., Checkland, K., Segar, J., McDermott, I., Harrison, S. and Peckham, S. (2014) 'Joining it up? Health and Wellbeing Boards in English Local Governance: Evidence from Clinical Commissioning Groups and Shadow Health and Wellbeing Boards'. *Local Government Studies*, 40, 4, 560–580. https://doi.org/10.1080/03003930.2013.841578

Crane, J. (2019) '"Save our NHS": Activism, information-based expertise and the "new times" of the 1980s'. *Contemporary British History*, 33, 1, 52–74. https://doi.org/10.1080/13619462.2018.1525299

Crane, J. (2022) '"Loving" the National Health Service: Social surveys and activist feelings', in J. Crane and J. Hand (eds) *Posters, Protests, and Prescriptions*. Manchester: Manchester University Press, pp 79–102. https://www.manchesteropenhive.com/view/9781526163479/9781526163479.00012.xml

Cribb, A. (2018) *Healthcare in Transition: Understanding Key Ideas and Tensions in Contemporary Health Policy*. Bristol: Policy Press.

Day, P. and Klein, R. (1987) *Accountabilities: Five Public Services*. London: Tavistock.

Day, P. and Klein, R. (2005) *Governance of Foundation Trusts: Dilemmas of Diversity*. London: Nuffield Trust.

Dean, R., Boswell, J. and Smith, G. (2019) 'Designing democratic innovations as deliberative systems: The ambitious case of NHS citizen'. *Political Studies*, 68, 3. https://doi.org/10.1177/0032321719866002

Department of Health (DH). (1999) *Patient and Public Involvement in the New NHS*. London: The Stationery Office.

DH. (2001) *Involving Patients and the Public in Healthcare: Response to the Listening Exercise*. London: The Stationery Office.

DH. (2003) *Strengthening Accountability: Involving Patients and the Public*. London: The Stationery Office.

Foot, M. (1973) *Aneurin Bevan 1945–1960*. London: Paladin.

Gilburt, H., Dunn, P. and Foot, C. (2015) *Local Healthwatch: Progress and Promise*. London: The King's Fund. https://www.kingsfund.org.uk/publications/local-healthwatch-progress-and-promise

Gillespie, A. and Reader, T.W. (2022) 'Online patient feedback as a safety valve: An automated language analysis of unnoticed and unresolved safety incidents'. *Risk Analysis*, early view https://doi.org/10.1111/risa.14002

Greer, S.L., Falkenbach, M., Jarman, H., Löblová, O., Rozenblum, S., Williams, N. and Wismar, M. (2021) 'Centralisation and decentralisation in a crisis: How credit and blame shape governance'. *Eurohealth*, 27, 1. https://apps.who.int/iris/bitstream/handle/10665/344946/Eurohealth-27-1-36-40-eng.pdf?sequence=1&isAllowed=y

Greer, S.L., Jarman, H. and Azorsky, A. (2014) *A Reorganisation You Can See from Space: The architecture of Power in the New NHS*. London: Centre for Health and the Public Interest.

Greer, S.L., Wilson, I., Stewart, E.A. and Donnelly, P.D. (2014) '"Democratizing" public services? Representation and elections in the Scottish NHS'. *Public Administration*, 92, 4, 1090–1105. https://doi.org/10.1111/padm.12101

Hagen, T.P. and Vrangbaek, K. (2009) 'The changing political governance structures of Nordic health care systems', in J. Magnussen, K. Vrangbaek and R. Saltman (eds) *Nordic Health Care Systems: Recent Reforms and Current Policy Challenges*. Maidenhead: Open University Press.

Healthwatch Network. (2021) *Are You Ready for Integrated Care Systems (ICSs)?* Healthwatch, 8 December. https://network.healthwatch.co.uk/guidance/2021-12-08/are-you-ready-integrated-care-systems-icss

Healthwatch England. (2022a) *Our History and Functions*. Healthwatch. https://www.healthwatch.co.uk/our-history-and-functions

Healthwatch England. (2022b) *Healthwatch Resourcing in the New Health and Care Landscape*. Healthwatch. https://www.healthwatch.co.uk/sites/healthwatch.co.uk/files/20220228%20Healthwatch%20resourcing%20in%20the%20new%20health%20and%20care%20landscape.pdf

Her Majesty's Stationery Office (HMSO) (2003a) *The Patients' Forums (Functions) Regulations*. London: HMSO.

HMSO (2003b) *The Patients' Forums (Membership and Procedure) Regulations*. London: HMSO.

Hodgkin, P. (2013) 'Five minutes with … The founder of Patient Opinion'. *The Guardian*, 13 December. https://www.theguardian.com/healthcare-network/2013/dec/13/paul-hodgkin-founder-patient-opinion

Hogg, C.N.L. (2007) 'Patient and public involvement: What next for the NHS?'. *Health Expectations*, 10, 2, 129–138. https://doi.org/10.1111/j.1369-7625.2006.00427.x

House of Commons – Health Committee. (2007) *Public and Patient Involvement in the NHS: Third Report of Session 2006–7* (HC 278-I). London: The Stationery Office.

Hunter, D.J. and Harrison, S. (1997) 'Democracy, accountability and consumerism', in J. Munro and S. Iliffe (eds) *Healthy Choices: Future Options for the NHS*. London: Lawrence & Wishart.

Hunter, D.J., Perkins, N., Visram, S., Adams, L., Finn, R., Forrest, A. and Gosling, J. (2018) *Evaluating the leadership role of health and wellbeing boards as drivers of health improvement and integrated care across England* (Policy Research Programme Project PR-X03–1113-11007). Durham: National Institute for Health Research.

Klein, R. (2010) 'The eternal triangle: Sixty years of the centre–periphery relationship in the National Health Service'. *Social Policy & Administration*, 44, 3, 285–304. https://doi.org/10.1111/j.1467-9515.2010.00714.x

Klein, R. and Lewis, J. (1976) *The Politics of Consumer Representation: A Study of Community Health Councils*. London: Centre for Studies in Social Policy.

Levitt, R. (1980) *The People's Voice in the NHS: Community health Councils After Five Years*. London: King Edward's Hospital Fund for London.

Marks, L., Cave, S., Hunter, D., Mason, J., Peckham, S. and Wallace, A. (2011) 'Governance for health and wellbeing in the English NHS'. *Journal of Health Services Research & Policy*, 16, 1_suppl, 14–21. https://doi.org/10.1258/jhsrp.2010.010082

Martin, G. (2008) ' "Ordinary people only": Knowledge, representativeness, and the publics of public participation in healthcare'. *Sociology of Health & Illness*, 30, 1, 35–54.

Martin, G. (2009) 'Whose health, whose care, whose say? Some comments on public involvement in new NHS commissioning arrangements'. *Critical Public Health*, 19, 1, 123–132.

Martin, G. and Carter, P. (2017) 'Patient and public involvement in the new NHS: Choice, voice, and the pursuit of legitimacy', in M. Bevir and J. Waring (eds) *De-Centred Health Policy: Learning from the British Experiences in Healthcare Governance*. Abingdon: Routledge.

Mazanderani, F., Kirkpatrick, S.F., Ziebland, S., Locock, L. and Powell, J. (2021) 'Caring for care: Online feedback in the context of public healthcare services'. *Social Science & Medicine*, 285, 114280. https://doi.org/10.1016/j.socscimed.2021.114280

Milewa, T., Harrison, S., Ahmad, W. and Tovey, P. (2002) 'Citizens' participation in primary healthcare planning: Innovative citizenship practice in empirical perspective'. *Critical Public Health*, 12, 1.

Mold, A. (2016) *Making the Patient-Consumer*. Manchester: Manchester University Press.

National Voices. (2022). *About Us*. National Voices. https://www.national voices.org.uk/about-us

Newbigging, K. (2016) 'Blowin' in the wind: The involvement of people who use services, carers and the public in health and social care', in M. Exworthy, R. Mannion and M. Powell (eds) *Dismantling the NHS?: Evaluating the Impact of Health Reforms*. Bristol: Policy Press, pp 301–322.

NHS England. (2022) *NHS Citizen*. https://www.england.nhs.uk/get-invol ved/get-involved/how/nhs-citizen/

NHS England and NHS Improvement. (2021) *Building Strong Integrated Care Systems Everywhere: ICS Implementation Guidance on Working with People and Communities* (No. PAR661). Leeds: NHS England. https://www.engl and.nhs.uk/wp-content/uploads/2021/06/B0661-ics-working-with-peo ple-and-communities.pdf

Ocloo, J.E. and Fulop, N.J. (2012) 'Developing a "critical" approach to patient and public involvement in patient safety in the NHS: Learning lessons from other parts of the public sector?'. *Health Expectations: An International Journal of Public Participation in Health Care and Health Policy*, 15, 4, 424–432. https://doi.org/10.1111/j.1369-7625.2011.00695.x

Peckham, S., Exworthy, M., Greener, I. and Powell, M. (2005) 'Decentralizing health services: More local accountability or just more central control?' *Public Money & Management*, 25, 4, 221–228. https://doi.org/10.1080/ 09540962.2005.10600097

Petsoulas, C. and Allen, P. (2021) 'Summary and commentary on the issue of accountability in the Health and Care Bill 2021'. Working paper, PRUComm. https://prucomm.ac.uk/uploads/PRUComm%20note%20 on%20accountability%20issues%20in%20bill%20nov%202021.pdf

Pickard, S. (1997) 'The future organization of community health councils'. *Social Policy & Administration*, 31, 3, 247–289.

Pushkar, P. (2018) 'NHS activism: The limits and potentialities of a new solidarity'. *Medical Anthropology*, 0, 0, 1–14. https://doi.org/10.1080/ 01459740.2018.1532421

Ryan, S. (2019) 'NHS inquiries and investigations: An exemplar in peculiarity and assumption'. *The Political Quarterly*, 90, 2, 224–228. https:// doi.org/10.1111/1467-923X.12703

Smith, J., Walshe, K. and Hunter, D.J. (2001) 'The "redisorganisation" of the NHS: Another reorganisation involving unhappy managers can only worsen the service'. *BMJ*, 323, 7324, 1262–1263. https://doi.org/10.1136/ bmj.323.7324.1262

Stewart, E. (2013) 'What is the point of citizen participation in health care?'. *Journal of Health Services Research & Policy*, 18, 2, 124–126. https://doi.org/ 10.1177/1355819613485670

Stewart, E., Dodworth, K. and Ercia, A. (2022) 'The everyday work of hospital campaigns: Public knowledge and activism in the UK's National Health Services', in J. Crane and J. Hand (eds) *Posters, Protests, and Prescriptions: Cultural Histories of the National Health Service in Britain.* Manchester: Manchester University Press, pp 79–99.

Tritter, J.Q. and Koivusalo, M. (2013) 'Undermining patient and public engagement and limiting its impact: The consequences of the Health and Social Care Act 2012 on collective patient and public involvement'. *Health Expectations*, 16, 2, 115–118. https://doi.org/10.1111/hex.12069

Warwick, P. (2006) 'The rise and fall of the patient forum'. Working paper. York: The University of York. http://www.york.ac.uk/management/resea rch/workingpapers/wp25warwick.pdf

Zoccatelli, G., Desai, A., Martin, G., Brearley, S., Murrels, T. and Robert, G. (2020) 'Enabling "citizen voice" in the English health and social care system: A national survey of the organizational structures, relationships and impacts of local Healthwatch in England'. *Health Expect*, 23, 1108– 1117. https://doi.org/10.1111/hex.13086

Zoccatelli, G., Desai, A., Martin, G., Brearley, S. and Robert, G. (2021) 'Finding the voice of the people in the pandemic: An ethnographic account of the work of local Healthwatch in the first weeks of England's COVID-19 crisis', in P. Beresford, M. Farr, G. Hickey, M. Kaur, J. Ocloo, D. Tembo and O. Williams (eds), *The Challenges and Necessity of Co-production: Volume 1: The Challenges and Necessity of Co-production.* Bristol: Policy Press.

Zoccatelli, G., Desai, A., Robert, G., Martin, G. and Brearley, S. (2022) 'Exploring the work and organisation of local Healthwatch in England: A mixed-methods ethnographic study'. *Health and Social Care Delivery Research*, 10, 32.

13

After 75 years, whither the NHS? Some conclusions

Martin Powell, Mark Exworthy and Russell Mannion

Introduction

We opened this book (Chapter 1) by observing that the NHS was in a parlous and unprecedented position. Now that the contributors have surveyed the period across a range of domains, there seems to be very little evidence to revise that verdict. Over its 75 years, the NHS has seen a number of 'big bang' reforms and many more, smaller incremental reforms (Tuohy, 2018). While there has been a great deal of analysis on the former (Robinson and Le Grand, 1994; Le Grand, Mays and Mulligan, 1998; Thorlby and Maybin, 2010; Exworthy Mannion, 2016), there is a danger that the smaller but cumulative changes of the latter may be missed (Powell, 2016).

Cumulative incremental changes are harder to detect and assess and receive less publicity than large-scale (big bang) reforms which are often heralded with much fanfare and public debate. Large-scale reforms of health systems such as the NHS may be somewhat constrained by its own logics (Tuohy, 1999) but they might also have a negative impact on the resilience of the NHS. Individual reforms (or a programme of them) may not necessarily lead to a loss of resilience at that time but repeated reforms may undermine the cohesion of its structures and processes. The rapidity of such change might only serve to weaken such cohesion further (Thorlby and Maybin, 2010; Exworthy and Mannion, 2016: 8; Timmins, 2012; Exworthy and Mannion, 2016: 8). Without a comprehensive and longitudinal evaluation programme, the cumulative impact of healthcare reforms will remain uncertain or unknown.

In this book, we have sought to offer a comprehensive analysis of the state of the NHS in its 75th year. The four analytical axes (governance; public/ private, central/local, and profession/state; introduced in Chapter 1 and reprised next) provided an overarching framework which applied, more or less, to the individual chapters. The subjects of these chapters enabled, we argue, a comprehensive coverage of the main dimensions of the NHS in its first 75 years. We note, however, the absence of topics, such as workforce wellbeing and diversity, and environmental sustainability (among others), from our analysis but we urge others to engage with these topics in future research.

It is often said that anniversaries are times to look backwards and forwards. The remainder of this concluding chapter places the 75th anniversary in the context of previous anniversaries. We then bring together some of the main threads from the diverse tapestries of the preceding chapters. This is followed by a section summing up the main themes arising from the chapters, including the analytical axes and perspectives on policy success. The next section takes stock of the current situation through the lens of the many recent commissions and inquiries. The final section then attempts to gaze into future anniversaries.

NHS anniversaries

The NHS has seen many 'big' anniversaries. For example, there have been many Parliamentary Debates each decade starting with the 10th anniversary in 1958. These have been explored through 'streams' such as problems (pressures, finance, structures), politics (principles and values) and policies (solutions) (Powell, 2019a), and themes such as creation, principles, stewardship, achievements and problems (Powell, 2019b).

We can examine these anniversaries in terms of content and character. First, Timmins (2008) suggested that most anniversaries focus on similar issues. He noted on the 60th anniversary of the NHS that his brief history of the big anniversaries demonstrated 'plus ça change' that many issues such as the longstanding pressures of medical technology, ageing populations and rising expectation had always been present.

However, Powell (2019b) suggested that interpretative content analysis suggested more nuanced conclusions. While most anniversary Parliamentary Debates have discussed most of the themes, their salience has varied over time. First, while Labour has always stressed that it created the NHS and the Conservatives voted against it, there is some evidence of an inverse relationship over time in that the further we get from the creation, the more important those become. Second, the debate on principles has continued, but they seem to be rather poorly defined and flexible, with the Conservatives stressing the minimalist version of comprehensiveness and *largely* free at the point of use. Third, the Conservatives stressed that they increased expenditure and activity more than Labour, while Labour claimed that Conservatives had not provided sufficient funding; introduced and increased charges; looked to the USA, and aimed to privatise the NHS. Fourth, discussion of achievements appeared in two broad ways such as temporal statistics of increased expenditure and activity and falls in deaths, and comparative claims of being the 'best in the world', largely without much evidence, and sometimes related to an apparent ignorance of other systems. Finally, many of the problems seemed to be 'hardy perennials': finance, demography, technology, waiting lists, staff shortages, staff morale, reorganisation and the 'Beveridge fallacy' of assuming that demand for healthcare would fall, with the term 'crisis' used in 1978 and 1988.

Second, the character of the anniversaries has varied. According to Paton (2018), since the British NHS reached its 40th anniversary in 1988, there has been a reckoning every 10 years. He considered that in 1988 the Thatcher Conservative government's latent hostility towards the NHS and resultant reforms brought skeletons to the birthday feast. The 50th anniversary in 1998 was much more upbeat, with the new Blair New Labour government having promised to save it but had not yet launched its own 'half-baked reforms'. The 70th anniversary in 2008 was less upbeat but nothing like as pessimistic as the 70th anniversary in 2018, which is borne on a wave of financial crisis and sparse care (2018: 291).

Examination of anniversary Parliamentary Debates and reports from around the anniversary years (Powell 2019a, b) confirmed many of these impressions. While most anniversaries have tended to display a mixture of optimism and pessimism, the 1978 and 1988 anniversaries tended to be pessimistic (see earlier), with perhaps (contra Paton) the most optimistic anniversary being in 2008. The sustained increases in resources following 'most expensive breakfast in history' (Timmins 2017: 610) had kicked in. On eve of the financial crisis, there were several reasons to be cheerful. Klein (2013: 268–270) pointed to low waiting lists, with public satisfaction in the 2009 'British Social Attitudes' survey higher than at any time since 1983 (2013: 270). He concluded that 'as the general election of 2010 approached, ministers had much to boast about the Labour government's stewardship of the NHS' (for example, Klein 2013: 268). Timmins (2017) also discussed similar issues of shorter waiting times, more staff and new or refurbished facilities, but was a little more wary. He pointed out that outcomes still lagged behind other nations, leading to an overall verdict of 'so much done, so much left to do' (2017: 651). He then posed the question of 'how much of this refurbished edifice would withstand the earthquake of the financial crisis' (2017: 655) or the 'fiscal ice age' (Klein 2013: 256). As we will see next, the answer must be 'not much'.

Analytical axes revisited

In Chapter 1, we presented four axes by which health policy in the UK might be interpreted:

- governance axis
- public/private axis
- central/local axis and
- professional/state axis.

Collectively, these axes define the institutional character of the NHS (Tuohy, 2022). Their dynamic nature and the interplay between them help to define the evolving narrative of the NHS and give indications of where it might be heading in the future. To varying degrees, each chapter in this book has considered the NHS across these four axes, thereby giving a comprehensive assessment of the state of the NHS as its reaches its 75th anniversary. In conclusion, this chapter is able to revisit these axes to provide a summative assessment of each, both individually and collectively.

The governance axis

The past decade or so has been distinctive in many ways for the NHS, not least the lack of a dominant policy narrative that had been apparent. The traditional narrative of the NHS moving from hierarchy to market and network did have some coherence to it but it was disingenuous in the sense that all co-exist to varying degrees. This could be evident from policy statements as well as organisational structures and processes. Since the HSCA (2012), the primacy of hierarchy remains but has been shifting away from the centre towards a more plural set of actors. Reliance on market-based reforms has eroded and new networks have emerged. The sedimented effect of these reforms is hard to assess given the interactive impact of reform upon reform. Indeed, it might be possible to discern a variant of these in the form of autonomy versus integration (Tuohy, 2022). For example, the Foundation Trust experiment of the 2000s in England has largely been overtaken by the drive towards integration. This nascent axis is less apparent in Scotland, Wales and Northern Ireland, as autonomy has been less prominent and integration more prevalent (Needham and Glasby, this volume).

The public/private axis

The public/private axis has been ever-present in the NHS thanks to the settlement between the government and profession, and to the permissive approach to pay beds since the outset of the NHS (Greener, 2016). However, for much of the past 75 years, this axis has been mostly latent. With the advent of NPM from the 1980s onwards, the principles and practices of the private sector have become more intrusive. Ideologies, interests and institutions related to the private sector have permeated all aspects of the NHS. The policy experiment of commissioning in England from April 1991 is perhaps the most distinctive expression of this axis at the time. It led to various related reforms including the self-governing status of NHS trusts (morphing later into Foundation Trusts), GP fund-holding and Any Qualified Provider, among others (Checkland et al, this volume; Allen and Sheaff, this volume). Arguably, the axis entered a new 'revolution' from 2014 onwards when the

'Five Year Forward View' was published by NHS England. Widely seen as the work of Simon Stevens, the then CEO of NHS England, it marked a transition towards more integration within the NHS. That said, many of the traits of the private sector remain. Many such (positive and negative) traits were evident during the response to the COVID-19 pandemic. Perhaps the most pervasive is the commodification and commercialisation of the NHS, such that its (human, material and financial) resources are managed in ways which mirror the private sector (Hodgson et al, 2021); this has been accelerated since the HSCA 2012. Tendencies towards public or social value seem to have had limited impact on this.

The years of austerity and, more recently, inflationary pressures have exacerbated existing tensions within the NHS – more prevalent chronic care, health inequalities, ageing population and so on (Powell and Exworthy, this volume). There appears to be no political or public appetite to move away from a publicly funded NHS but media voices in the post-COVID-19 crisis of 2022–2023 (calling for co-payments or a model of social insurance) seem to be louder than before. The private medical insurance market remains hovering around 10 per cent (as it has done in recent years) but the rise in out-of-pocket health expenditure is significant (Charlesworth et al, this volume). Patients are responding to what they perceive as a lack of access and/or comprehensiveness of care by paying themselves (Checkland et al, this volume).

The central/local axis

This axis has been a fundamental part of the DNA of the NHS (Greer, this volume). The political and organisational settlement of 1948 has ensured an oscillation between the centre and the periphery (however defined). Sometimes conceived as a pendulum (Klein, 2013), there is a cyclical nature to this oscillation. Indeed, Klein (2003) likens the 'discovery' of localism to a revolving door.

In any case, the central–local axis involves a tension between different conceptions of the NHS. For example, the public has a strong connection with their 'local' hospital and yet subscribe to a notion of a 'national' health service. The public still subscribe to a standard NHS model of care (Buzelli et al, 2022). Yet the sense of what is 'local' is in flux; the nearest emergency room or maternity department have strong resonances in public debates but the evidence-based approach has directed the centralisation of services, invariably away from local provision to more remote locations or even online.

The central–local axis has been re-structured by the political devolution since 1999. To varying degrees, Scotland, Wales and Northern Ireland have assumed their powers to varying extents (John Stewart, this volume). While there had been some form of administrative devolution previously, political devolution has shifted the debate as to what policies are possible. Responses to the COVID-19 pandemic illustrated this (Greer et al, 2021). Similarly, a regional (administrative) structure in England has been reformed several times, largely in response to politically-inspired re-organisations of the NHS. It is unlikely that the strategic planning of the English NHS could be effective without some form of regional structure. However, what form this would take is specific to the political and organisational context at the time.

The professional/state axis

This axis concerns professional (here, clinical) interest groups, especially the medical profession. It is not simply the re-creation of the central-local axis for various reasons. First, professional interest groups span the centrality and locality. Second, it cannot be assumed that managers are necessarily acting on behalf of the governments as 'local agents of the state' (Harrison, 1988). Third, over the past two decades, the rise in the number of hybrid clinical managers has been dramatic, with implications for the local implementation of national policy (see Kirkpatrick, this volume) and adoption of quality improvement (Millar, Waring and Lalani, this volume).

So what of the state of the metaphorical 'double bed' (Klein, 1990) between the government and medical profession? Doctors have long been central to the formulation and implementation of national policy; note the approach of clinically-led commissioning since 1991 as one example. Indeed this may have a strong evidential basis, given the association between clinically-led organisations and their performance (for example, Goodall, 2011). Yet, the medical profession cannot be conceived as homogenous. While health policy has sought to 'play off' one group against another (such as GPs and hospital consultants), other developments have shifted the intensity of this axis; these include physician associates, salaried and locum doctors as well as role delegation and substitution to other (clinical) staff. Digital technologies, especially those delivered during the COVID-19 pandemic, have intensified pre-existing developments still further. Doctors still retain significant power within the NHS but their position vis-à-vis others has shifted. For example, nurses and paramedics have become more vocal. Indeed, the strikes of late 2022 were the first taken by the members of the Royal College of Nursing in over 100 years.

A major inimical effect of the COVID-19 pandemic has been the cumulative effect of work-related pressures upon individuals. This has long been evident in terms of staff vacancies (exacerbated by the lack of a national workforce plan) but more recently in terms of workforce wellbeing, viz. burnout, morale and job satisfaction. The ongoing recruitment of international clinical staff has not offset the vacancies or done much to ameliorate staff wellbeing; besides there remain serious ethical concerns about recruitment from health systems in low- and middle-income countries. The Brexit referendum led to the abolition of free movement of clinical staff which has hampered recruitment still further.

The NHS at 75: taking stock

This section examines 'stock takes' of the NHS in the period since its 70th anniversary, set within the longest financial squeeze in the history of the NHS and widespread concerns of a 'crisis' (for example, House of Lords Committee on the Long-term Sustainability of the NHS, 2017).

To mark the NHS' 70th anniversary, the *BMJ* (2018) conducted a poll of its greatest achievements, resulting in 'providing care based on need and free at the point of delivery' just ahead of 'limiting commercial influence on patient care' and 'general practice as the foundation for patient care'.

Four independent health 'think tanks' – The Health Foundation, the Institute for Fiscal Studies, The King's Fund, and the Nuffield Trust – collaborated to produce a series of five reports which examined (the then) state of the NHS and social care (Dayan et al, 2018; Thorlby et al, 2018; Syoye, 2018; McKenna, 2018; Castle-Clarke, 2018). The largest of the five reports assessed how good the NHS was compared to other health systems (Dayan et al, 2018; see also Greener, chapter 11). It concluded that although the NHS has many good qualities, in particular being relatively efficient and in providing equal access to care irrespective of wealth, it was not as good at delivering health outcomes as many of its peers, and saying that it is hard to argue that the NHS is 'the envy of the world'. A second report that reviewed social care provision was more damning (Thorlby et al, 2018). It highlighted that the social care system was 'riddled with holes' and unlike NHS services which are free at the point of use, means-testing for social care services 'remains a fundamental source of inequity and unfairness today'. The third report explored NHS financing (Stoye, 2018). The report noted that although spending on the NHS was just below the European average, spending would need to be increased by an average of at least 3.3 per cent a year up to 2033–2034 to maintain the status quo and by 4 per cent a year to address key priorities such as mental health, cancer and general practice. The fourth report looked at public satisfaction with and support the NHS (McKenna, 2018). It noted that although the NHS has historically received a high level of support among the general public and likened to a 'national religion', public satisfaction for the organisation is starting to waiver, in particular with regard to GP services due to ongoing staff shortages, long waiting times, lack of funding and government reforms. Finally, the fifth report outlined four technological advances that had the potential to transform how the NHS organises and delivers care: genomics and precision medicine, remote care, supported self-management and artificial intelligence

(Castle-Clarke, 2018). It concluded that although there was great potential for developments in information technology to improve the delivery of care to patients, the NHS does not have a strong track record in implementing technological advances at scale and pace and needs to get better at assessing the feasibility and challenges of implementing new technological innovations.

A joint LSE–*Lancet* Commission on the future of the NHS was launched in 2017 with a remit to investigate the main opportunities and challenges facing the NHS and to propose a set of targeted policy recommendations framed around a long-term vision for the NHS. This took a little longer to report, with the final report published in May 2021 (Anderson et al, 2021) making seven key recommendations. First, it proposed the need for increasing investment across the NHS, social care and public health and advocated that annual increases in funding of at least 4 per cent, in real terms is required for the provision of these services. Second, that there was a need for improved resource management across health and care at national and local levels. Third, it would be important to develop a sustainable, skilled and fit for purpose health and care workforce to meet changing health and care needs. Fourth, an imperative to strengthen prevention of disease and preparedness to protect against major threats to health. Fifth, a need to improve diagnosis to improve outcomes and reduce inequalities. Sixth, a need to develop the culture, capacity and capability to become a so-called learning health and care system And finally, improve integration between healthcare, social care and public health across different providers, including the third sector.

A review of health and care services led by Lord Darzi and supported by the Institute for Public Policy Research (IPPR) was published in 2018 (Darzi, 2018). This called for greater public investment in health and care services and set out a 10-point plan of investment and reform to improve the health and care system during the 2020s. Key recommendations in the action plan included the need to embrace a 'health in all policies' approach across government; a focus on developing a digital infrastructure to support the delivery of care services; ensuring that social care is free at the point of need; simplifying commissioning arrangements into a single structure at the regional level; creating a coherent quality strategy for health and care; and ensuring that health and care services are properly staffed and remunerated. In April, 2022, yet another commission was launched. The IPPR Health and Prosperity Commission is co-chaired by former Health Minister Lord Ara Darzi and former Chief Medical Officer Dame Sally Davies with a remit to work for a period of two years on gaining a better understanding of the interconnections between health and the economy and to set out a blueprint to harness the potential of better health for all.

There seem to be some common strands linking these reports. First, most stress the importance of 'birthday presents' of increased resources. Second, it is broadly considered that the NHS can't be 'fixed' without 'fixing' social care. Third, while the NHS generally compares well to other healthcare systems in some terms such as equity, it does seem to lag other systems in outcomes. Finally, there needs to be more stress on issues such as public health and prevention. While these conclusions emerged from reports set out in connection with the NHS' 70th anniversary, most could have been said for much of the period of the service's history.

We conduct a more recent stock take on one of the main underlying issues, and focus on a closely linked issue that perhaps did not emerge as clearly as might be expected of the workforce.

Relative performance and health spending

Although international comparisons should be treated with caution, a comparison of health system performance published in 2021 by the Commonwealth Fund ranked 11 high-income countries on the basis of 71 performance measures across five domains (Greener, this volume). The UK was ranked fourth overall with only Norway, Netherlands and Australia achieving a higher overall score (Schneider, Shah, Doty et al, 2021). Previously the NHS had been the top-rated system in the previous reports published in 2014 and 2017. In the latest report, the UK performed comparatively well in terms of Access to Care (4th); Administrative Efficiency (4th) and Equity (4th). However, the UK was ranked only ninth in terms of Health Outcome, which is a measure of how well patients recover following treatment (Schneider, Shah, Doty et al, 2021).

Over the last decade, health spending in the UK has been consistently lower than the EU average and the cumulative effect is that the NHS has less capacity to respond to addressing the backlog of care since the pandemic (Charlesworth, Shembavnekar and Stevenson, this volume). The Health Foundation conducted a recent review of how UK health spending compared with 14 EU countries in the decade preceding the COVID-19 pandemic, with the aim of assessing how cumulative trends in spending have impacted healthcare resilience (The Health Foundation, 2022). Their analysis found that the average day-to-day health spending in the UK between 2010 and 2019 was £3,005 per person – 18 per cent below the EU14 average of £3,655. By their calculations, if UK spending per person had matched the EU14 average, then the UK would have spent an average of £277 billion a year on health between 2010–2019. This is £40 billion higher than the actual average annual spending during this period (£187 billion) (The Health Foundation, 2022). For capital spending, matching the cumulative EU14 average over the past decade would have resulted in the UK investing £33 billion more in health-related buildings and equipment. The authors conclude that, if UK spending had kept up with its European neighbours, it would be fair to assume the NHS would have been more resilient and had greater capacity to provide care during the pandemic and in a better position to reduce the large backlog of care.

Workforce issues

While the government has provided more funding for the NHS, over the last two decades government responses have been limited to 'stop-gap' measures with no national NHS workforce strategy since 2003 (but see Chapter 3). Yet workforce-related issues such as recruitment, retention, staff and wellbeing represent a major challenge for the NHS, particularly in the current context of growing waiting lists and the substantial elective care backlog. Recent analysis (Shembavnekar et al, 2022) has highlighted an overall workforce supply-demand gap in 2021–2022 of around 103,000 FTE across the NHS hospital and community health services and general practice in England (around 7 per cent of estimated FTE workforce demand). Workforce shortages are also endemic in adult social care in England, with recent data suggesting there are over 100,000 vacancies in the sector on an average day in 2020–2021 (Shembavnekar et al, 2022). Unfilled vacancies increase the pressure on staff which can lead to higher levels of stress, absenteeism and a high staff turnover. The 2021 NHS staff survey highlighted growing concerns about working conditions in the NHS (NSS, 2022). In 2021, only 59.4 per cent of staff would recommend their organisation as a place to work – a decline of more than 7 per cent percentage points from 66.8 per cent in 2020, and lower than at any point in the last five years. A key area of concern compared to the previous survey undertaken in 2020 survey was in the proportion of staff who reported that there were enough staff in their organisation for them to do their job properly. This fell from 38.4 per cent in 2020 to 27.2 per cent in 2021. The drop was even steeper in ambulance trusts, where only one in five staff answered positively (20.3 per cent in 2021 vs 36.7 per cent in 2020 – a drop of more than 16 per cent points). Moreover, only 52.5 per cent of NHS staff said in 2021 that they look forward to going to work – a decline of more than 6 per cent points from 58.8 per cent in 2020. The UK has been highly reliant on recruiting clinical trained outside the UK. For example, about 15 per cent of registered nurses in the UK are trained outside the UK – more than double the OECD average.

Looking to the future

Writing at the time of its 70th anniversary, Klein (2019: 1) suggested that perhaps the most remarkable aspect of the NHS was its survival in an institutional form that would still be recognised by its original architect, Nye Bevan. However, Hunter (2019) noted that Klein overlooked a notable weakness that the focus on curing ill-health has been at the expense of wider health and wellbeing, and that 'his preoccupation poses a greater threat to the NHS's future than privatisation' (2019: x) and that 'it may be that the NHS is finally running out of road unless it chooses a different route' of a 'whole health systems place-based approach' (2019: 13).

At the time of writing, there is a growing sense of crisis in the NHS. Powell (2015) pointed out that it has been claimed that the NHS has been in crisis at some point in each of its 67 years of its existence, and – like Mark Twain – accounts of its death have been exaggerated. By 'crying wolf at the cat with nine lives' it is possible that the wolf is now at the door of the NHS, but alarmed cries may no longer be heeded' (2015: 268).

The House of Lords Committee on the Long-term Sustainability of the NHS (2017) report stated that the NHS was in crisis and the adult social care system was on the brink of collapse, with many witnesses portraying an NHS at breaking point. It noted that while the NHS had seen previous crises, 'this crisis is different from the other crises'. The period since has given few reasons for greater optimism. The 75th anniversary may be a turbo-charged extension of the 70th anniversary, with the current crisis seeming to have changed into the 2022 'word of the year' of 'permacrisis' with additional steps of ABC (austerity, Brexit, and COVID-19) (Powell, forthcoming). The 'perfect storm' of 'endogeneous' factors such as prolonged austerity and lack of workforce planning and 'exogeneous' factors such as workforce issues associated with Brexit, COVID-19 backlogs, industrial action in a 'Winter of Discontent' linked to inflation appear to result in the 'Narnia' of 'always Winter' in the NHS.

Looking to the future, it may be argued that perhaps the only sensible prediction is that predictions will generally not be correct. For example, on the NHS' 50th anniversary, Berwick (1998) set out some predictions in a message on the 75th anniversary, noting that 'today, unlike in 1998, the NHS is almost waitfree. At a cost that has been held for 20 years at 7 per cent of gross domestic product, your citizens can get the help they need, day or night, when they need it' (1998: 57).

He explained this by pointing out that 'shortly after the 50th anniversary celebration in 1998, the NHS reached a historic turning point as the secretary of state, the NHS Executive, and the royal colleges ... settled wholeheartedly on a new set of eight principles ... sometimes called the Langlands Eight' [named after the Chief Executive of the NHS] (1998: 57). While the NHS did not get the 'Langlands Eight', it got a Constitution, and this Constitution and funding well above Berwick's 7 per cent of GNP has not delivered his optimistic prediction. He appears to have been equally incorrect in another prediction that 'by the early 21st century, the NHS was becoming a truly patient centered clinical care system. ... Shared decision making, incorporating every patient's values and circumstances, is now the norm' (1998: 61).

On the NHS' 70th anniversary, Stephen Powis (2018, p 51), National Medical Director of NHS England, predicted that 'by its 80th anniversary, the NHS will be very different to today, and by its 100th anniversary it will be almost unrecognisable'.

Filochowski (2018), imaging the NHS in 2028, got very close with some of his predictions (a disastrous flu pandemic in 2019, a grand coalition government in 2021, more funding, a dedicated health and social care tax [a speedily withdrawn levy]) but was far off track with others (the virtual disappearance of crisis, surplus provision, reductions in taxation). In other words, he was very accurate with the 'turning point' part of crisis, but not with the response. It seems that the NHS was not for turning.

It is perhaps best, then, not to try to predict the future, and follow the words of Nye Bevan, the founder of the NHS: 'why look in the crystal ball when you can read the bloody book'. In 2023, the NHS is faced with enduring issues which would be familiar at (almost) any other time in the history of the NHS. While the language might change and the context be different, the fundamental challenge of balancing access, cost and quality of care – the so-called triple aim – persists (Berwick, Nolan and Whittington, 2008). The fourth aim – staff wellbeing – has lacked sufficient emphasis in recent years (Bodenheimer and Sinsky, 2014) but this now lies at the heart of understanding the NHS. Workforce planning has been neglected in recent years but the NHS is not unusual; many health systems have overlooked the salience of workforce (Charlesworth, Shembavnekar and Stevenson, this volume).

In short, Klein (2013) likens the NHS to operatic melodies whereby actors on the stage move but familiar refrains can be heard. We argue that the melodies have changed in tone and the actors are more numerous and influential, but also that the NHS' form and function remain familiar. Specifically, the dramatic state of the NHS in 2023 is ultimately a political crisis, Populist politics have shaped the NHS in recent years (such as the claims made on the side of the bus in support of leaving the EU during the Brexit referendum, and misleading media about COVID-19) (Speed and Mannion, 2017, 2020). Recent political leadership has also failed to ensure that relevant interests (including patients and staff) are engaged in the ongoing process of improvement, rather than large-scale, top-down reform.

Demographic and technological change is accelerating the need to address improvement strategies within the NHS. In other words, the quadruple aim remains salient but how each of the individual aims is achieved needs to adapt and evolve. For example, there is, however, an increasing need to engage patients in co-production with the advent of the internet, the 'expert patient' (linked to the rise of chronic conditions) and a more consumerist approach to healthcare (Stewart, Desai and Zoccatelli, Chapter 12). This is most relevant in prevention and public health. Such contextual factors will inevitably place a tax-funded health system under further strain but social and private insurance health systems will also face the same challenges.

Predicting the future is futile but it is possible to discern trends which will shape the evolution of the NHS in the next decade (and beyond). First, technology is already re-casting professional working life, clinician-patient interactions and changing public expectation of what the NHS can and should do. We have seen some initial signs of this with telemedicine and video consultations (inter alia) in recent years. However, personalised (genomic) medicine will stretch the very conception of the NHS, challenging the notion of delivering a comprehensive service. Second, climate change and sustainability will shape health policy and health service delivery. This is perhaps most pressing in terms of the response of the NHS to extreme weather conditions (and a consequent rise in 'excess' deaths) but also the climatic factors which shape health (such as damp housing). Certainly, the NHS is already addressing the 'net zero' challenge (from single use devices to patient transport); reporting on progress in this challenge is underway. Businesses can also aid this through their EHSG – environmental, health, social and governance – activities. Yet, the salience of the issue has not figured much in health policy debates so far. With over 10 per cent of GDP spent on healthcare, it follows that the NHS has much to contribute to achieving net zero, especially in improving public health with its partner agencies. Third, a new settlement between the centre and locality (or more precisely, localities) need to provide adequate (central) funding while also ensuring sufficient (local) autonomy to drive innovation and implementation. Diverse local leadership will facilitate the latter. The difficulty will be in holding the performance of central and local actors to account, without delving into mutual blame.

It is often claimed (somewhat erroneously) that Bevan argued that 'the NHS will last as long as there are folk with faith left to fight for it'. While the NHS has constantly evolved over its 75 years, it has also been subject to political and/or ideological challenge. Yet, many continue to fight for its original principles of being centrally funded and free at the point of delivery. It has often been the interpretation of these principles which has been and continues to be contentious. It is not simply the public support through the COVID-19 pandemic (as witnessed only three years ago via public clapping or chalked messages on streets) but it is also the space that it continues to occupy in the public space (through newspapers, social media and TV media) which suggests that the NHS will survive to another anniversary. However, the balance between (public and political) support for the model of the NHS (that is, centrally funded, free at the point of delivery and open to all) and its operationalisation (viz. its practices and procedures as well as patient experience) will crucially determine its form and function in the future. In 2023, support for the former remains strong while the latter is under unprecedented strain.

Yet, as we write these concluding words, the state of the NHS in 2023 feels like a watershed moment. It is hard to say what state the NHS will be in at its 80th or even 100th anniversary. That said, although the future is likely to look quite different from the past, we can discern much from looking at its evolution over its first 75 years.

References

Anderson, A., Pitchforth, E., Asaria, M., Brayne, C., Casadei, B., Charlesworth, A. et al (2021) 'LSE–Lancet Commission on the future of the NHS: Re-laying the foundations for an equitable and efficient health and care service after COVID-19'. *The Lancet*, 397, 1915–1978.

Berwick, D. (1998) 'The NHS: Feeling well and thriving at 75'. *British Medical Journal*, 317, 57–61.

Berwick, D.M., Nolan, T.W. and Whittington, J. (2008) 'The triple aim: Care, health, and cost'. *Health Affairs*, 27, 3, 759–769.

Bodenheimer, T. and Sinsky, C. (2014) 'From triple to quadruple aim: Care of the patient requires care of the provider'. *Annals of Family Medicine*, 12, 6, 573–576.

Buzelli, L., Cameron, G., Duxbury, K., Gardner, T., Rutherford, S., Williamson, S. and Alderwick, H. (2022) *Public Perceptions of Health and Social Care: What the New Government Should Know*. London: Health Foundation (https://doi.org/10.37829/HF-2022-P11).

British Medical Journal (BMJ) (2018) 'Providing care based on need and free at point of delivery is NHS's greatest achievement, say *BMJ* readers'. *British Medical Journal*, 361: k2770. https://doi.org/10.1136/bmj.k2770

Castle-Clarke S. (2018) *The NHS at 70: What Will New Technology Mean for the NHS and its Patients?* London: Health Foundation, Institute for Fiscal Studies, King's Fund, Nuffield Trust.

Darzi, A. (2018) *Better Health and Care for All: A 10 point-plan for 2020s*. London: The Institute for Public Policy Research.

Dayan, M., Ward, D., Gardner, T. and Kelly, E. (2018) *The NHS at 70: How good is the NHS?* London: Health Foundation, Institute for Fiscal Studies, King's Fund, Nuffield Trust.

Exworthy, M. and Mannion, R. (2016) 'Evaluating the impact of NHS reforms: policy, process and power', in M. Exworthy, R. Mannion and M. Powell (eds) *Dismantling the NHS? Evaluating the Impact of Health Reforms*. Bristol: Policy Press, pp 3–15.

Filochowski, J. (2018) 'The NHS at 80? How it might look in 2028'. *British Medical Journal*, 361, k2106. https://doi.org/10.1136/bmj.k2106

Goodall, A.H. (2011) 'Physician-leaders and hospital performance: Is there an association?'. *Social Science & Medicine*, 73, 4, 535–539,

Greener, I. (2016) 'An argument lost by both sides? The Parliamentary debate over the 2010 NHS White Paper,' in M. Exworthy, R. Mannion, and M. Powell (eds) *Dismantling the NHS? Evaluating the Impact of Health Reforms.* Bristol: Policy Press, pp 105–124.

Greer, S., King, E.J., da Fonseca, E.M. and Peralta-Santos, A. (eds) (2021) *Coronavirus Politics: The Comparative Politics and Policy of COVID-19.* Ann Arbor: University of Michigan Press.

Harrison, S. (1988) *Managing the NHS: Shifting the Frontier?* London: Chapman Hall.

Health Foundation. (2022) *How Does UK Health Spending Compare Across Europe Over the Past Decade.* London: The Health Foundation.

Hodgson, D.E., Bailey, S., Exworthy, M., Hassard, J., Bresnan, M. and Hyde, P. (2021) 'On the character of the new entrepreneurial NHS in England: reforming health care from within?' *Public Administration*, 100, 2, 338–355.

House of Lords Select Committee on the Long-term Sustainability of the NHS. (2017) *The Long-term Sustainability of the NHS and Adult Social Care*, HL Paper 151. London: TSO.

Hunter, D. (2019) 'Looking forward to the next 70 years: From a National Ill-Health Service to a National Health System'. *Health Economics, Policy and Law*, 14, 11–14.

Klein, R. (1990) 'The state and the profession: The politics of the double bed'. *British Medical Journal*, 301, 6754, 700–702.

Klein, R. (2003) 'The new localism: Once more through the revolving door?' *Journal of Health Services Research and Policy*, 18, 4, 195–196.

Klein, R. (2013) *The New Politics of the NHS* (7th ed). London: Radcliffe Publishing.

Klein, R. (2019) 'The National Health Service (NHS) at 70: Bevan's double-edged legacy'. *Health Economics, Policy and Law*, 14, 1–10.

Le Grand, J., Mays, N. and Mulligan, J-A. (1998) *Learning from the NHS Internal Market: A Review of the Evidence.* London: King's Fund.

McKenna, H. (2018) *The NHS at 70: Are We Expecting Too Much from the NHS?* London: Health Foundation, Institute for Fiscal Studies, The King's Fund, Nuffield Trust.

NHS Staff Survey 2021. (2022) London: NHS.

Paton, C. (2018) 'Editorial – the NHS at 70: National treasure or threadbare antique?'. *International Journal of Health Planning and Management*, 33, 291–293.

Powell, M. (2015) 'Who killed the English National Health Service?'. *International Journal of Health Policy and Management*, 4, 267–269.

Powell, M. (2016) 'Reforming a health care system in a big way? The case of change in the British NHS'. *Social Policy and Administration*, 50, 2, 183–200.

Powell, M. (2019a) 'Seventy years of the British National Health: Service: Problem, politics and policy streams'. *Health Economics, Policy and Law*, 14, 29–39.

Powell, M. (2019b) 'Parliamentary debates on the anniversaries of the British National Health Service 1958–2008: "plus ça change?"'. *Revue Française de Civilisation Britannique*, XXIV-3, http://journals.openedition.org/rfcb/4133. DOI: 10.4000/rfcb.4133

Powell, M. and Exworthy, M. (2016) 'Never again? A retrospective and prospective view of English health reforms', in M. Exworthy, R. Mannion and M. Powell, (eds) *Dismantling the NHS?* Bristol: Policy Press, pp 365–380.

Powell, M. (forthcoming) 'Health,' in H. Bochel, and M. Powell (eds) *The Conservatives and Social Policy*. Bristol: Policy Press.

Powis, S. (2018) 'Editorial: The NHS at 70,' *BMJ Leader*, 2, 51.

Robinson, R. and Le Grand, J. (eds) (1994) *Evaluating the NHS Reforms*. London: King's Fund Institute.

Royal Commission on the National Health Service (NHS). (1979) Report, Chairman: Sir Alec Merrison, Cmnd 7615. London: HMSO.

Schneider, E. Shah, A., Doty, M.M., Tikkanen, R., Fields, K. and Williams, R.D. (2021) *Mirror, Mirror 2021 – Reflecting Poorly: Health Care in the U.S. Compared to Other High-Income Countries*. New York: Commonwealth Fund.

Shembavnekar, N., Buchan, J., Bazeer, N., Kelly, E., Beech, J., Charlesworth, A. et al (2022) *NHS Workforce Projections 2022*. London; Health Foundation (https://doi.org/10.37829/HF-2022-RC01).

Speed, E. and Mannion, R. (2017) 'The rise of post-truth populism in pluralist liberal democracies: challenges for health policy'. *International Journal of Health Policy and Management*, 6, 5, 249–251.

Speed, E. and Mannion, R. (2020) 'Populism and health policy: Three international case studies of right-wing populist policy frames'. *Sociology of Health and Illness*, 42, 1967–1981.

Stoye, G. (2018) *The NHS at 70: Does the NHS Need More Money and How Could We Pay For It?* London: Health Foundation, Institute for Fiscal Studies, King's Fund, Nuffield Trust.

Thorlby, R. and Maybin, J. (eds) (2010) *A High Performing NHS? A Review of Progress 1997–2010*. London: King's Fund.

Thorlby R. Starling, A., Turton, C. and Watt, T. (2018) *The NHS at 70: What's the Problem with Social Care, and Why Do We Need to Do Better?* London: Health Foundation, Institute for Fiscal Studies, King's Fund, Nuffield Trust.

Timmins, N. (ed) (2008) *Rejuvenate or Retire? Views of the NHS at 60*. London: Nuffield Trust.

Timmins, N. (2012) *Never Again? The Story of the Health and Social Care Act 2012: A Study in Coalition Government and Policy-making*. London: King's Fund/Institute of Government.

Timmins, N. (2017) *The Five Giants*, 3rd ed. London: William Collins.

Tuohy, C.H. (1999) *Accidental Logics: The Dynamics of Change in the Health Care Arena in the United States, Britain and Canada*. Oxford: Oxford University Press.

Tuohy, C.H. (2018) *Remaking Policy: Scale, Pace and Political Strategy in Health Care Reform*. Toronto: University of Toronto Press.

Tuohy, C. (2022) 'Anniversary narratives of the healthcare state: Institutional entrenchment in retrospect.' *Journal of Health Politics, Policy and Law*. 10234212. DOI: https://doi.org/10.1215/03616878-10234212

Index

References to figures appear in *italic* type; those in **bold** type refer to tables.
References to endnotes show both the page number and the note number (85n1).